"*Life Support* belongs in the august company of *Silent Spring, The Other America, The Feminine Mystique*, and other pivotal works with the power to shift the nation's consciousness. . . . It needs to be read by every medical student, practicing physician, medical educator, health care policy maker, insurance executive, hospital administrator, and health journalist; by every American who will ever either be or know a patient; and by every one of us who will die. I cannot praise it highly enough."

— Beryl Lieff Benderly, *Washington Post*

IF YOU ARE A NURSE

you'll probably find some of your own experiences (and frustrations) reflected in this account of three registered nurses at Boston's Beth Israel Hospital. The book offers confirmation that you are not alone in working both within and — too often today — against America's health care system to provide quality care to those who are sick.

Your friends who read *Life Support* will likely gain new insight into your work, its special importance, why you chose to become a nurse, and how your work helps make you the person you are.

IF YOU ARE NOT A NURSE

Life Support will help you understand why, when you're sick, you will want — and will be lucky to find — a nurse to help care for you.

"*Life Support* is a gripping description of how crucial well-trained nurses are to the well-being of patients in hospitals and elsewhere. . . . The next time you are scheduled to be hospitalized, this book will help you raise questions that may save your life."

— Sidney Wolfe, M.D., Public Citizen's Health Research Group

"*Life Support* is medicine at its most thrilling. Gordon's moving prose demystifies the profession of nursing and justifiably glorifies it. We all have been — or will be — their patients. And that truth makes *Life Support* must reading for every one of us."

— Michael Palmer, M.D., author of *Extreme Measures*

"Suzanne Gordon has written a compelling book uncovering hidden truths about health care reform. This book is a clarion call."

— Patricia Benner, R.N., Ph.D., F.A.A.N., Professor of Nursing, University of California, San Francisco

"Gordon's demonstration of the value of nursing is done with moving, and sometimes teeth-gritting, realism. It makes you not want to fall seriously ill — and to have a nurse on your side if you do."

— Bruce Ramsey, *Seattle Post-Intelligencer*

"What Gordon does accurately and passionately is to present an unfamiliar view of the health care system from the point of view of the educated registered nurse — a perspective all too rarely heard. . . . For patients, physicians, nurses, and health policy analysts, Gordon's passionate and accessible account of the impact of managed care on skilled nursing provides clear grounds for concern."

— Elizabeth Fee and Mary E. Garofalo, *Health Affairs*

"I work with nurses every day, but it took Suzanne Gordon to open my eyes to see all they do and how important — and underappreciated — their work is. *Life Support* should be required reading for all doctors, health policy decision-makers, and anyone else who cares about the future of our health care system."

— Timothy McCall, M.D., author of *Examining Your Doctor*

"Suzanne Gordon shows us why nursing matters. That is a profound achievement in a world in which most 'women's work' is still invisible, marginal, or misunderstood. Pass it on!"

— Laurel Thatcher Ulrich, Professor of Early American History and Women's Studies, Harvard University

LIFE SUPPORT

Three Nurses on the Front Lines

SUZANNE GORDON

Foreword by

Claire M. Fagin,

R.N., Ph.D., F.A.A.N.

ILR Press

AN IMPRINT OF CORNELL UNIVERSITY PRESS

Ithaca and London

A VOLUME IN THE SERIES

The Culture and Politics of Health Care Work
Edited by Suzanne Gordon and Sioban Nelson

Assisted Living for Our Parents: A Son's Journey, by Daniel Jay Baum

From Silence to Voice: What Nurses Know and Must Communicate to the Public,
Second Edition, by Bernice Buresh and Suzanne Gordon

*Differential Diagnoses: A Comparative History of Health Care Problems and Solutions
in the United States and France*, by Paul V. Dutton

Nobody's Home: Candid Reflections of a Nursing Home Aide, by Thomas Edward Gass

*Nursing against the Odds: How Health Care Cost Cutting, Media Stereotypes, and Medical Hubris
Undermine Nurses and Patient Care*, by Suzanne Gordon

Nurses on the Move: Migration and the Global Health Care Economy, by Mireille Kingma

The Complexities of Care: Nursing Reconsidered
edited by Sioban Nelson and Suzanne Gordon

Code Green: Money-Driven Hospitals and the Dismantling of Nursing
by Dana Beth Weinberg

First published in cloth 1997 by Little, Brown and Company
First paperback edition, Back Bay Books, 1998
First printing, Cornell Paperbacks, 2007

Printed in the United States of America

Library of Congress Cataloging-in-Publication Data

Gordon, Suzanne, 1945–
Life support : three nurses on the front lines / Suzanne Gordon ; foreword by Claire M. Fagin. — Cornell
ed.
p. cm. — (The culture and politics of health care work) (Cornell paperbacks)
Originally published: Boston, MA : Little, Brown and Co., 1997.
ISBN 978-0-8014-7428-6 (pbk. : alk. paper)
1. Nursing. 2. Nurses—Social conditions. I. Title. II. Series. III. Series: Cornell paperbacks

RT82.G67 2007
610.73—dc22   2007033208

Cornell University Press strives to use environmentally responsible suppliers and materials to the fullest
extent possible in the publishing of its books. Such materials include vegetable-based, low-VOC inks and
acid-free papers that are recycled, totally chlorine-free, or partly composed of nonwood fibers. For further
information, visit our website at www.cornellpress.cornell.edu.

Paperback printing   10   9   8   7   6   5   4   3   2

It seems a commonly received idea among men and even some women themselves that it requires nothing but a disappointment in love, the want of an object, a general disgust, or incapacity for other things to turn a woman into a good nurse. This reminds one of the parish where a stupid old man was set to be schoolmaster because he was "past keeping the pigs." . . .

The everyday management of a large ward, let alone of a hospital — the knowing what are the laws of life and death for men, and the laws of health for wards (and wards are healthy or unhealthy, mainly according to the knowledge or ignorance of the nurse) — are not these matters of sufficient importance and difficulty to require learning by experience and careful inquiry, just as much as any other art?

FLORENCE NIGHTINGALE

Of course, the story of nursing would be different if it was not "women's work." Founders of modern nursing, in both Great Britain and the United States, often reminded their colleagues that the future of women and the future of nursing were the same. Societal values associated with giving care were, and still are, largely identified with women. The real question for the future is whether we will ever so desire a civil, sympathetic society that we attach higher value to this "women's work." Will we come to see one another as valuable human beings to the point where we all, whether men or women, will feel both free and obliged to take care?

JOAN LYNAUGH

Contents

Contents

Foreword to the Cornell Edition

In 1996, when I wrote the introduction to the first edition of this book, I began with an example of the media's coverage of nursing. At the time, a young woman had been brutally attacked in Central Park, and the papers were full of the story. In particular, the *New York Times* and *New Yorker* ran excellent articles on the plight of this woman, who was unidentified in the *Times* and called Urgent Four in the lengthy *New Yorker* profile. Accounts in the *New York Times* highlighted the care and concern of this woman's nurses. But as she began to recover, the tone of the stories changed. Instead of quoting nurses and describing the complexity of the actions that kept this woman alive and helped her to recover, the focus shifted entirely to physicians and the surgical procedures being performed. When it came to the more "serious" matters of the mechanics of her treatment and recovery, only physicians were quoted and appeared in the narrative. The *New Yorker* described her maverick and superb brain surgeon and the high-tech procedures used in her cure. What the article failed to mention (but what Judy Dillworth, Director of Nursing, Critical Care Services, NYU Hospitals Center, has shared with me) was that the nurses were sensitive to the fact that Urgent Four was a pianist, and they were highly motivated to insure that her care, from admission to discharge, would utilize a multidisciplinary team for the achievement of her highest recovery possible. In this definitive article, nurses and their contributions to cure were entirely invisible. Because of nursing's invisibility, I felt Suzanne Gordon's new book about three nurses and their knowledge and skill was a critical contribution to our ongoing societal conversation about the present state and future of health care not only in the United States but globally.

That was over ten years ago. Have things changed for the better since *Life Support* first appeared? Sadly, no. As I write this foreword, the United States suffers from one of the longest-lasting and most serious nursing shortages of its history. Many hospitals are having great difficulty recruiting nurses and a terrible time retaining them. Some suffer from 20 percent turnover rates and equally high vacancy rates. This means patients will not get the lifesaving attention of nurses. The U.S. Bureau of Labor Statistics, among other sources, predicts that the shortage will continue and even worsen. Because the average age of the nurse is now forty-seven, many will be retiring within the next decade. If we do not produce enough nurses to replace them, we will have a shortage of over 800,000 RNs by the year 2020.

Meanwhile, shortages of faculty are limiting admissions of thousands of qualified applicants to nursing programs, and the climbing average age of faculty currently employed presages even greater problems ahead as retirements occur. While baccalaureate and higher-degree programs are changing degree requirements, associate degree programs remain the major producers of first-level nurses. Few of these nurses go on to pursue the higher degrees that are mandatory for faculty and advanced clinicians alike.

One would think that the media would be concerned about how they portray nurses—after all, editors and journalists get sick, too, and need nursing care. While the media have written extensively about the nursing shortage, contemporary articles reflect the same medical bias that was present in the *Times* and *New Yorker* coverage of the Urgent Four case. The *New Yorker*—unarguably one of the most influential magazines in the United States—continues to regularly profile the work of physicians. Two of its staff writers—Jerome Groopman and Atul Gawande—are respectively an internist and surgeon. Although they are excellent writers and their stories riveting, nurses rarely make an appearance in their articles, and when they do, they don't enhance the reader's understanding of the vital role nurses play. In my many years as a faithful *New Yorker* subscriber I have rarely read an article about a nurse of any stripe or encountered a review of some of the many nonfiction or fiction books written about or by nurses. And as a nurse educator, I find it fascinating that newspapers such as the *New York Times* publish accounts of the vicissitudes of physician education yet rarely, if ever, devote attention to the highly controversial issue of nursing education.

Things are even worse on television. After years of watching countless medical dramas that downplay the contributions of nurses, I can barely stand tuning into shows such as *Grey's Anatomy* where there are no nurses taking care of the sick. Patients recover because the doctors do all the doctoring—and also all the nursing. "Women" in these shows may demonstrate nursing skills, but these women portray physician characters.

The fact that our media culture seems awash in ignorance about nursing explains why, even a decade after the first edition appeared, Suzanne Gordon's book is so relevant today. By focusing on the knowledge and skill of these three nurses she gives nursing practice the sustained attention it deserves. Today, we need many more nurses in hospitals, clinics, rehabilitation facilities, nursing homes, schools, and other settings. We need many more doing the nursing research on which quality care depends. We need more nursing educators to prepare an expanded nursing workforce for tomorrow's needs.

Gordon's book explains just why we need these nurses and what it is they do. Her three nurse portraits show the rewards and challenges of work that is as dynamic as that of any physician and rewards the practitioner with incredible satisfaction and feelings of self worth. I should know. I have been a nurse for over fifty years, and the satisfactions of providing direct nursing care, counseling, preparing future nurses, and helping patients and families respond to their illness and life adjustments have outweighed the ego problems that could be caused by the challenges I have just mentioned. Suzanne Gordon guides us through a world that few of us understand and even fewer can articulate. In spite of global attention to a serious international nursing shortage, why is it that so few people understand the work of nurses when so many of us come in contact with them during our own or another's health or illness crises?

Some nurses, like me, have tried to explain this vacuum of public understanding in various ways.

The nursing scholar Donna Diers and I have commented on the paradoxical fact that a group educated and valued because they give comfort seems to make some of the very same people they care for and with whom they work closely socially uncomfortable. We attribute this discomfort to metaphors such as mothering, nurturing, social class, and intimacy, which turn nurses into an uncomfortable reminder for patients of their vulnerability and, for physicians, the limits of their practice and their fallibility. (See our "Nursing as Metaphor," *New England Journal of Medicine* 309 [July 14, 1983]: 116–117.)

In this book Suzanne Gordon explores these metaphors in great detail and explains the various aspects of nurses' contribution to patient care. Many nurses will be grateful for this in-depth depiction of their work. But nonnurses—particularly patients and their families—should also be grateful for a vivid look at three nurses and what they, through their profession, bring to the health care system as a whole and to their patients in particular.

Why should we be grateful? Because the kind of care so many of us value and want when we are sick is always in jeopardy. Cries of a serious nursing shortage are often followed by lulls in attention, particularly when improving the conditions of nursing work costs money and, perhaps even more important, requires changes in the power structure of institutions and changes in attitude.

We cannot protect nurses' work unless we understand it and act to preserve it when we are healthy. When we, as patients, are at our most vulnerable, it is too late to worry about the lack of expert nursing care. And in the coming years, millions of baby boomers will become vulnerable and need that care in hospitals, at home, in the community, and in many other facilities where people access health care. I worry that nursing will disappear from the radar screen again and that quality nursing will not be available unless something is done, and soon. That is why *Life Support* remains as important—perhaps even more important—today than it was a decade ago. What Gordon gives us is the knowledge and awareness we need to be smart consumers and health policy advocates. Smart consumers need to act before noxious events occur. Smart consumers need to be prepared and to know about the services they will be using—in this case services on which their very lives depend. In the health care field, this means that smart consumers need to know about and understand what is involved in quality nursing care, how to get it, and how to protect it. Consumers cannot depend on the health policy community for their protection because many of its members often understand too little about or undervalue the role of nursing, the largest profession in the health care field.

Suzanne Gordon addresses not only public and health policy issues in this book. She also makes an argument that the medical profession has neglected for too long the importance of doctor-nurse relationships and health care teamwork. Ten years after the first publication of *Life Support*, teamwork in health care is a mantra, heard by all, but little practiced. This is another reason that Gordon's work remains relevant. She explains and explores what happens when people invoke the concept of the team and contend that patient care relies on teamwork yet fail to build the teamwork infrastructure on which quality care depends. What we see is that people fail to share information, goals, and insights. This, in turn, ensures that lack of open communication about patients' conditions and their needs prevails, and patients subsequently suffer.

Gordon depicts many physicians in this book. We meet young, inexperienced interns, more-experienced residents, as well as attending physicians and researchers, all focused on their part of the patient-provider interaction. In some cases Gordon describes doctors who understand care and who have positive relationships with nurses, medical colleagues, and others. In other cases, however, she highlights the negative and demeaning experiences nurses confront in their day-to-day interactions with physicians. All of these negative experiences, implicitly or explicitly, have some kind of effect on patients.

Because of these dramatic stories, some readers may conclude that Suzanne Gordon is antiphysician and, despite being a doctor's daughter, started her investigation with a negative bias. But that is far from the truth. If anything, the reverse was the case when she was growing up in a loving environment that cherished the medical profession. It was in her journalistic career and personal experiences that she began to take close notice of and interest in the work of nurses in hospitals. Her stories are real, and she got them by being there and by looking and listening to what went on in the patient-care situation.

Some years ago, when I was dean of the School of Nursing at the University of Pennsylvania, a colleague in the School of Medicine suggested that nursing faculty were inculcating hostility toward physicians by talking about their own negative experiences with doctors and by preparing students to expect the same. This, I was told, made a sham of our efforts to design courses in which nursing students and medical students might learn together, and hopefully, go on to develop collaborative relationships in the work setting.

In my own conversations with physicians, I was always cheered by their comments about our students and graduates and how much they valued them and their contributions. So I decided to investigate this charge since it concerned and troubled me. In talking with students I learned that it was not the faculty who were making them hostile. What they talked to me about was the clinical experiences they were having at a major teaching hospital. No matter what their age or gender, when they worked in the hospital with medical students and physicians, they experienced some of the same arrogance and insults that Gordon describes. Yes, they had many positive, friendly relationships with physicians, and perhaps these were occurring in a greater number than their negative experiences. Yet for the students, the positive experiences were outweighed by the negative ones. The students defended the faculty and said repeatedly, "We did not need the faculty to make us hostile." In other words, physicians and medical students were doing that themselves.

This was deeply disappointing to me, to say the least. The University of Pennsylvania School of Nursing is one of the top nursing schools in the world, and its admission standards are on a par with those of the most selective American universities. Yes, I had heard stories from nurses all over the world about their relationships with physicians that are similar to those described in this book. Still, in the Penn context, where educational background and social class are not dividers, the ubiquitous nature of the problem presents itself dramatically. Ten years later the vast majority of medical and nursing students still don't learn together nor do most doctors and nurses act as team members throughout their careers.

The kinds of experiences nurses described have made me more impatient with the rigidity of attitudes among the most powerful providers. Significant demographic changes in our country have led to an increased number of people of all ages who need chronic and maintenance care. Consumers are interested in self-care. Cost restraints are already having an impact on our use of technology, and questions of who needs what at what cost will only multiply. Nurses and doctors must combine their collective talents to answer these questions together, to improve and protect patient care, and to serve society better. But this will require major changes in the way they think about themselves, their roles in the health care delivery system, and their power, authority, and domains.

Looking at the health care needs of people from the perspective of one powerful discipline has always been dysfunctional for patients and for the other players on the health care stage. Today, however, complexities and constraints on the health care system make this traditional approach dysfunctional for physicians as well as for all of those who depend on health care for their lives and work. For patients to be at the center of the health care experience, the health care professions must move to a broader shared perspective that focuses more on patients than on protecting their own hegemony.

One of Gordon's major themes in the book, the care of the dying, illuminates the centrality of patients. Today, how we deal with death is still a subject of intense public concern. Many patients fear that doctors have been trained to torturously prolong their lives. Others, including ethicists, health care professionals, clergy, and many family members, are increasingly concerned with the apparent growth of a movement advocating legally assisted suicide. Gordon's account of how Nancy Rumplik, Jeannie Chaisson, and Ellen Kitchen take care of people who are dying and help them die with comfort and dignity should be case studies for these contemporary discussions. Nurses have been far in the lead, though without recognition, or in many cases of recognition being attributed to physicians, in introducing innovations and trying to deal constructively with patients who are dying and in pain.

Nurses' work means being there over time with patients and helping them deal with their illness and its ramifications. It is only natural, therefore, that concern should lead to seeking palliative measures to alleviate pain and suffering. The hospice movement came about because of such concerns. Gordon's discussion of hospice and palliative care can help patients and families make better choices and teach them that solutions to their pain and suffering may lie within the medical and nursing community.

Although *Life Support* is a work of journalism, a sense of history pervades its pages. Some find it comforting to believe that the work of nursing has changed dramatically. This seems to make it more "respectable" to be a nurse. Yes, nurses' work has changed dramatically to incorporate new knowledge and technical skills. Yet, the essential aspects of the "tapestry of nursing" remain the same. Throughout its history, the profession of nursing has woven all that nurses know and do into an integrated and seamless tapestry of care and competence. This is strikingly exemplified in the home care nurse practitioner Ellen Kitchen's work. Reading Gordon's descriptions, I was reminded of early tales of the Henry Street Settlement Visiting Nurses, "invented" by Lillian Wald to meet the needs of the poor on the Lower East Side of Manhattan. Certainly the roles and activities of nurses in home care have evolved along with advancing knowledge, skills, and the increased acuity of patients' conditions because of earlier discharges from hospitals. However, the basics of home care nursing—the concerns for the patient's environment, nutrition, daily routines, and activities for helping the patient achieve and maintain the highest degree of independence—are among the constants of nursing in the home throughout nursing's professional history.

Suzanne Gordon brings us into the hospital, the community, and the home. She brings us into the lives of patients with complex, debilitating, life-threatening, and fatal conditions. Our guides to what frightened, anxious, vulnerable patients experience are the eyes, minds, and hearts of nurses. Gordon's goal is to improve patient care and help us all recognize that we cannot reach this vital goal without the help and insight of nurses.

Suzanne Gordon describes in the preface to this book how she became passionate about nursing, and *passionate* is about the most fitting word I can find. The key to Gordon's advocacy is passion that is linked to the critical understanding that patients cannot be served without superior nurses and superior nursing care. Thus, she is not advocating for nurses qua nurses, but for patients. Without nurses, there is no care that can be described with any sense of satisfaction, admiration, or safety. This she learned not only by watching nurses but also by experiencing the value of that care herself when she had her own children and when she experienced the death of her father and friends. For her memory, awareness, sensitivity, and talent, all of us—nurses and nonnurses alike—must be grateful.

Claire M. Fagin
Dean Emerita, University of Pennsylvania
School of Nursing

Preface

A poster decorates the wall of my study. In tones of sepia, faded teal, rust, and pewter, it depicts a medieval woman, worried and attentive, holding on her lap a pale, glassy-eyed child. At her side sits an earthenware pitcher that, we assume, holds a medicinal potion. The painting, by Gabriel Metsu (ca. 1660), is called "The Sick Child." Below it is announced an exhibition and book: *Nursing: The Oldest Art.*

Nursing may be the oldest art, but in the contemporary world, it is also one of the most invisible. One of the most invisible arts, sciences, and certainly one of the most invisible parts of our health care system.

For years, nursing was also invisible to me. I grew up with nursing quite literally all around me and yet nowhere noticed. My father was a famous ophthalmologist, researcher, and surgeon. One of the wizards of cure, he helped develop the use of ACTH and cortisone for inflammatory eye diseases. When I was a child, I was at home racing through the halls of the New York Hospital–Cornell Medical Center, where he practiced and taught. I remember the doctors in their white coats strolling confidently through the wards and the imposing portraits of distinguished "medical men" staring down at me from their honored perches in the medical school corridors.

There was the nurse in my father's office: a roly-poly, fairy godmother–like lady. But I have no idea what she did or knew. Nor did I ever inquire.

When I was a young woman coming of age as a feminist, nurses were similarly alien to my political universe. I devoted much reflection to the injustices perpetrated by patriarchy against almost every other female group. Had I given it much thought, I suppose, like so many feminist activists I would have vaguely imagined that women's problems in health care, and the medical system in general, would be remedied when more women became doctors.

My first experience as a hospitalized patient began to alter my preconceptions. I had my first child in a small suburban community hospital outside Boston. My labor was intense and seemed unendurable. Although my friend who was also my obstetrician came in every couple of hours to check on me, administered an epidural, and finally pulled the baby out, my nurses — two in particular — were with me every minute during that twelve-hour ordeal. Afterward, my friend popped in to check my stitches and write orders. But my nurses were the ones who furnished the confidence a thirty-nine-year-old professional with no brothers or sisters, nieces or nephews, no experience at all with babies, needed to begin her career as a mother.

In the middle of the night, after a labor that included three and a half hours of pushing, an episiotomy, and a forceps delivery, one of my nurses — who happened to be one of the few male nurses at the hospital — came in to pack my aching groin with ice and give me medication to ease my pain. The next day, he arrived with a small baby food jar containing a dark amber liquid. What was that, I wanted to know. It was a strong infusion of tea, he replied. Then he handed me a supply of Q-Tips and told me to apply this potion to my nipples after each breastfeeding. "It will toughen them up so they won't be so sore," he guaranteed. And it did.

Over the next few days, my nurses helped me control the myriad unexpected side effects of labor. I needed pain medication, but the drugs made me constipated. Because of the pushing and pulling, I couldn't urinate. Would my plumbing ever readjust, I wondered frantically. The nurses were immensely reassuring: to them all this was purely routine. They managed to sort through this array of side effects and get me back to normal.

Their most invaluable aid came in the form of education. They helped me learn that I could actually be a mother to this fragile life suddenly entrusted to me. I remember watching one nurse bathe my child, burp her, diaper and swaddle her. It was comforting to realize that what to me was a terrifying prospect was to her an everyday experience. At night, I walked down the silent hospital corridor and stood outside the nursery window awestruck as the nurses scooped up a howling newborn with one arm while they rocked a calm baby in the other. I began to see that these tiny creatures were not as brittle as I had imagined and that caring for them was a skill I could actually learn.

Although I could not find the words to describe these initial glimpses, I began, during those four days in the hospital, to understand the caregiving relationships I have since come to value so much. The power of the nursing expertise I experienced lay in more than the concrete information those nurses passed on to me. I could never have learned all that they taught me through the impersonal techniques that have become so popular today as hospitals, insurers, and employers cheat new mothers and newborns of nursing care. Bathing or diapering a plastic doll would not have helped me. Nor would I have benefited from watching a video of some anonymous nurse caring for someone else's equally anonymous infant. After all, I wasn't afraid of dropping a doll or someone else's baby. I was afraid of dropping my own.

I began to build on these initial encounters during the writing of my last book, *Prisoners of Men's Dreams*. For it, I interviewed nurses about the highly publicized national nursing shortage of the mid-1980s. These nurses opened the door into a world about which so many of us are ignorant.

This book is the product of almost a decade of studying and writing about nurses. I have spent years watching nurses practice, and I have also talked with their patients and with the physicians and social workers they work with. (To protect the confidentiality of patients, I have given them pseudonyms, indicated after each name by an asterisk, and have also changed some relevant details about their cases and their lives.) The book is written in the present tense to convey a sense of immediacy. But a number of small details have changed since I started work on the book.

I have also spoken with hundreds of other nurses in hospitals all across the country. Staff nurses from dozens of nursing specialties, clinical nurse specialists, nurse practitioners, nursing researchers, scholars, and administrators have spent hours teaching me about their profession, as well as sharing their feelings about the public's and the media's failure to value and respect their work. They have generously devoted hour upon hour helping me to understand what it means for human beings to become sick and vulnerable and what happens when they get older, become weaker, or face death. These nurses have helped me comprehend not only the essence of nursing, but the essence of the human activity of caregiving, and I want to thank all of those who have shared their work and thoughts with me.

Through my own work with nurses, I have come to appreciate very personally how much better patient care can be when it's structured so that nurses can respond to the physical and emotional needs of patients and their families. Twenty-five years ago, my father was diagnosed with pancreatic cancer and died within three months. At the time, I was too young and emotionally immature to help either of my parents deal with this situation. Distraught, afraid, and at odds, my mother and I were never able to *be with* my father, so that, with him, we could acknowledge our real feelings about his impending death and allow him to express his.

And there seemed, sadly, no one else in the hospital who could assist us. The physicians who cared for my father at the beginning of his illness gradually disappeared as his case clearly became "hopeless." Nurses, moreover, were unable to give us the kind of support physicians were unable to provide. At New York Hospital, circa 1970, nursing was an invisible, instrumental activity. Under the nursing models of that era, no one seemed to be accountable for a patient's care, and nurses had difficulty getting to know patients and their families. There seemed, thus, no expert nurses who could assume responsibility for my father's care on a continuous basis and establish a relationship with his stricken wife and daughter. So with no one to coach us, guide us, or help us confront our fears, we were unable to support each other or him. As a result, my father spent his last days in a state of terrible emotional isolation — a condition that may have been as painful as the disease that killed him.

A quarter of a century later, I've learned from the nurses in this book that there's a different kind of caregiving available today — at least in those institutions where nursing has expanded and maintained its critical role. The nurses I have gotten to know have helped me respond to sickness and terminal illness in a way I was unable to when my own father was dying.

While I was following Nancy Rumplik at the Beth Israel Hospital, a close friend was diagnosed with lung cancer. He spent months receiving aggressive curative treatments. But nothing helped. At the end, he was cared for at home by his hospice nurse and his wife. All through his illness, Nancy Rumplik was my coach. She told me how to interpret his symptoms, talk to him about his illness, tolerate his feelings of loneliness and terror, and nourish his hope. She encouraged me to talk with him about my feelings, and tell him how much I loved him and would miss him.

Several weeks before he died, I went to visit him at home. He was tethered to an oxygen machine, listless, sedated to keep the pain at bay, barely able to keep his eyes open. We sat in the pale, filtered sunlight of his living room while he dozed in a reclining chair. I had learned from Nancy Rumplik that at this point in the dying process just sitting with a dying human being is important. My friend could not bear to eat or drink, so even the offer of a glass of water was unwelcome. He did not have the energy to carry on a conversation, so there was nothing to say. Every once in a while, he would open his eyes and apologize for nodding off.

A year before I would have felt that I had to "do something." I would perhaps have found it too painful to be in a situation where there was literally nothing to be done. But I was undergoing my own apprenticeship in caregiving, and I could now tolerate simply being with someone in pain, trying as much as possible to share that pain or temper it with a human presence. I sat with him for several hours, watching him sleep, feeling that just being with him was a privilege, something I would be able to remember when he was gone. My friend died several weeks later when I was away on vacation, and I will always cherish the memory of that afternoon.

The three nurses in this book, Nancy Rumplik, Jeannie Chaisson, and Ellen Kitchen, have taught me that you can never totally comprehend the experience of illness unless you have gone through that experience yourself. To say "I understand," "I am with you," "I can help," they acknowledge, is to make the simplest of assertions. Yet, they are also some of the most profound. They bear witness to the possibility of caregiving from this distance — even within an overwhelming sense of confusion and powerlessness — which is one of the most important lessons people who will have to give care may ever learn.

I cannot sufficiently express my gratitude to Nancy Rumplik, Jeannie Chaisson, and Ellen Kitchen for sharing their lives and work with me. I also want to thank the Beth Israel — and in particular Joyce Clifford and Kathy Horvath — for facilitating this work and helping me find the expert nurses who are the focus of this book. The Beth Israel has always been an institution remarkable for its courage in helping journalists understand some of the more controversial areas of health care. I also want to thank Mitchell T. Rabkin, its president, for his help and support.

Many others have contributed to this book. I want to thank Peggy O'Malley, the first nurse I ever interviewed, for opening up a new world to me. Her devotion to nursing is an inspiration. For years, Joan Lynaugh — one of the sagest observers of health care — has been an enormous influence on my view of nursing in particular and health care in general. Patricia Benner and Nel Noddings have helped me understand the complex work of caregiving. Claire Fagin and Ellen Baer have been wonderful guides and colleagues. I also am indebted to Ellen Baer for the concept of the tapestry of nursing. We originally wrote about the tapestry of nursing in a coauthored article in the *American Journal of Nursing*. I also thank Trish Gibbons for her knowledge and support and Nancy Valentine for our numerous discussions. My good friend Beth Grady has talked with me for hours over the years helping me better understand nursing. I would like to thank nurse managers Patty Lydon, Ellen Powers, and Karen Dick. Emergency nurse Gail Lenahan also gave great suggestions. Thanks also to oncology nurses Gretchen Denoyer and Janice Marienze for their time. Karen Buhler-Wilkerson and Charlene Harrington were kind enough to go over important sections. Judith Shindul-Rothschild has also added to my knowledge.

I want to thank Geraldine Zagarella, John Jainchill, and Michael Cahalane — three of the most caring physicians I have met — for helping me understand the physician's mission and perspective and for their unstinting advice and guidance. To Glenn Bubley in particular, I owe a debt for his unstinting help with medical details. Eduardo Bruera and Declan Walsh helped educate me not only about palliative care but about oncology, and Emily Lowry and Timothy McCall were invaluable in contributing their medical knowledge to this project. Alan Sager has helped me understand the economics of the health care system, and David Himmelstein and Steffie Woolhandler have given advice about health policy and the waste of valuable health care resources on administration.

Initial conversations with David Mehegan were very productive. There is no gift that can repay my friends Bernice Buresh and Judy Dugan for their suggestions. Patricia Smith knows that I am forever in her debt for her editorial consultation and knowledgeable caring. Patients aren't the only ones who need the caregiver's art. This writer struggling at her desk could not have produced this book without so many excellent suggestions and so much nurturance.

Again, my agent, Anne Borchardt, has been with me and given me her heart, and Denise Shannon has shared with me the insights that stem from a layperson's love of nursing. And thanks for insightful comments and suggestions of my editor, Frederica Friedman, her assistant, Jacqueline Miller, and copyeditor, Betty Power, all of whom have greatly improved the final product.

My always supportive husband, Steve Early, spent many long hours on his vacations poring over my manuscript. His obsessive-compulsive tinkering with the text, while not always appreciated at the moment, has definitely been for the best. What's more, in a wonderful role reversal, he also types and babysits. Finally, I want to thank my two daughters, Alexandra and Jessica, for putting up with a mother often preoccupied with phone calls, interviews, and endless word processing. They have both promised not to avoid a career in nursing because of my lengthy immersion in this project.

LIFE
SUPPORT

Chapter 1

The Tapestry of Care

It is four o'clock on a Friday afternoon. The Hematology / Oncology Clinic at Boston's Beth Israel Hospital is quiet, almost becalmed. Paddy Connelly and Frances Kiel, two of the eleven nurses who work in the unit, sit at the nurses' station, an island comprising two long desks equipped with computers and constantly ringing phones. They are encircled by thirteen reclining blue leather chairs in which patients may spend only a few minutes for a short chemotherapy infusion, or an entire afternoon when they receive more complicated chemotherapy or blood products. The two nurses write the results of their day's work in various patient charts. Across from where they sit, Nancy Rumplik is starting to administer chemotherapy to a man in his mid-fifties who has colon cancer.

Nancy is forty-two and has been a nurse on the unit for the past seven years. Her brown, straight hair is cut in a short bob. Her eyes are a pale, almost indistinguishable hazel, the bridge of her nose a wide track that crooks slightly to the left at its tip. Her soft voice is muted by the weariness of a long day.

She stands next to the wan-looking man and begins to hang the intravenous chemotherapy that will treat his cancer. Dressed in black jeans and a black T-shirt that accentuates his pallor, he seems apprehensive about the treatment but does not verbalize his concerns. Nancy, who wears a white lab coat with a stethoscope dangling around her neck, reminds him of the purpose of every drug that is going into his system. As the solution drips through the tubing and into his vein, she sits by his side, watching to make sure that he has no adverse reaction.

Although she is primarily responsible for this particular patient, today she is acting as triage nurse. Each week, one of the clinic's eleven nurses serves as the person responsible for any patients who walk in without an appointment, for any patients who call with a problem but can't reach their primary nurse, for the flow of the unit, and, of course, for emergencies. Even though she concentrates on her own patient, Nancy's eyes thus constantly sweep the room to check on the remaining patients. She focuses for a moment on a heavy-set African American woman who is sitting in the opposite corner. The woman, in her mid-forties, is dressed in navy slacks and a brightly colored shirt. Her sister, who is notably younger and heavier, is by her side. The patient seems fine, so Nancy returns her attention to the man next to her. Several minutes later, she looks up again, checks the woman, and stiffens. There is a look of anxiety on the woman's face she did not see before. Leaning forward in her chair, she stares at the woman.

"What's she getting?" she mouths to Kiel.

Looking at the patient's chart, Frances Kiel names a drug that has caused a number of severe allergic reactions. In just that brief moment, as the two nurses confer, the woman suddenly clasps her chest and her look of anxiety turns to terror. Her mouth opens and shuts in silent panic. Nancy leaps up from her chair, as do Kiel and Connelly, and sprints across the room.

"I can't breathe," the woman sputters when Nancy is at her side. Her eyes bulge and she grabs for Nancy's hand; she tightens her grip and her eyes roll back as her head slips to the side. Realizing that the patient is having an anaphylactic reaction — her airway swelling and closing shut — Nancy immediately turns a small spigot on the IV tubing to shut off the drip. At the same instant, Kiel calls a physician and the team responsible for responding to medical emergencies in the hospital. By this time, the woman is struggling for breath.

Kiel next slips an oxygen mask over the woman's head and places a blood pressure cuff around her arm. Connelly administers an antihistamine and cortisone to stop the allergic reaction and to decrease the inflammation blocking her airway. An oncology fellow arrives within minutes. He assesses the situation and then notices the woman's sister standing, paralyzed, watching the scene. "Get out of here!" he furiously commands.

The woman moves away as if she has been slapped. Then, with practiced synchronicity, no one leading or following, Nancy continues to work with the nurses and physician to stop the reaction and stabilize the patient.

Just as the emergency team arrives, the woman's breathing returns to normal and the look of abject terror fades from her face. Grasping Nancy's hand, she looks up and repeats, "I couldn't breathe. I just couldn't breathe." Nancy gently explains that she has had an allergic reaction to a drug and reassures her that it has stopped.

After a few minutes, when he knows the patient is stable, the physician and emergency team walk out of the treatment area, but the nurses continue to comfort the terrified woman. Nancy then crosses the room to talk with her male patient who is ashen-faced at this reminder of the potentially lethal effects of the medication he and others are receiving. Responding to his unspoken fears, Nancy says quietly, "It's frightening to see something like that. But it's under control."

He nods silently, closes his eyes, and leans his head back against the chair. Nancy goes over to the desk where Connelly and Kiel are breathing a collective sigh of relief. One of the nurses comments about the physician's treatment of the patient's sister. "Did you hear him? He just told her to get out."

Wincing with distress, Nancy looks around the room to try to locate the patient's sister. She goes into the waiting room, where the woman is sitting in a corner, looking bereft and frightened. Nancy sits down next to her. She explains what happened and suggests that the patient could probably benefit from some overnight company. Then she adds, "I'm sorry the doctor talked to you like that. You know, it's a very anxious time for all of us."

At this gesture of respect and recognition, the woman, who has every strike — race, class, and gender — against her when dealing with elite, white professionals in this downtown hospital, smiles solemnly. "I understand. Thank you."

Nancy Rumplik returns to her patient.

*   *   *

2:00 P.M.

Ellen Kitchen, a nurse in Beth Israel's Home Care Department and a geriatric nurse practitioner for the past seven years, spends her workday in some of Boston's most ramshackle neighborhoods visiting poor and elderly patients. There is the crotchety old African American man who lives alone in a tattered one-bedroom apartment. He is trapped in those two rooms because his ancient lungs have been damaged by emphysema. Then she visits an elderly woman with diabetes and congestive heart failure who tries, despite her many ailments, to care for the grandchildren her daughter has abandoned. Next comes the ninety-two-year-old woman with coronary artery disease and arthritis who lives with her yelping dogs and is at constant risk for falls and other serious medical problems.

The forty-year-old nurse is slender and of medium height. Her blunt-cut brown hair is going gradually gray. A self-described optimist, her demeanor is so friendly as to be at times almost perky. She generally rides her bike to work and home visits. To make her last visit of the day, Ellen, who dresses casually in slacks and a windbreaker, parks her bike in a lot of an apartment building. As she passes the staff in their offices, they wave her in. An apartment door on the third floor has been left ajar so she can enter.

The tall black man who lives here is dressed nattily in slacks and a navy-blue-and-white plaid cardigan. At age eighty-eight, however, his legs are weak and he must grasp the end of a table to haul up his lanky frame and greet Ellen. He smiles and welcomes her with a barrage of personal questions about her upcoming move to another apartment, her husband's work, and the health of her two-year-old son. Then he settles back into his chair.

For the past five years, Ellen Kitchen has been a constant in the life of Theodore Cousins.* She originally cared for his wife, who after a stroke was wheelchair-bound until she died three years ago. On weekly, sometimes even biweekly, visits, Ellen has traveled the short distance from the Longwood Avenue medical area — home to many of Boston's major teaching hospitals, Harvard Medical School, and the Harvard School of Public Health — to this neat, compact apartment. Here she watched with increasing respect as Cousins devoted himself to his wife's care. His children had long ago left home, and it was the former waiter who cooked, cleaned, and shopped and bathed, dressed, and fed his wife during her long illness.

When Cousins himself grew increasingly frail and ill, Ellen began taking care of both husband and wife. Since the death of his wife, Ellen has been the primary-care provider and coordinator of the services "Mr. C." receives from the homemaker who cleans his house, the neighbor who cooks his meals, and his social worker and physical therapist.

Unloading the backpack that contains her medical paraphernalia — rubber gloves, blood pressure cuff, syringes, tourniquets, prescription blanks, and medical charts — she appraises her patient. "How are you, Mr. C.?" she asks. Then, without once being prompted by his medical chart, she inquires about the arthritis in his right shoulder, the injured tendon in his leg, and mentions, in passing, the aortic aneurysm he suffered from — and to everyone's surprise survived — many years ago.

"How's the cold you had last week?" she continues. "Did you have any more pains in your chest? Have you needed to take your nitroglycerin?" She checks a plastic pillbox stationed under a sign she has posted — Take Your Heart Pills! — and frowns as she scans the contents.

"It looks like you've missed one pill," she observes and then checks more carefully. "No, two. Let's see. You didn't take a pill Tuesday and Wednesday." Patiently, without condescension, she reviews each medication. "Remember, Mr. C., there's the nitroglycerin — that's a vasodilator for your heart — the digoxin for your congestive heart failure and atrial fibrillation, and the enteric-coated aspirin to thin your blood since you had the stroke last summer."

Mr. C. points a wrinkled hand at his crotch and complains about vague urinary symptoms. So she asks him to give her a urine specimen "just to see if anything's cooking." She wants to prevent a repeat of an undetected urinary tract infection that put him in the hospital last fall. He lurches up out of his chair, goes into the bathroom, and comes out with a vial full of urine to offer her.

Then Ellen takes his blood pressure while he's sitting and standing and escorts him into the bathroom to weigh him, all the while continuing to chat about his week. The conversation inevitably turns to a major concern — monitoring the prostate cancer that was diagnosed a year ago. "Before all this, I never even knew what a prostate was," Mr. C. jokes.

The cancer is slow-growing and appears to be stable. But Mr. C. brings up the subject of his refusal to have the operation — the orchiectomy, or removal of the testicles — his doctors had originally recommended. Instead, Mr. C. received monthly injections that lower testosterone to treat his prostate cancer. As they chat about his decision, the old gentleman suddenly slaps his thigh and reveals a powerful boyhood memory.

When he was a boy, he lived on a farm in the South. There he was a spectator to a horrifying ritual. Although it took place decades ago, the memory is still vivid. He would stand outside the large pen and watch as farmers corralled their hogs. With the animals squealing and wriggling, they took their huge knives, grabbed a hog, and with a swift motion sliced off its testicles. The animals spurted blood and bellowed in agony as the farmers smeared tar over the bleeding wounds before setting them loose.

"You know, I can't get that out of my mind. I remember those hogs, cut and tarred, running off squealing and bleeding."

Ellen flinches at the description. "Mr. C., that would never happen to you," she assures him. Although she makes no attempt to persuade him to have an operation he clearly does not want, she does express surprise that he has never before confided this story. "Why didn't you tell me this when we talked about the operation a year ago?" she inquires.

Looking sheepish, he confesses. " I guess I didn't want to tell that to a woman."

Then he smiles slyly and winks. "But I found out women know a damn sight more than I thought they did."

6:00 P.M.

Today, clinical nurse specialist Jeannie Chaisson arrived on her general medical unit at seven in the morning and cared for patients until 3:30 in the afternoon. Before leaving at 4:30, she wrote notes in their charts and reported on their condition to the nurses who would replace her. Then she made the forty-five-minute commute from Boston to her home in suburban Auburndale. As soon as she enters her home, she makes herself a pot of coffee and, cradling a fresh cup, sits down in her living room. She has only a few moments to relax before her kids return home from their after-school activities. Jeannie takes off her burnished copper wire–rimmed glasses and rubs her opalescent blue eyes. Her brown hair, lightly filamented with gray, is cut in a hairdo that varies only slightly — a modified bob that falls either just below her ears or somewhere above her shoulders.

Just as she is shedding the strain of the day, the phone rings.

It's the husband of one of Jeannie's patients — a sixty-three-year-old woman suffering from terminal cancer. She has metastases in her bones. When she left the hospital, Jeannie knew the family was in crisis. After having the cancer for several years, the woman was exhausted from the pain, the effects of the disease and failed treatments, and the pain medication upon which she had become increasingly dependent for any peace. Jeannie knew she was ready, willing to let death take her. But her husband and daughter were not.

Now, the crisis that was brewing has exploded. The caller is breathless, frantic with anxiety. "She says she wants to die, that she is prepared to die," explains the husband, relaying his wife's pleas. "She says the pain is too much. This isn't her," he insists. "It can't be. She's such a fighter. It's not like her to give up, to abandon us like this." He insists that it's the disease talking, or maybe the pain, or the painkilling drugs.

"You've got to do something," he implores Jeannie. "Keep her going, stop her from doing this."

Jeannie knows that it is indeed time for her to do something — but, sadly, not what this anguished husband wishes.

"Be calm," she tells him, "please hold on. We'll all talk together. I'm coming right in."

Leaving a note for her family, she gets into her car and drives back to the hospital.

When Jeannie arrives on the floor and walks into the patient's room, what she finds does not surprise her. Seated by the bed is the visibly distraught husband. Behind him, the patient's twenty-five-year-old daughter paces in front of the large picture window that looks across Boston. The patient herself is lying in a state somewhere between consciousness and coma, shrunken by pain and devoured by the cancer's progress. Jeannie has seen scenes like this many times before in her fifteen-year career as a nurse. A patient who has tried to fight his or her disease for months, perhaps years, is reconciled with death. But the family and / or medical team are unable to let go.

As she looks at the woman, she can understand why her family is so resistant. Her child and husband remember her as she first appeared to Jeannie three years ago. Then she was a bright, feisty, sixty-year-old woman — nails tapered and polished, hair sleekly sculpted into a perfect silver pouf. Jeannie remembers the day, on that first of many subsequent admissions to a medical unit on the sixth floor of the Feldberg Building — a building of the hospital named after a wealthy donor — when she asked the woman if she wanted her hair washed.

"Wash my hair?" the woman replied in astonishment. Then she announced in a clearly enunciated staccato, "I do not wash my hair. I have it done. Once a week."

Now that hair is unkempt, glued to her face with sweat. Her nails are no longer polished. Their main work these days is to dig into her flesh when the pain becomes too acute. That immaculately tailored frame has crumbled under her. The disease — like the dirt and stones that pit and burrow into winter snow, eroding its pristine surface — has slowly bored through her bones. Simply to stand evokes pain and could even be an invitation to a fracture. The doctors have done everything to try to shore her up and beat back the disease — operated and pinned disintegrating bones, treated every infection, given her narcotics to try to offset the excruciating pain.

To no avail. Her pelvis is disintegrating. The nurses have inserted an indwelling catheter because the simple act of slipping a bedpan underneath her causes agony. But she has developed a urinary tract infection. Because removing the catheter will make the infection easier to treat, doctors suggest this course of action. Yet, if the catheter is removed, the pain will be intolerable each time she has to urinate.

When the residents and interns argued that to fail to treat the infection could mean the patient might die, Jeannie responded, "She's dying anyway. It's her disease that is killing her, not a urinary tract infection," and they relented.

Now, it is the family's moment to confront reality.

Jeannie goes up to the woman's bed and gently wakens her. Smiling at her nurse, the woman tries to muster the energy to explain to her daughter and husband that the pain is too great, she can no longer attain that delicate balance between fighting off pain and remaining alert for at least some of the day that is so crucial to dying patients. Only when she is so drugged that she is practically comatose can she find relief. Using Jeannie as an intermediary to relay the words that were too painful for her to tell her family herself, she apologizes because she no longer has the strength to continue fighting.

That isn't living, she tells them. "I am ready to die," she whispers weakly.

But they interrupt, try to contradict her, and promise that there is still hope.

Jeannie Chaisson stands silently during this exchange and then intervenes, asking them to try to take in what their loved one is telling them. Then she repeats the basic facts about the disease and its course. "At this point we have no treatment for the disease," she explains. "But we do have treatment for the pain, and we can make her comfortable and ease her suffering." Jeannie spends another hour simply sitting with them, answering their questions and allowing them to feel supported. The family finally is able to heed the wishes of the patient — to leave in the catheter, not to resuscitate her if she suffers a cardiac arrest. Give her enough morphine to stop her from feeling pain. Let her go.

The woman visibly relaxes, lies back, and closes her eyes. Jeannie approaches the daughter and husband with whom she has worked for so long and with a look of great sympathy and affection, hugs them both in turn. Then she goes out to talk to the medical team.

Before leaving for home, Jeannie again visits her patient. The husband and daughter have gone for a cup of coffee. The woman is quiet. Jeannie sits down at the side of her bed and takes her hand. The woman opens her eyes. Too exhausted to say a word, she merely squeezes Jeannie's hand in gratitude. For the past three years, Jeannie has helped her to fight her disease and live as long as possible. Now she is here to help her with her most difficult work. She is helping her to die.

When we hear the words "hospital," "medicine," "health care," images of technology and scientific invention often spring to mind. Mechanical ventilators, dialysis machines, intravenous pumps, biomedical research, surgery, medication. These, many believe, are the life supports in our health care system. It is this science and technology that keeps people alive, that helps them cure and heal.

In fact, there are other equally important life supports in our health care system. These are the 2.5 million nurses in America who make up the largest profession in health care, the largest female profession in America, and the second-largest profession. These women — and men — weave a tapestry of care, knowledge, relationship, and trust that is critical to patients' survival.

This book is the story of three of those nurses practicing on the front lines of nursing, of technology, and of the many changes in our health care system.

Nancy Rumplik, Jeannie Chaisson, and Ellen Kitchen have, between them, more than five decades of experience caring for the sick. They work in an acute care hospital — one of Harvard Medical School's teaching hospitals. The Beth Israel is not only known for the quality of its patient care, it is also world renowned for the quality of its nursing staff and its institutional commitment to nursing. Inside the BI, Nancy Rumplik, Jeannie Chaisson, and Ellen Kitchen are also recognized for their expertise. Nancy Rumplik is an outpatient nurse who works in an ambulatory cancer clinic; Jeannie Chaisson is a medical clinical nurse specialist on a general medical floor; and Ellen Kitchen is a nurse practitioner who delivers home care services. Their work thus spans the spectrum of what nurses do on inpatient hospital wards, outpatient services, and in the home and community.

As you watch these nurses work with patients, it might be easy to conclude that the knowledge, skill, and empathy they display are extraordinary. In fact, there are hundreds of thousands of expert nurses like them working in hospitals, nursing homes, rehabilitation facilities, psychiatric institutions and mental health clinics, rural and urban health clinics, public health, home care and hospice care all across the nation. Without their care of the body, patients would not recover and heal. Without their care of the soul, patients would be unable to withstand the arduous high-tech treatments upon which our modern medical system depends. Without their acceptance of death, our death-denying medical system would exact even more suffering from patients and their families.

Although nurses are some of the most cost-effective professionals, the for-profit, market-driven health care that is sweeping this nation — and many others — is threatening this valuable resource. To gain an advantage in the competitive new health care marketplace, hospitals all over the country are trying to cut their costs. One popular cost-cutting strategy is laying off nurses.

Three-fourths of all American hospitals are engaged in or developing plans for "restructuring," and many are laying off more than 20 to 50 percent of their nursing staff. For the first time in a decade, many nurses feel their patients are in danger. With great sadness and distress, they say that hospitals and insurers will not allow them to deliver the kind of quality care they have been educated to give patients and families.

Yet this very restructuring and downsizing of health care institutions is touted as one of the ways to cure our system's serious defects. The latter are well known. The American health care system suffers from lack of access, too much fragmented, expensive, high-tech treatment, not enough attention to health maintenance and disease prevention, and failure to attend to patients' emotional and social needs as well as their pain and suffering.

Reducing the number of experienced, educated nurses hardly solves these problems.

Although American hospitals already use about 20 to 40 percent fewer nurses than a number of other industrialized countries, hospital administrators and some nursing executives now argue that units staffed with educated, experienced nurses are a luxury we can no longer afford. Yet, in 1992, the average staff nurse earned a little less than $33,000 a year, the average clinical nurse specialist earned about $41,000 a year, and the average nurse practitioner earned slightly less than $44,000 a year. (At a major teaching hospital like those in Boston, staff nurses in a union bargaining unit can earn up to $67,000, while a clinical nurse specialist or nurse practitioner can earn more than $80,000.) Nurses' salaries and benefits compose only about 16 percent of hospitals' total costs.

Compare this with the average income of physicians. According to *Modern Healthcare*'s 1996 physician compensation report, physicians' compensation in internal medicine is $135,755, in family practice $128,096, in anesthesiology $193,242, in oncology $164,621, and in general surgery $199,342. Some specialist physicians earn up to several million dollars a year.

A survey conducted in 1995 by *Hospitals & Health Networks*, the magazine of the American Hospital Association, stated that the average base salary and total cash compensation for hospital CEOs was $188,500. In a large hospital that went up to $280,900. And in a for-profit chain it's far higher. In 1995, at age forty-three, Richard Scott,

CEO of Columbia / HCA Healthcare Corporation received a salary of $2,093,844. He personally controls shares in Columbia / HCA worth $359.5 million.

Nurses' salaries seem particularly paltry when compared with some of the most egregious waste in the system — the income of the CEOs of for-profit HMOs. In 1994, the executive compensation packages of the CEOs of the seven largest for-profit HMOs averaged $7.9 million. Even CEOs of not-for-profit insurers make startling sums. John Burry Jr., chairman and CEO of the nonprofit Ohio Blue Cross Blue Shield was paid $1.6 million. According to a report in *Modern Healthcare*, a proposed merger with the for-profit Columbia / HCA Healthcare Corporation would have paid him $3 million "for a decade-long no-compete contract . . . and up to seven million for two consulting agreements."

Nurses are clearly not the cost escalators in the system. Quite the contrary. Their care saves not only lives but money.

Over the past twenty years, this fact has been confirmed in study after study. In major studies conducted in 1976, 1986, 1989, 1994, and 1995, medical and nursing researchers linked the number and educational qualifications of registered nurses on hospital units to lower mortality rates and decreased lengths of hospital stay.

Reducing the number of expert nurses in the hospital, community, and home needlessly endangers patients' lives and wastes scarce resources.

Nurses have also helped to increase access to our health care system. Many provide services to some of the 41 million Americans who have no health insurance or to Americans who live in areas that physicians tend to avoid. It is Ellen Kitchen and her colleagues who give health care to poor minority women and their newborns, who staff rural health clinics in which few doctors choose to practice, or who go into the homes of the elderly and homebound, allowing them to live on their own for as long as possible. Again, by helping elderly citizens to live at home, rather than in a nursing home, this kind of care saves billions.

Choosing to save money by reducing nursing care aggravates the impersonality and inhumanity of a medical system that tends to turn human beings into their diseases and the doctors who care for them into sophisticated clinical machines. When they're sick, patients do not only ask what pills they should take or what operations they should have. They are preoccupied with questions like, Why me? Why now? How can I deal with this? How can we, as a family, cope? Where is hope? Is there meaning? Is there God?

Because of their history, and their daily work, nurses live through this day-by-day, minute-by-minute attack on the soul. They know that, for the patient, there is not only a sick or infirm body, but a life, a family, a community, a society that has been disrupted and that needs to heal.

Although nurses help us live and die, in the public depiction of health care, patients seem to emerge from hospitals without ever having benefited from their assistance. Whether patients are treated in an emergency room in a few short hours, or on a critical-care unit for months on end, we seem certain that physicians are responsible for all the successes — or failures — in our medical system. In fact, we seem to believe that they are responsible not only for all of the curing, but for much of the caring.

Nurses, on the other hand, remain shadowy figures moving mysteriously in the background. On television series, nurses often appear as comic figures. In TV shows like the short-lived *Nightingales*, the sitcom *Nurses*, or the medical drama *Chicago Hope*, nurses are far too busy pining after doctors or racing off to aerobics classes to actually care for patients. The new hit *ER* gives nurses more prominence than many other doctor shows. Nonetheless, doctors on *ER* are constantly barking out the simplest commands — get a blood pressure, a Chem-13 (blood chemistries), type and cross, and call the OR, or call respiratory therapy — to experienced emergency room nurses.

In reality, these nurses would have thought of all this before the doctor. In an emergency room as busy and sophisticated as the one on *ER* (this is, after all, a level one trauma center), the first clinician a patient would see is a triage nurse, who would assess the patient and dictate what he or she needs, who will see him or her, and when. Experienced nurses will, in fact, direct less-experienced residents, suggesting a medication, test, consultation with a specialist, or transfer to the operating room. The great irony of *ER* is that Carol Hathaway, the nurse in charge — and thus one of the key figures in any real emergency room — is generally relegated to comforting a child or following a physician's direction rather than helping to direct the staff in saving lives.

Not only do doctors dominate television, they are also the focus of most hard-news health care coverage. Reporters rarely cover nursing innovations, use nurses as sources, or report on nursing research. When reporters and politicians consult with health care experts and report on their recommendations or their responses to reform proposals, they invariably interview physicians, representatives of physician organizations, or health care policy specialists who tend to look at health care either through the prism of medicine or through economics. Thus, a 1990 study, "Who Counts in News Coverage of Health Care?" of the health care coverage in three American newspapers of record — the *New York Times*, the *Los Angeles Times*, and the *Washington Post* — documented that out of 908 quotes that appeared in three months' worth of health care stories, nurses were quoted exactly ten times.

Conventional wisdom has held that when more women entered the nation's newsrooms, they would pay greater attention to the varied contributions of women in society. This hasn't helped those women who are nurses. Of the 119 articles women journalists clearly authored, there was a larger percentage of female main sources (23.53%) than in those authored by men (16.01%). Female journalists tended to quote more female physicians, hospital administrators, organizational spokespersons, politicians, and policymakers. But female reporters did not seek out nurses for sources of information or expertise any more frequently than their male counterparts.

Today, the revolution in health care has become big news. Occasionally reporters turn their attention to the phenomenon of nursing layoffs. But the story is rarely framed as an important public health issue. Rather it is generally depicted as a labor-management conflict. Nursing unions are battling with management. Nurses say this, hospital administrators claim that. Whom can you believe?

Worse still, this issue may be couched in the worst stereotypes of nursing / women's work. A typical example ran on NBC's *Nightly News*. The show did a story about problems of substituting aides for nurses: the anchor introduced it as "a new and controversial way of administering TLC." Imagine how reporters would play the issue if 20 to 50 percent of physician staff were eliminated in thousands of American hospitals. Would it not be front page news, a major public health catastrophe? Patients all over the country would be terrified to enter hospitals. Yet, we learn about the nursing equivalent with only a minimum of concern. If the only problem with laying off thousands of nurses is the loss of a little TLC, what difference does it make if an aide replaces a nurse?

But nursing is not a matter of TLC. It's a matter of life and death. In the hospitals where 66 percent of nurses work, nurses are the ones who monitor and evaluate a patient's condition before, during, and after high-tech medical procedures. It is the nurse who adjusts medications, manages pain and side effects of treatment, acts instantly to intervene if there are life-threatening changes in a patient's condition, or alerts physicians so that they can protect their patients.

Nurses like Nancy Rumplik, Jeannie Chaisson, and Ellen Kitchen are constantly engaged in what appear to be simple interactions — administering a medication, giving a bath, emptying a bedpan, checking a patient's medication box, making sure his home refrigerator is well stocked. But there is nothing simple about these exchanges. They are some of the threads with which their tapestry of care is woven and are critical to nurses' knowledge of and relationships with patients. These encounters allow nurses to develop a sense of patients that they refer to as the patient's "baseline." This permits them to know, often at a glance, when an important change in a patient's condition has occurred even before that change is registered in a falling blood pressure, rising temperature, or labored breathing.

In a cancer ward, nurses catch a serious reaction to medication almost before it happens. In an operating room, nurses make sure the right patient is being operated on, or that the right procedure is being performed on the right limb or organ. On an ICU or in home care, nurses question why a patient is getting another painful diagnostic test that may reveal little useful information; why adequate pain medication is not given following surgery; why a patient is being discharged too quickly; whether someone is available to take care of the patient in the home; and at the end of life, why expensive, heroic treatment that will only prolong death is presented as the only option.

In the self-enclosed world of the high-tech hospital, where ordinary men and women and children are confronted with people who wear alien costumes, adhere to peculiar customs, and even speak their own language, nurses help patients deal with their fear and anxiety — not only of their diseases but of the people who are supposed to cure them. Watch Nancy, Jeannie, and Ellen, and you see how important this is to frightened patients and family members.

In our high-tech medical system, nurses are the ones who care for the body and the soul. No matter how sensitive, caring, and attentive physicians are, in both the hospital and home nurses are often closer to patients' needs and wishes than physicians. That's not because nurses are inherently more caring than doctors, but because they spend far more time with patients and know them better. This investment of time and knowledge allows nurses to save lives. But nurses also help people adjust to the lives they must live after they have been saved. And when death can no longer be delayed, nurses help patients confront their own mortality with at least some measure of grace and dignity.

The tapestry of care that nurses weave would be much strengthened if physicians and nurses constructed it together and if both groups had an equal voice in health care institutions and in the health care system as a whole. In many instances, both in this book and in the health care system, doctors and nurses do cooperate effectively. But, in general, the history of medicine and nursing and contemporary physician-and-nurse relationships preclude genuine collaboration. In spite of their important work, nurses — members of a quintessentially female profession (95 percent of all nurses are female) — have long been subordinated to the quintessentially male profession of medicine. In the American medical system, rigid, gender-ridden hierarchies make it difficult for doctors and nurses to relate as colleagues. Thus, today, many doctors — male and female alike — still consider nurses to be their handmaidens.

This has serious consequences for patients and for the health care system as a whole. When doctors don't listen to nurses, they can't hear their patients. In 1995, the *Journal of the American Medical Association* (*JAMA*) released the highly publicized SUPPORT study (the Study to Understand Prognoses and Preferences for Outcomes and Risks of Treatments) focused on patients' suffering at the end of life. Over the course of five years, the study tracked the experiences of 9,105 dying patients in five major medical centers. To help patients die with less-aggressive treatment and in greater comfort, doctors were provided with up-to-date information on patient prognoses. Expert nurses communicated with patients and families and relayed information about patient wishes to physicians, and great attention was paid to pain control. Yet the results were abysmal. Physicians did not understand or heed patients' wishes, too many patients spent too much time on ICUs, and too many died in pain.

Why did this well-intentioned project go wrong? As Bernard Lo, who wrote a *JAMA* editorial on the study, told the media (and one of the nurses involved in the study told me), doctors are notoriously unwilling to listen to nurses. Should we be surprised, then, when the result for patients is less than satisfactory? We must do more than teach doctors how to listen to patients. We must teach them how to learn from and collaborate with nurses. And in an era when more and more members of the public are worried about how they will die, they must understand the role nurses can play in helping them cope with pain and suffering and finding a good enough death.

There is another reason nurses' work so often goes unrecognized. Even some of the patients who have benefited the most from nurses' critical care are unable to publicly credit its importance. Because nurses share and cushion what Oliver Sacks has called human beings' "radical fall into sickness," nurses are a living reminder of the pain, fear, vulnerability, and loss of control adults find it so difficult to tolerate and thus openly discuss. A man who has just had a successful bypass operation will boast of his surgeon's accomplishments to his friends at a dinner party. A woman who has just survived a bone marrow transplant will extol her oncologist's triumph in the war against cancer to her friends and relatives.

But what nurses did for those two individuals will rarely be mentioned. It was a nurse who bathed the cardiac patient and comforted this grown man while he struggled with the terror of not knowing if he would live or die. It was a nurse who held the plastic dish under the cancer patient's lips as she was wracked with nausea and who wiped a bottom raw from diarrhea. As Claire Fagin and Donna Diers have explained in an eloquent essay entitled "Nursing as Metaphor," nurses are a metaphor for intimacy. They are our secret sharers. Even though they are patients' lifelines during illness, when control is restored the residue of our anxiety and mortality clings to them like dust and we flee the memory.

Because we would prefer to forget the realities of illness, we grasp the fantasy that medicine can triumph over the human condition. In defining health care as medical care, we've come to think of illness as an event. You get sick. You go to a doctor. He or she gives you a diagnosis and treatment plan. You follow it and hopefully you are cured.

But illness is a process, not an event — one that requires care both before, during, and after the medical encounters that punctuate it. Rather than forcing nursing into the biomedical model of diagnosis, treatment, and cure, think of nursing as a tapestry of care woven from countless threads into an intricate whole. At one moment, a nurse like Nancy Rumplik, Jeannie Chaisson, or Ellen Kitchen may be involved in a sophisticated clinical procedure that demands expert judgment and advanced training in the latest technology. The next moment, or even at the same time, she may do what many people consider trivial or menial work, such as emptying a bedpan, giving a bed bath, administering medication, feeding or walking a patient.

The fact that nurses' work is interspersed with many so-called menial tasks that don't demand total attention is not a reason to demean their work or, as is happening today, to replace nurses with less-skilled workers. It's this hands-on care that allows nurses to explore patients' physical condition *and* register their anxiety and fear. It's this that allows them to save lives *and* to ascertain when it is appropriate to help patients die. And it is only in watching them weave the tapestry of care that we grasp its integrity and intent.

Chapter 2

The Care of Strangers

NANCY RUMPLIK

The first patient of Nancy Rumplik's day is Deborah Celli.* I think of Debussy's melancholy refrain from "The Girl with the Flaxen Hair" when I first meet her. Her thick blond hair falls across her face as if it were a shield. Her head forlornly bends into the cascade.

She is waiting in Hematology / Oncology Clinic's so-called family room — an office that has been temporarily equipped with a couch and upholstered metal office chair — for her nurse, Nancy Rumplik, to administer her chemotherapy. But it takes Nancy a few extra moments to reach Deborah. That's because the young woman is not receiving her chemo in the main treatment area of the Hematology / Oncology Clinic, which is housed on the third floor of an older building — the Kirstein Building — across the narrow hospital driveway from the main hospital area. Patients ride up a creaky elevator to the third floor and exit directly into the clinic's waiting room, which is furnished with rows of comfortable chairs, up-to-date magazines, a large urn of steaming coffee for patients, friends, or family members, and a reception station.

A series of exam rooms where physicians meet with patients is scattered along a narrow corridor off to the left. A phlebotomist's station stands at the head of this corridor. There, patients stop for their first exercise at most visits — a blood draw. For patients currently on treatment, the phlebotomist permanently assigned to the unit does a finger stick. This provides enough blood for the complete blood chemistries (CBCs) that will show if a patient's white blood and / or platelet count is high enough to permit chemotherapy (patients with low white cell counts or low platelet counts are susceptible to infection and bleeding and administration of chemotherapy may not be safe). If other blood tests are necessary, the nurse will draw blood prior to giving chemotherapy. The blood is taken down to the end of this corridor, where the unit's lab tech has a small laboratory in which she does blood counts (any other, more sophisticated blood work is done in the main hospital lab). The unit's health assistant is also stationed here. She weighs patients and takes their vital signs — temperature, pulse, and blood pressure.

To get to the unit's treatment area, patients walk through a small hallway off the waiting room into a brightly lit space containing the nurses' station with the reclining chairs that encircle it. At the far end are two private patient rooms equipped with hospital beds for patients who are very sick and thus too weak to sit in treatment chairs, patients who have low white counts and are thus vulnerable to infection, patients who are themselves infectious because of decreased resistance resulting from chemotherapy, or those who are in particular need of privacy. Off to one side is a narrow, cramped coffee room where patients and staff can get juice, coffee, tea, or ginger ale (in great demand by patients who are often nauseous), and next to it is the pharmacist's station. The unit has its own pharmacist. After receiving physicians' orders, he prepares the chemotherapy drugs in a room with a modern fume hood that ventilates and filters any residues of the toxic chemicals he uses.

To get to the family room, Nancy must walk out of the main treatment area, down the exam room corridor, past the lab, out a set of double doors leading to the rest of the building, and past the physician conference room with its many microscopes and x-ray view boxes where the unit's fellows meet with attending physicians for formal and informal teaching rounds. Several doors past the conference room is the makeshift family room.

Nancy wheels an IV pole beside her and carries loops of plastic tubing, a plastic sack containing saline solution, and a small tray with several vials of drugs. As Deborah hears Nancy enter, she stirs and seems to move in slow motion, lifting her neck, then her head, then parting the hair in front of her face. Finally, with only a faint smile, she acknowledges the nurse's presence.

Nancy is accustomed to her patients' anxiety and depression. But Deborah's sense of dejection is even more acute than that of many cancer patients. And it is no wonder. From an Italian working-class family from outside of Boston, she was diagnosed with Hodgkin's disease eighteen years ago when she was only twelve. This cancer of the lymphatic system can often be cured. For Deborah, cure came at a terrific price. Over the course of six months, she underwent mantle radiation — radiation of her entire sternum — followed by six cycles of MOPP, an arduous chemotherapeutic cocktail made up of nitrogen mustard, Oncovin (vincristine), procarbazine hydrochloride, and prednisone.

In any era chemotherapy is difficult to tolerate. Because cytotoxic drugs — drugs that attack cancer cells — are physiologically "blind," they attack not only fast-growing cancer cells, but all fast-growing cells. That's why patients on cancer chemotherapy often lose their hair and suffer from mouth sores and diarrhea. Hair follicles and mucous membranes are fed by fast-growing cells. Cytotoxic drugs also directly affect the vomit center in the brain.

Today, there are a number of drugs that are effective in blocking nausea. But when Deborah had Hodgkin's disease there were far fewer. The uncontrollable nausea and vomiting were not well tempered.

But Deborah did not die.

For thirteen years she was fine. She married Richard Celli,* had two children, now toddlers, and then a few months ago discovered a lump in her breast. She was diagnosed with infiltrating, multifocal breast cancer, grade III — the highest grade, a very negative prognostic factor. It means that the cancer has more likely spread to other organs and is therefore likely to recur.

Doctors recommended a mastectomy. This was followed by breast reconstruction. She is also receiving what is called adjuvant chemotherapy — chemotherapy that tries to eliminate any stray cancer cells that might migrate through the body. Deborah's oncologist prescribed a regimen called CMF.

This treatment lasts for about six months and includes six cycles of cyclophosphamide (Cytoxan), methotrexate, and 5-fluorouracil. The two latter drugs are given by what is called IV (intravenous) push in the clinic on day one and day eight. From day one to day fourteen, the Cytoxan is taken orally. The cycle lasts twenty-eight days, involves two visits to the clinic spaced seven days apart, with two weeks off all chemotherapeutic agents before it begins again. During that two-week period, Deborah will, however, need to have a CBC.

Nancy works in the clinic from Monday to Friday and follows about two hundred primary patients. When she first learned about this new breast cancer patient, she envisioned her role as helping the young woman through the chemotherapy by administering the treatment and monitoring the side effects. Then she read the patient's chart and talked with the doctor and social worker. Nancy realized Deborah would be a far more complicated patient to care for than a woman who had just been diagnosed with cancer for the first time.

"You always dread it when you learn that a patient had Hodgkin's disease over a decade ago, because you know how sick their treatment made them," Nancy explains. "Many cancer patients currently undergoing chemotherapy suffer from anticipatory nausea and vomiting. The medications they take make them nauseous, and so they sometimes get sick before a treatment, just in anticipation. But because of her history, Deborah is even worse. She only has to walk into the main treatment area of the clinic to throw up."

Just getting Deborah through one or two good cycles of chemotherapy, Nancy believed, would be a major challenge. Deborah's emotional response to the prospect of chemotherapy was, for example, what led to the family room. Most patients do not get their chemotherapy in an antechamber. They sit in the treatment area in reclining blue leather chairs arranged in a semicircle around the nurses' station in the middle of the clinic. The smell and sight of chemicals is all-pervasive. So is the vision of their impact on the human body and soul.

In this treatment area, privacy is the most ephemeral of commodities. The two small patient rooms shelter those who must discuss highly sensitive issues — the fact that the cancer is not responding to chemotherapy, or that a patient's family is unable to cope — while getting treatment. But when patients are in the main treatment area, they observe an unwritten code of etiquette. They try not to stare at one another, concentrating instead on their magazines, books, or the small televisions that jut out from wall attachments in front of their chairs.

When a patient begins to retch, breaks down in tears, has a sensitive conversation with a physician, nurse, or social worker, or suffers a more serious medical crisis, plaid cotton curtains are hastily drawn to create the illusion of privacy. But it is often too little too late. Others have captured that burst of sorrow or terror and can hear the whispers, sobs, or in the case of an emergency, the frantic comings and goings of the medical staff.

Unwritten rules nonetheless stipulate the pretense of ignorance. Like a judge who advises a jury to disregard what a witness has just said, patients try to filter out the distressing evidence of the disease and its treatment. They struggle to make inadmissible the emaciated man who is clearly dying of AIDS; the elegant, sophisticated thirty-something woman with breast cancer; the old woman huddled in the arms of her daughter; or the woman going into respiratory arrest and gasping for air.

It is no wonder that nursing scholar Patricia Benner says that one of the main things nurses do is keep hospitals from scaring patients to death.

Deborah Celli has known too much about hospitals in her short life. She is unable to feign disregard. All she has to do is remember her first encounter with cancer to feel defeated by this one.

When Nancy joined Deborah's doctor and was introduced to Deborah, the issue of the first incidence of cancer was, thus, everyone's paramount concern. For Deborah, it was the reason not to endure another course of chemotherapy. Deborah simply could not believe that chemotherapy would increase her chances for a cancer-free life. That was what the medical experts had said so many years ago, and here she was. This was not supposed to happen. Why should she believe it would not happen again? How could she be convinced that it wasn't the first chemo and radiation therapy that actually brought on the breast cancer? Her concerns are, in fact, understandable. For people who have had chemotherapy or radiation before, there is an increase in second malignancies.

"The very first issue we had to deal with was getting her the chemotherapy," Nancy says. "She has so many terrible associations with chemotherapy, which is why we went to the family room. The major thing was to get her through one cycle at a time."

Because Deborah couldn't face going into the main clinic, Nancy assured Deborah that she could enter the main door to the Kirstein Building, walk through the narrow first-floor corridors, turn right, and take the elevator leading directly to the corridor outside the family room. The only visible evidence of the clinic would be the sign outside its entrance. Nancy would join her there. Nancy would even do the blood draws for Deborah's blood counts herself. As far as was possible, the team would try to erase the clinic from her mind.

Deborah agreed, and Nancy could start on her first priority — administering Deborah's drugs.

Today Nancy is giving Deborah her treatment. The actual administration of Deborah's chemotherapeutic drugs is only the last phase of the multistep process that Nancy engages in with every patient to whom she gives medication. Both legally and ethically, nurses are responsible for the medications and treatments they administer. Nurses are patients' last line of defense in a system that is supposed to protect patients from potentially harmful or lethal human errors.

Before Nancy even approaches Deborah with her medication, she has checked it against the physician's written order. "According to an old-fashioned saying in nursing, we check the Five Rights — Right Patient, Right Drug, Right Dose, Right Method (intravenous versus intramuscular, to be swallowed versus dissolved under the tongue), and Right Time," Nancy explains.

When it comes to chemotherapy drugs, Nancy looks at the physician's order and then does her own calculations to make sure it is correct. "First, of course, you make sure it's the right drug. All nurses are educated in a general knowledge of pharmacology. But when you specialize, as I have in oncology, then you add specialized knowledge of the specific drugs used in the field. For example, you have to know that you wouldn't give a breast cancer patient CHOP [a chemotherapy regimen for patients with lymphoma] or a lymphoma patient CMF. Then you have to check the dose. To do this I calculate the patient's BSA — body surface area."

Nancy goes to the computer and enters the patient's height and weight to calculate the correct BSA. The computer program determines the body surface area in metered square. Deborah, for example, is five feet two inches tall and weighs 110 pounds. This makes her 1.5 meters squared. To calculate Deborah's dose of Cytoxan, which is 600 milligrams per meter squared, Nancy multiplies 600 times 1.5.

This method of calculation is used because weight itself is not an accurate measure in determining the dosage of chemotherapy drugs. What is critical is the actual volume in which the drug will be distributed. If, for example, a patient is very thin and very tall, his or her body weight alone would lead to an underdose of medication. Conversely, if a patient is short and fat, using body weight alone to calculate the dose might lead to a fatal overdose.

"You have to check everything yourself," Nancy says. "Although it's rare, sometimes the recorded weight is incorrect. Also sometimes patients lose weight and you have to recalculate their BSA. If I think there is a question about body surface area, I will weigh the patient again and recalculate. And believe me, sometimes the dose needs to be recalculated."

Then Nancy makes sure it is the right time to give the drug. "If the patient is supposed to receive their drugs every three weeks, you have to check and make sure they have come in to the clinic at three weeks, not two weeks. Again, there are mistakes. I've sent people home because they've come in at the wrong time to take their drugs."

Besides making sure she is giving the right dose of the right drug to the right patient at the right time with the right method, she must also make sure the patient's blood counts are in the right range. Nancy thus checks Deborah's white counts to make sure it's safe to administer the chemotherapy at this particular moment. "Most chemotherapeutic agents make white counts drop. To avoid neutropenia — a state in which patients' white counts are dangerously low and they don't have enough neutrophils [mature white cells] to fight infection — you have to make sure their counts are okay." (Nancy and the doctors are aware that patients can still become neutropenic even though they receive chemotherapy with normal white counts.)

Once all this is checked, Nancy gives the medication order to the clinic pharmacy and the pharmacist mixes the drugs. When Nancy comes back to get them, she checks the vials — the patient's name, drug name, and dosage are all marked clearly on the label — and then, with the top copy of the physician's order, she goes to the patient to give the drugs. At this point, she also pays attention to any questions or reservations the patient may have. "You always listen to a patient. If someone says, 'I've never taken a blue pill before,' then I never give them that blue pill without checking." As Nancy adds, her motto is "The patient is always right."

After a final check of the drugs against the orders, she gives the drugs.

Today, before inserting the IV and hanging Deborah's medication, Nancy sits down next to her and asks her how she is. The young woman mutters that she is okay. Nancy then reaches for a rectangular plastic hot pack, hits it with her fist to release the heat, and wraps it carefully around the back of Deborah's hand.

When the heat makes Deborah's vein swell, Nancy places a tourniquet around her upper arm and then gently massages the back of her hand. Deborah averts her eyes and winces as Nancy smoothly inserts a finely honed needle with a blue butterfly-shaped handle into the vein. Then she hangs a transparent coil of tubing, which is attached to the IV. Into it she will inject saline and the anticancer agents. The latter will attack, and hopefully destroy, any cancer cells that cling to Deborah's chest wall despite her mastectomy or that have migrated through her body during the period before her breast cancer was removed.

Finally, she adjusts the rate of the saline drip. After the saline drips into the vein, she will add the anticancer drugs one after another. The saline drip, she explains to me later, is a clinic staple. It serves to dilute the IV push drugs so they are less traumatic to the vein. "If Deborah went to some other doctor's offices, she might have been given the drugs without the saline and they would have been delivered much more quickly — perhaps in forty-five minutes. I give them to her over about a two-hour period very deliberately."

Some might argue that giving the drugs more slowly — which means nurses can administer chemotherapy to fewer patients — is too costly. In fact, as we shall see, the time Nancy devotes to a patient like Deborah actually makes it possible for the patient to continue her therapy and follow her physician's recommendations as well as deal with other significant problems that emerge.

For Deborah, as for so many cancer patients, the relationship to her nurse becomes a powerful therapeutic tool. "From the very beginning," Nancy says, "it became clear that my objective was to have time with her because I knew how much she needed to talk."

And talk Deborah does, during each session as well as during telephone calls to Nancy in between sessions.

Not surprisingly, one of Deborah's main concerns is controlling her nausea. A number of antinausea medications are tried, but none seems to work well. The most effective medication for her turns out to be Marinol, the brand name for THC, or delta-9-tetrahydrocannabinol, the active ingredient of marijuana in pill form. Unfortunately, in spite of the drug's efficacy, getting an adequate supply proves to be a problem. Not many pharmacies regularly stock Marinol and the pharmacy chain closest to Deborah's house not only has difficulty getting it, but seems reluctant to do so.

This becomes clear one Friday early in Deborah's treatment. In the midst of a busy day in the clinic Nancy is called to the phone. She sits on a swivel chair at the nurses' station and rolls up to the wide desk she shares with her colleagues. It's Deborah, in tears. The patient explains that after she left the clinic that Friday morning, she took her prescription for Marinol directly to her pharmacy as Nancy had advised. The pharmacist told her he could not get the pills until the next day. Although this was a day late for Deborah, she had another, less effective, antinausea drug on hand and felt she could tough out the nausea for that one day. Assured that she would have the Marinol on Saturday, she left off the prescription.

But she had just received a call from the pharmacist saying that he could not get the pills until Monday. What was worse, and most humiliating, Deborah sobs, was the fact that the pharmacist gave her the distinct feeling that he didn't really believe she needed the Marinol. "He thinks I only want it so I can get legally stoned," she cries. She says he seemed completely unaware that she has cancer and needs the medication for legitimate reasons.

"It's too much," Deborah exclaims. "I can't deal with this."

Frowning, Nancy listens to the story. Effective symptom management is central to Deborah's continued treatment. To control her nausea, Deborah will have to take the Marinol at consistent intervals coordinating with her medication. Which in turn means that her pharmacist will have to provide those pills expeditiously. Yet, this pharmacist is apparently an obstacle, rather than an adjunct, to treatment.

In a calm voice, Nancy tells Deborah she would like to call the pharmacy. "I have to talk to him, because I really have an issue with this. If they can't find the drug, they're supposed to notify us. More to the point, you need this drug now, not on Monday. It's their job to find it for you now, not four days after it's ordered. I need to explain that you needed it yesterday and that it was their job to get it for you."

Deborah agrees and hangs up. Nancy stands by the phone shaking her head in disbelief. She has heard many similar tales in her long career as a nurse, but she has never become accustomed to such unsympathetic responses to the suffering of her patients. She turns and relays the story to one of her colleagues, Paddy Connelly. How, she asks, could a pharmacist lay such a guilt trip on a woman who has had not just one, but two bouts of cancer. Then she dials the chain pharmacy to convey her instructions — in strong but measured tones — to the pharmacist. After explaining the urgency of the matter, she also puts in a call to an independent pharmacy to ask if they stock the drug. They do. She explains that a patient might be coming in to pick it up later that afternoon. This druggist is immensely helpful and says he will have the drug for Nancy's patient. Turning to me, Nancy explains that she was not surprised at this reaction. "If you work with an independent pharmacist, they'll break their back to get you stuff. If you go to a big chain, it's such a warehouse that they really don't try very hard."

Several minutes later, Deborah calls again. She had just spoken to the chain's pharmacist, who, prodded by Nancy's terse comments, explained that he could not, in fact, get the drug. He had, however, found another nearby pharmacy that could, perhaps, have it for her later that afternoon.

"Listen, Deb," Nancy advises, "what you have to do is call that pharmacy and see if they can have the drug by three this afternoon. If they can't you have to go back to the chain and get the prescription and then come into Brookline to Pelham Drug." She pauses to commiserate with Deborah about the inconvenience of such a course of action but adds that it is the only way to make sure she will get what she needs.

"We used to be able to call in narcotic prescriptions to the phar-

macy," she explains. "But now we either have to give patients the prescription when they're here or mail it to them. So when something
like this happens, it's very hard on a patient or their family member."
The patient is already sick, she adds, and it's unconscionable to make
them drive from pharmacy to pharmacy picking up prescriptions and
trying to get them filled, or for them to have to drive an hour back to
the clinic for another prescription. But that is what happens all too
often.

Finally, Deborah gets the drug. A week later, as she receives her IV
chemo, Nancy asks if the Marinol helped and how Deborah is coping. Deborah lifts her head and whispers bleakly, "Each time I feel
the nausea in the morning, it reminds me of the MOPP."

"I know." Nancy nods. "That's why it's so important for you to
keep taking the medication at the right time."

Deborah seems not to register this and continues. "I hear all these
stories about how people do so well with chemotherapy these days.
And look at me. I just can't seem to cope. Everything just seems to be
going wrong. I'm so sick I can't do anything. I'm so tired I can barely
take care of my kids. I'm getting fat. And now, this," she laments,
running her hands through her straight hair and pulling out the
strands. "I'm losing my hair."

Bending into her grief, she cries quietly.

Nancy leans in to her as Deborah continues to draw her fingers
through her hair like a child picking furiously at a festering scab and
moans, "It's coming out. It used to be so thick, and now it's coming
out."

She looks up at the nurse. "You know, Nancy, it's funny. The only
thing I have ever liked about myself is my hair. When everything else
was bad, I would think, well at least I have nice hair. And now," she
pauses, peering at the golden filaments, "I'm losing it all."

Nancy's face fills with empathy. "It's as if your hair were your self-
esteem," she suggests.

"I can't do anything right," Deborah says with growing frustration. "Nothing. Not even this. Look at me. I've done nothing with
my life. Nothing."

Struck by the brutality of her patient's self-deprecation, Nancy
shifts back in her chair. Then she moves forward, puts her hand
under Deborah's chin and lifts her head so that Deborah is looking
straight at her.

"Deborah," she says emphatically, "you have to understand that all these feelings are perfectly normal. Everybody who undergoes this kind of treatment has them. Everybody. But everybody did not have cancer when they were so young. You have to remember that. You have to remember that you have spent half of your life trying to save your life, and that's an incredible accomplishment." Nancy presents this analysis gently, but in the firmest tones.

A flicker of hope seems to light Deborah's eyes. "But why don't other people understand this, Nancy?" she asks. "My mother-in-law comes over and sees me in my bathrobe and gets right on my case. 'Why am I in bed, why aren't I doing more in the house, how can I let the kids run wild?' My father took me home the other day from the clinic and started at me when he saw that I had left some meatballs on the stove overnight. 'What a waste,' he said. I tried to tell him that I have more important things to worry about now than meatballs. But he doesn't seem to understand."

After she catalogs her parent's and in-laws' responses, she gets to the most acute problem. "Rich [her husband] tells me he doesn't understand all this. The other day when I was feeling so sick, he said, 'I don't want to hear about the cancer. Don't talk to me anymore about the cancer!' He just doesn't get it. Neither he nor his mother or even my father. They just don't understand because none of them have ever been sick."

"It sounds like — and tell me if I'm wrong — that the people who are surrounding you don't know how to help you and support you," Nancy interjects. "They bring you in to the clinic, but there seems to be a breakdown afterwards."

"They all expect so much," Deborah agrees. "I do the best I can. I try so hard," she adds, desperately pleading for reassurance. Nancy puts her arms around the young woman and allows her to cry.

"I know you do, Deborah. I know you do, and I think you're doing great. We all do. But you can't get through this alone. You need support."

"I feel like I have to scrounge up every ounce of understanding." Deborah sobs.

Nancy waits a few moments and then proposes, "I think you might want to talk to Hester. Why don't I call her and see if she has time to talk to you today."

With a halfhearted nod, Deborah acquiesces, and Nancy leaves the room. When she returns, she explains that the social worker is booked up for the day but has requested that Deborah call tomorrow.

"Will you call, Deborah?" Nancy asks pointedly.

Despondent still, Deborah replies, "Probably not." The tears well up again as she explains, "When I call, it just brings the whole thing up again. Sometimes I just don't want to think about all this again — about being sick, about Richard. I just don't want to talk about it."

Nancy says calmly, "I think you told me enough. I'll call Hester and she'll reach you tomorrow."

Nancy leaves the room.

It happens this way each session. The conversation leads from Deborah's treatment to her side effects and then from those side effects to her personal history. Fix me, she seems to beg Nancy. Not just my cancer. Help me, please, to fix my life.

Nancy Rumplik, with a four-year degree in nursing and a master's in nursing administration and family nursing, is the epitome of the modern nurse. And the hospital she works in is clearly a state-of-the-art facility. Modern as she and her workplace may be, the critical role she, as a nurse, plays for her patients is nothing new. For well over a hundred years, nurses like Nancy Rumplik have been heeding the pleas of patients like Deborah Celli and have been central to their care. Not only have their activities transformed the lives of patients, they have transformed the entire health care system.

Nursing's transformation of health care began in the nineteenth century when advances in science helped to re-create the hospital as a more desirable place to care for the sick. Until the mid-1800s, the sick were almost exclusively cared for in the home. For those with no other alternative, the hospital offered a place of last resort. The hospitals were dreadful, filthy asylums whose patients were the poorest of the poor or sailors or wayfarers who were far from home. The "nurses" who delivered care to these patients were untrained women desperate for employment and willing to work under difficult circumstances. They might even have been former patients. Religious orders and institutions also maintained hospitals, often staffed by nuns.

It was the British involvement in the Crimean War of 1854 that changed all of this by giving the woman who is credited with founding modern nursing — Florence Nightingale — her great opportunity.

Far from being a shy and retiring "lady with the lamp," Nightingale not only launched a new profession, she was also the foremost hospital reformer of her day, one of the first nurse researchers, and one of the earliest health statisticians. She was an astute political operator who actually pushed, prodded, cajoled, threatened, and charmed whatever establishment figures blocked her way or whose patronage was necessary to achieving her goals.

Nightingale was born in 1820 to wealthy parents. Although she was very well educated, she was raised to marry well and fulfill the traditional family role of the wealthy Victorian woman. The young Florence Nightingale refused, however, to spend her days chatting at teas and her nights dancing at society balls. Before her seventeenth birthday, Nightingale had a mystical experience and determined to devote her life to God's service. She later decided that she was called to nursing the sick. Nightingale herself had often cared for sick relatives and villagers who lived near her parents' large estate. But she felt such efforts yielded insufficient knowledge of the sick and no systematic approaches to their care. She felt that a formal apprenticeship in nursing would be more useful. Thus, Nightingale proposed a term of study at an infirmary run by a friend of her family's and located near her home.

Rather than supporting this idea, Nightingale's family was aghast. The notion that a young aristocratic woman would spend her days working in such a place was beyond consideration. Thwarted, at least temporarily, Nightingale continued to pursue her dream of becoming a full-time nurse. That dream was fueled as much by her desire to escape the confines of the Victorian family as it was by her desire to care for the sick.

Nightingale was not one of the typical nineteenth-century feminists who fought primarily for women's suffrage. Nonetheless, in the early 1850s, while she was struggling to become a nurse, she wrote one of the most powerful feminist texts of her era. This essay on the position of women was a section of Nightingale's *Suggestions for Thought*. Privately published in 1860, this 829-page, three-volume work tried to articulate her spiritual philosophy. In passages like the following, Nightingale laid the foundation for Virginia Woolf's widely known argument against patriarchy articulated in *A Room of One's Own*. "In many families, there is one with a great dramatic talent, another with a genius for music, and a third one equally remarkable for the pencil; a fourth writes like Coleridge. Yet we know perfectly well that these will be neither Michael Angelos, nor Beethovens, nor Mrs. Siddonses, nor Miltons. Why? Mrs. A has the imagination, the poetry of a Murillo, and has sufficient power of execution to show that she might have had a great deal more. Why is she not a Murillo? From a material difficulty, not a mental one. If she has a knife and fork in her hands during three hours of the day, she cannot have a pencil or brush."

Impassioned by these sentiments, Nightingale refused to renounce her dream of professional nursing. In 1850, on one of her family's European tours, Nightingale visited Kaiserwerth, a hospital, penitentiary, and orphanage in Germany that taught working-class and peasant women to perform basic nursing services. A year later, she was able to persuade her parents to allow her to stay there for a period of three months to study its nursing service. When she and her family visited Paris in early 1853, Nightingale also advanced her career as one of the first health statisticians, gathering information on the organization of European hospitals and their nursing services.

Finally, in April 1853, Liz Herbert, the wife of Lord Sidney Herbert — a powerful aristocrat who soon became one of Nightingale's closest allies and sponsors — recommended her for the position of superintendent of a charity hospital in London known as the "Institution for the Care of Sick Gentlewomen in Distressed Circumstances." This served as a convalescent facility for governesses who fell ill and had no one to care for them at home, but who were a cut above those in the lower classes consigned to the squalid hospitals of the era. At age thirty-three, much to the displeasure of her mother and sister but aided by a five-hundred-pound annuity from her father, Nightingale took up her new job and an independent life.

Had it not been for one of the most disastrous campaigns in British military history, all of this might have been only a footnote in the development of modern nursing. But in 1854, England and France, in an alliance with Turkey, declared war on Russia. Their aim was to keep Russia from gaining control of the eastern Mediterranean. Like all wars, the conflict was supposed to end quickly with a minimum of casualties. Instead, it became a quagmire. For the first time in the history of war, a special correspondent — William Howard Russell, of the *Times* — sent home dispatches from the front that vividly described the horrors of war to the English populace.

What Russell reported was that cholera and other enteric diseases — not artillery fire — were responsible for the fact that 20 percent of the expeditionary force had been hospitalized. Yet, conditions in military hospitals were abominable. Unlike the French, Britain provided no nurses to care for its sick and wounded soldiers.

When Nightingale learned of this, she contacted her friend Lord Sidney Herbert — who was then Secretary at War and in charge of finances and accounting for the War Office. After much negotiating, Florence Nightingale left Britain for the Crimea with a force of thirty-eight nurses.

Although the battles of the Crimean War were largely fought near Sevastopol (now part of Ukraine), ships transported wounded British soldiers across the Black Sea to a hospital at Scutari across from Constantinople. The young Englishwoman was appalled by what she found there. Scutari had no beds, no clean laundry, no food, no source of clean water, not even an operating table. The sick lay huddled on filthy, damp floors, with no mattresses or blankets. The system of supplying the army hospital was so Byzantine that orders for supplies would be given and then disappear, as if into an abyss of bureaucratic irresponsibility.

Rather than welcoming Nightingale and her ministering band, British army surgeons viewed them as uppity, meddlesome women. Although the wards were filled with war casualties — as well as casualties of army neglect — the surgeons refused to ask for the nurses' assistance. Shrewdly, Nightingale waited for days before these doctors finally recognized that they could not deal with the sick without her. But they accepted the nurses' help only after a major entanglement, the Battle of Inkerman, flooded military hospitals with new patients.

"Oh, you gentlemen of England who sit at home in all the well earned satisfaction of your successful cases, can have little idea, from reading the newspapers, of the horror & misery in a military Hosp'l, of operating upon these dying exhausted men," Nightingale wrote in anger to surgeon William Bowman. "We have had such a sea in the Bosphorus, and the Turks, the very men for whom we are fighting are carrying our wounded so cruelly, that they arrive in a state of agony — one amputated stump died two hours after we received him, one compound fracture just as we were getting him into bed, in all 24 cases on the day of landing. We have now 4 miles of beds & not 18 inches apart."

When she was finally allowed to deliver the care she had come to provide, it was not simply to the soldiers' wounds that she attended, but to the hospital environment itself. She ordered workmen to construct new wards that were well ventilated, clean, and had a source of pure water. She set up a kitchen and installed her own chef to prepare the kind of special food men suffering from dysentery and fever would require. She ordered the shirts and trousers to clothe them. She arranged for the soldiers to set aside pay to send home to their families, created a reading room in which they could learn, and generally countered the conventional wisdom that the British soldier was fit to do little but drink and die.

It was these manifold activities that endeared her to the British public and allowed her to return home to be the most famous woman of her era. In 1861, with the help of the Nightingale Fund, she financed the Nightingale School of Nursing at St. Thomas' Hospital in London. This was the first school of nursing that was not aligned with a particular religious order or denomination. She also continued to fight for the reform of British hospitals and the reform of military hospitals, and to address the plight of the British army in India. Her fame and influence soon spread to America and all over the world.

In the United States, the growth of nursing shared many parallels. American medicine followed the advances of European science. The Civil War played a great role, as did immigration and industrialization. With men, women, and children forced to work in factories, few workers could afford to take time off to care for their sick family members. Immigrants without families who lived in crowded tenements far from their nearest relatives were also unable to utilize the traditional caregivers of the sick — women in the home. No wonder then, that between 1880 and 1920, religious orders, charities, and other private organizations filled the resulting void by establishing over 7,000 hospitals (a century later, America has 6,500 hospitals).

The sick were, however, understandably reluctant to enter these forbidding new institutions. During the latter part of the nineteenth and early twentieth centuries, it was not only the development of medicine but of professional nursing that made hospitals acceptable to the public and to the charitable patrons and community leaders who supported their growth. What nurses did was to make sure the hospital was clean, well ventilated, and orderly and to ensure that patients actually received care in them. As medical science and thus the hospital developed, physicians began to recognize that nurses were central to their own success and began to support the creation of rudimentary nursing schools within hospitals.

"No single change transformed the hospital's day-to-day workings more than the acceptance of trained nurses and training schools," says America's premier hospital historian, Charles Rosenberg.

Nancy Rumplik's journey into nursing recapitulates its long and sometimes tortuous history. Nancy laughs whenever someone asks her why she became a nurse. It seems like such a tired cliché, she tells me as we sit in her small office. Ask that question and you expect a stereotypical response, such as I used to love to play nurse with my dolls. I came to life when my rabbit broke his leg. I read a children's book about Nurse so and so, and was fascinated by the Band-Aids, stethoscope, and pictures of that cheerful-looking woman in a white uniform and cap.

She has heard those clichés over and over again. But that's exactly what happened when she was a child. She did indeed read a book about a nurse. Along with text and illustrations, it contained a kit with all the requisite paraphernalia — a packet of Band-Aids and a plastic stethoscope. But the thing that sticks in her mind was its title. As if it had been designed to send a message especially to her, it was called *Nurse Nancy.*

Then there was also her visit, when she was five or six, to her great-grandmother in the hospital. She can't recall ever meeting her great-grandmother before that. Sadly, she believes this was her first and last visit. The sick old woman lay in the hospital bed, and a nurse — Nancy doesn't remember her name — cared for her. She remembers the nurse's kindness and attentiveness. This encounter made a lasting impression on the child that remained with her as she grew older and carried with her the determination to become a nurse.

Of course, when Nancy Rumplik was a child and adolescent, nursing was one of the only professions legitimately available to a woman, along with teaching and social work. In those days there were no *Doctor Nancy* books. But when she reflects on it, she feels she wouldn't have chosen Doctor Nancy over Nurse Nancy had that choice been offered. It was nursing — the *care* of the sick — that appealed to her and, after almost thirty years, continues to move her.

In her home in the western Massachusetts town of West Springfield, she was certainly encouraged in her ambition. She was one of five children. Her father — who died in 1977 — was an engineer and her mother a housewife who had worked as a sales development manager before she had children. As a child she attended parochial schools — St. Thomas of the Apostles for elementary school and Cathedral High School. She has two sisters and two brothers, all of whom are married. The only unmarried member of her family, she surrounds herself on long weekends and holidays with her nieces and nephews.

In 1967, when she applied to nursing school, it seemed that all the young women in her class had read the same childhood stories. Along with her, they applied to two-year community college nursing programs. Nancy had every expectation that she would get into one, if not all, of the schools to which she had applied. She had good grades — particularly in math, which was her second love. She'd briefly flirted with the idea of becoming a math teacher but decided that she did not want to teach.

Then came the unwelcome surprise. That year, students who were applying to two-year nursing programs were asked to take a special exam put out by the National League for Nursing — the organization that accredits nursing schools. The exam centered on nursing practice and skills — none of which Nancy Rumplik had. Nor had she been told she would have to prepare for this exam. Not surprisingly, she did not do well on it. In spite of her school record, the NLN exam turned out to be the deciding factor. The young woman who would eventually become one of the most respected nurses at the Beth Israel Hospital eagerly rushed to her mailbox day after day to collect letters of what she thought would be acceptance. And day after day she burst into tears as she read the "I regret to inform you" that seemed to shut the door firmly on her dream.

"I was devastated," she recalled. "It was the only thing I wanted to do, and they were telling me I couldn't do it. I decided to forget it. If I couldn't be an RN, I thought, I wouldn't be anything.

Nancy's father intervened. Seeing his daughter become more and more distraught, he sat her down and told her she should simply go to practical nursing school. Her grades were excellent. She would have no trouble getting into a one-year licensed practical nursing program, like one that was offered at Springfield Technical Community College, and then being licensed by the state of Massachusetts to become an LPN. There would be no NLN exam to take. It was a shoo-in.

Nancy resisted.

Being a practical nurse, she told him, was like being a glorified aide. That was not what she wanted to be. She wanted to be a registered nurse. "I'll never forget his next words," Nancy recalls. "He said, 'That's not the point. The point is, you get your foot in the door and you continue.' If it wasn't for my father, I wouldn't have done that." Nancy applied to the program, breezed through the one-year course, and graduated as the most outstanding practical nurse in the class. But this success did not entirely erase her sense of early disappointment, which was, she postulates, the beginning of a drive to prove herself.

When she got her first job, she had to *prove* she was better than an LPN. When she became an RN, she had to *prove* she was an excellent RN. "I had to be the best, because I couldn't get into nursing school. I had to prove to everyone that I could be the best. I think I still do that."

Nancy Rumplik's educational struggles are not unique. For nurses, education is a continuing obstacle course. For the profession, the setting of the educational standards that determine who is a registered nurse is a continuing source of conflict. One hurdle is overcome and then another appears.

Although they are all called nurses, there are, in fact, four categories of educated women — and some men — who take care of the sick. Licensed practical nurses, or LPNs — a category of nursing personnel developed during World War II — usually have a year of post–high school education. The state licenses them to perform less-skilled caretaking tasks like uncomplicated dressing changes, administering some routine medications, giving baths, and helping patients to eat and walk and perform other activities of daily living, under the supervision of a professional nurse or physician. Then come registered nurses, or RNs. A registered nurse may have graduated from an associate-degree program in a two-year community college, from one of the increasingly rare hospital schools that grant a three-year diploma, or from a four-year program in a college or university. The latter grant a baccalaureate degree. In pursuing the baccalaureate, students devote 50 to 60 percent of their coursework to the liberal arts and sciences and 40 to 50 percent to a professional curriculum.

Most health care institutions have exploited this fragmented educational model and have refused to pay nurses on the basis of their education as well as their experience. Hospitals generally pay four-year graduates exactly the same amount they pay a nurse with a two-year or three-year diploma.

For decades, nurses have struggled against this system. That struggle is yet another example of the gender politics that have dominated nursing. Indeed, the history of nursing education is one of the longest-running feminist struggles in any profession in America. Sadly, however, nursing's battle for a room of its own — in this case educational institutions of its own — has been largely invisible.

At the turn of the century, the status of nurses relative to doctors was far less inferior than it is today. Physicians were able to create a coherent system of academic medical training and gain control of medical practice. Nurses were unable to do the same.

In the early 1900s, nurses were trained in schools — which were wholly owned and operated by hospitals — and which were adamantly not educational institutions. Offering young women room and board and a rudimentary introduction to physiology, pharmacology, and other scientific principles, they viewed student nurses as a cheap source of labor, not as learners. Members of this cheap labor force would be expected to log twelve- to fourteen-hour days and then remain awake for a few classes at night. Hospitals limited nurses' occupational mobility by tying their educational credentials to a particular institution, that is, a hospital school or training program and its needs. Hospitals also successfully gained and maintained control over the money used for nursing education. Thus, nursing was effectively tethered to the institutions that purchased nursing services.

Some nursing leaders rebelled against this system and fought for university education. But hospitals' need for a cheap labor force and societal attitudes toward women's work stood in the way of this goal. Women, male civic and medical leaders alike argued that women did not need a college education to care for the sick. Only a small number of nurses were university graduates in the earlier decades of the twentieth century. In spite of a number of important reports in which prominent nursing leaders argued for a four-year academic education, organized nursing received little public support for its professional aims. Thus the hospital school — with its three-year diploma program turning out nurse after nurse to work mainly on private duty in patients' homes — became the de facto standard.

This changed only during World War II, when for the first time there was an infusion of federal money into nursing education, and after World War II, when the community college system was developed and gave rise to two-year community college nursing programs. In 1964, the passage of the Nurse Training Act gave all schools of nursing money for capital expansion and funding for students studying nursing. This helped expand four-year school enrollment, but two-year degree programs still grew faster. Although there has been a major expansion of four-year schools, today about 40 percent of nurses in practice hold a four-year degree.

In 1965, all the major nursing organizations endorsed a position paper stating that all professional nurses should have a four-year degree to enter practice. While promising to grandfather in all associate and diploma graduates until 1985, from thence forward, these two-year and three-year nurses would be known as technical nurses and would be licensed to do fewer activities than registered nurses. Nurses spent the next twenty years trying to pass bills implementing this entry into practice into state legislatures across the country. Because of opposition from hospitals and many of the schools graduating two- and three-year nurses — as well as from these nurses themselves — the only state to pass such legislation was North Dakota.

Nancy took and easily passed the LPN boards and then got a job working on a medical / surgical floor in a small hospital in Springfield. After a few months, she decided to move to Boston. She originally wanted to work in pediatrics and intended to apply to Children's Hospital. But her confidence had been shaken by the experience of rejection. "I panicked," she recounted. "I didn't have any experience working with kids."

Practicing in an acute care hospital with adult medical patients seemed a more secure option. She went to talk with personnel at the Beth Israel and several other hospitals. They all used LPNs and all seemed eager to hire her. But to her there was only one choice: the Beth Israel. It was the only hospital she knew of in which nurses didn't have to work three different shifts within the very same week. She started in a stepdown unit from the Surgical Intensive Care Unit (SICU), where she cared for patients who had been discharged from the ICU into a less-intensive but nonetheless highly specialized nursing setting.

Although she worked harder than she ever had, Nancy explained, it seemed like heaven. She was finally near nurses — nurses who were her mentors and who would nurture her and encourage her to go to school to become an RN. From 1969 to 1979, she worked as an LPN. During that time, she entered the associate degree program at Northeastern University. While she took basic science courses, and then moved on in the curriculum, she worked rotating shifts and on weekends. In 1977 she finally graduated from Northeastern with her associate degree.

"Before the nursing boards," she recounted, "I was a nervous wreck. I had a cold and high fever." She entered the exam room flushed, sweating, coughing, desperate for a glass of water, wishing she could be anywhere but in that giant, impersonal auditorium. For the next few hours, she hunched down into her chair and wrote her exam. "They wouldn't even let me have a glass of water," she recalled. But when it was over, she was a registered nurse.

In spite of her success, when Nancy first worked as an RN at the Beth Israel its nursing department was extremely undistinguished. Although they may have had better schedules, nurses at the Beth Israel were, for the most part, an unhappy, demoralized lot. Like most nurses across the country, their working lives were rigidly regulated by a centralized nursing hierarchy, and they practiced under one of two nursing models — functional (task) or team nursing. The administrators who supervised nurses, the hospitals who employed them, the patients they cared for, generally viewed nursing as a series of tasks that almost anyone — at least anyone female — could perform. The reigning philosophy was, A nurse is a nurse is a nurse. Nancy didn't need much educational preparation or expertise to do her job and received little encouragement from her employer to get more of either once on the job.

As they have for over a century, hospitals seemed to view nursing as a frustrating necessity — a source of expense that they would try to reduce through whatever means possible. In the postwar era, the majority of nurses were the products of either hospital schools or the community college system. Even though far cheaper to educate and employ than registered nurses with a four-year degree, registered nurses with two-year degrees from community colleges were still far more expensive than the student nurses of the prewar period, who were little better than indentured servants. So hospitals tried to avoid the expense of hiring too many RNs of any variety by assigning direct patient care to nurses' aides or LPNs.

Joyce Clifford, Beth Israel's vice president of nursing and nurse in chief, recalls that era. "Much of the patient care provided was done by members of the staff with the least educational preparation: nursing assistants and licensed practical nurses. Registered nurses were giving medications, checking doctors' orders and being 'in charge,' which meant that they were constantly checking on the nursing assistant and LPN to see what he or she was doing, or more likely, doing those things that these positions were unable to do in the care of patients."

This was the legacy of earlier hospital nursing. Organized around the principles of efficiency and productivity promoted by the scientific management movement of the 1920s, nurses were trained like industrial machines to perform a discrete set of tasks. On a thirty-bed unit, one nurse might spend her whole day giving baths, emptying bedpans, or distributing medications. Consider the *task* of the bath. Two nurses might start at one end of a unit and proceed to the other. Carrying water and linen in and out of patients' rooms, they performed their chores in rote fashion.

This system of functional nursing endured until the late forties and early fifties, when "team nursing" was developed. This was yet another attempt to reduce nursing costs. Hospitals believed that they could "extend" the better-educated and more expensive registered nurse by hiring only a few RNs on any particular ward and deploying cheaper labor — LPNs and aides — to work under them. The RNs would oversee these less-skilled workers while they provided most of the direct patient care. Grouping lower-paid workers around the better educated RN, hospitals created a so-called team — one with very few registered nurses on it.

RNs on such "teams" were left with little time to devote to "knowing" patients. They didn't have much opportunity to collectively develop any new approaches to nursing that would enhance continuity of care or promote collaboration between physicians and nurses. Because they often lacked a clear and coherent picture of the patient, they were rarely asked to communicate that picture to physicians. Responsibility for communicating important patient information was given to the head nurse, who became the de facto case manager but who was unable to really get to know patients because she didn't give hands-on care. In this system, administrators did not believe it was necessary for nurses to make their own notes in patient charts, to make rounds with physicians — except to learn what "orders" they were to carry out — or to spend time conferring with patients and family members about medications, life activities, and any postdischarge issues.

Nancy Rumplik flinches visibly when asked to describe what the hospital was like when she first went to work there in 1969. "It was totally chaotic. From day to day, you didn't know which unit you were going to work on. Especially on the weekends. You would be floated from unit to unit. On Saturday, for example, you might be floated to a neuroorthopedic unit with twenty patients, none of whom could walk on their own. There were never enough nurses. Nurses were so demoralized that they were always calling in sick or leaving. You'd be taking care of twelve or thirteen patients, all by yourself. You worked with coworkers — aides — but that didn't make a dent."

Nor could nurses get the kind of education Nancy, Jeannie, and Ellen now take for granted. Nursing departments did not tend to offer any advanced educational seminars for nurses because nurses were in the hospital to serve as the handmaidens of doctors — not as skilled professionals with their own approach to patient care. The teaching hospital's mission was supposed to be, in great part, an educational one. But medicine and hospital administration dictated that there was only one set of learners within it — doctors and doctors-in-training.

Much of this changed in the years after Mitchell T. Rabkin became CEO of the Beth Israel in 1966. Rabkin had trained at the Massachusetts General Hospital and was teaching and caring for patients at Mass. General when he was asked to lead the BI in 1966.

A small, slight man, with jet black hair and an attentive and kindly demeanor, Rabkin had always been deeply committed to patient care and had learned the value of collaboration with nursing early in his career, when he was an intern. When he came on board at the BI, at age thirty-six, he knew that he could not turn it into a world-class hospital without transforming its nursing service.

As quickly as he could, Rabkin hired a nursing administrator who believed, as did he, that the nurse-patient relationship should be central to patient care. Joyce Clifford, a nursing administrator who had been at the University of Alabama, was his choice.

Clifford — a tall, imposing woman with a demeanor that is genial but very much in charge — has become a legend at both the BI and in nursing. Clifford immediately set about replacing "the fragmented, uninformed, and depersonalized care" with a new system that kept nurses at the bedside, and helped them better know and understand their patients. To help her she hired Trish Gibbons, then a staff nurse at Boston City Hospital, to take part in the new reorganization of nursing.

Clifford and Gibbons determined that the vehicle for their realization was the newly developing model of primary nursing. As in the physician model, each patient would be assigned a primary nurse when he or she came to the hospital. That nurse would be responsible for creating a nursing plan of care for that patient and would be able to effectively manage that care because she had time to develop a relationship with the patient. This would give her intimate knowledge not only about the patient's disease but about his or her life. She would be responsible and held accountable for patient care management decisions. She would work with associate nurses, who would share that responsibility and who would be able to alter the care plan in an emergency. To assure continuity of care, when a patient was readmitted to the hospital he or she would, whenever possible, be admitted to the unit on which his or her primary nurse worked.

Over the next several years, the top management team of the hospital began to transform its nursing department. Joyce Clifford's title — vice president of nursing and nurse in chief — reflected this change. The first part of the title underlined the fact that the hospital now viewed its chief nurse executive as a powerful figure — a top administrator and part of the hospital's management team. In those days, nursing administrators typically had no contact with hospital boards of trustees. Clifford, however, would attend all planning board and committee meetings and have access to the hospital's board of trustees. Her other title — nurse in chief — highlighted the fact that a nurse would be viewed as a clinical chief like the surgeon in chief or physician in chief.

Physicians at the Beth Israel were not uniformly happy about these changes in the nursing department. Primary nursing would mean that physicians could no longer rely on collecting information from a unit's head nurse, but would have to get to know individual nurses. "I remember one physician asking me if I seriously meant that he would now have to come up and talk to all sorts of different nurses about his patients rather than going to the head nurse," Trish Gibbons recalls. "This would mean, he said, that he would have to know all of their names."

Clearly troubled by the prospect of having to attach individual identities to the nameless, faceless mass of females that had previously been at his disposal, this doctor eagerly offered Gibbons what he considered a helpful suggestion. Why not have a billboard on each unit, with the nurses' photographs displayed like mug shots, with their names underneath? This would save him all kinds of trouble, he averred. When a doctor needed to contact a particular nurse, he could quickly scan the mug shots until he found the RN he was searching for.

Gibbons shakes her head with incredulity at the recollection. "I held my temper, sympathized with his dilemma, and then asked him if he realized how many different physicians nurses had to deal with and how many different names they had to know. Did he think we should have mug shots of physicians as well?" She assured him that, over time, it would be possible to get to know the different nurses.

After Gibbons successfully piloted primary nursing on two units, it was integrated into the entire hospital. The hospital decided to hire only nurses with four-year college degrees — which has increasingly become the standard in tertiary care hospitals and academic medical centers — for their staff-level positions. Nurses who, like Nancy Rumplik, had a two-year associate degree were thus encouraged to get their four-year degree. "The Beth Israel helped me to get more and more education," Nancy says with obvious gratitude for the hospital's financial contributions and moral support.

The Beth Israel also began hiring clinical specialists; encouraging nurses like Jeannie Chaisson, who already had a Bachelor of Science in Nursing, to get further education so they could serve as educational resources to their colleagues in the hospital, and it began to establish formal avenues that rewarded experienced nurses who remained at the bedside. This helped to address one of nursing's perennial problems. Nursing has suffered from wage compression — salaries of nurses have tended to be very flat. If hospitals do not have career ladders, the only way nurses can advance in the profession is to leave the bedside for a career in education or administration. This inevitably deprives patients, novice nurses, and physicians of experienced nurses as caregivers, mentors, and colleagues.

The BI instituted a system of career ladders that allows bedside nurses to advance through four levels of what is called clinical nursing. Expert nurses earn more money and gain more respect without leaving the bedside. Jeannie Chaisson and Nancy Rumplik, for example, are both clinical nurse fours.

"I can't imagine going back to what nursing was like when I first came to the BI," Nancy Rumplik says, almost shuddering at the thought. "There would be no autonomy and no relationship with the patient because there would be no room for it to develop. Nurses and patients would lose. And so would other professionals who have come to respect the work of nursing. Nursing would become just a paycheck instead of something that's so enriching because you're always helping people — people in crisis — as best as you can."

When primary nursing was instituted at the BI, Nancy and her patients began to experience what nurses can do when they have time to get to know their patients and have more institutional support. She was then working on a neurological unit with chronically ill and often desperate patients, many of whom had temporal lobe epilepsy (TLE) — a very debilitating neurological disease. Patients with TLE may be afflicted with both grand mal and petit mal seizures. In grand mal seizures, out-of-control electrical impulses go off and patients lose consciousness, flail their arms and legs, roll back their eyes, and are in danger of biting their tongue. When they wake up, they are disoriented and confused. In petit mal seizures, patients abruptly lose contact with reality in the middle of a conversation or activity, as if they are no longer of this world. Because seizures can occur anytime during a hospital stay, patients require extensive monitoring to keep them safe. Some of Nancy's patients were so depressed they became suicidal. "You turned around and they'd make a break for a window seven floors up," Nancy says. Which was why all the windows in the unit were locked.

While Nancy worked on this unit, the Beth Israel initiated primary nursing. Nancy thus worked with the same patients over and over again as they came to the hospital on repeated admissions. Here she was also offered one of her most exciting cases at that time. Howard Bloom, a doctor on the unit, was pioneering a new surgical procedure for patients with temporal lobe epilepsy that promised to dramatically reduce their seizures. He asked her to be primary nurse for his first surgical patient — whom she calls Jesse Wallace.*

Nancy's patient Jesse had been experiencing seizures for over twenty years. He'd spent much of his life as a patient at Children's Hospital, located a block from the BI. The other children on the unit at that hospital adored him. He had grown accustomed to their attention and to that of the staff. When, as a young man, he was admitted to an adult hospital unit, there were no more adoring children around him, just other depressed adults like himself.

Each day, he had one generalized motor (grand mal) seizure and at least ten petit mal seizures. He was on a variety of antiseizure medications and as a result was so drowsy that he had to drink coffee nonstop just to stay awake. He had had one surgery that failed and was admitted to the Beth Israel for the new operation. Although he seemed indifferent to the upcoming surgery, Nancy and the other nurses who worked with him knew his nonchalance had to be a facade. How could it be anything else? If this surgery didn't work, Jesse would be doomed to a life of relentless disruption.

During the two- to four-week pre-and postoperative period, Jesse would have to remain on the neuro floor. Both preoperatively and postoperatively nurses were crucial to the procedure's success. The operation would locate and then remove the area of Jesse's brain that was causing erratic electrical activity. To do this, Bloom had to pinpoint the correct area. Because normal electroencephalograms (EEGs) monitor only surface brain activity, the surgeon performed an initial craniotomy in which he bored a number of holes into Jesse's shaved skull. Through these, he inserted deep electrical leads.

Jesse's head was then covered with a sterile dressing that protected the holes in his scalp. His antiseizure medication was reduced, and he returned to the neuro unit, where he was attached to a large mechanical telemetry machine that would record his seizure activity. Once the location of seizure activity was correctly ascertained, he would again go into surgery for the final part of the procedure.

While Jesse waited for technology to discover the part of his brain that was malfunctioning, Nancy and her colleagues had to keep his dressing clean to prevent infection. The decrease in his antiseizure medications put him at significant risk for a fall and injury. He had to spend most of his day in a hospital bed, with its padded rails up. If he moved around the unit or hospital, he had to be strapped into a wheelchair with a safety belt and he had to wear a helmet. Because of the fire hazard, he could smoke only with a staff member present, and he could not go to the bathroom unaccompanied.

No one nurse could be with Jesse every minute of the day. Nancy and her colleagues tried to help him understand the need for all these precautions. For a young man like Jesse, it all seemed too much. The nurses' instructions seemed to be only an invitation to bend the rules. The very evening on which she explained these restrictions, Nancy was sitting quietly in the nurses' station when she and her colleagues heard a loud thump coming from Jesse's room. Certain that he had fallen out of bed, they rushed in. The room was empty. Jesse was on the floor of the bathroom, wedged into the tiny space between the sink and toilet, unconscious, his chin bleeding profusely from a deep cut. Trying to protect his head from further injury, Nancy and her colleagues squeezed into the cramped space to dislodge him, secure his head, and make sure his airway stayed open. He gradually revived and was rushed down to x-ray to make sure no further harm had been done.

Nancy knew she could not allow this kind of accident to happen again. To make sure it didn't, she sat down with Jesse and reviewed all the safety instructions. Much chastened, Jesse agreed to cooperate with all but one. The helmet. To wear a helmet in a wheelchair when he circulated through the unit, he said, was just too demeaning. So they reached a compromise. If he promised to wear his seat belt, the helmet could go.

"The trick with Jesse was compromise," Nancy explained. "He needed to feel he had some control. He was in an institution which gave him very little. He lived with a disease that ruled his life." By allowing Jesse to wear his own clothes rather than hospital johnnies, and by giving him unlimited cafeteria privileges — provided he was accompanied by a nursing assistant — Nancy did just that.

Even with these compromises, Jesse's care still required continuing reevaluation. Small things like daily trips to the cafeteria brought unexpected problems: for example, excessive coffee drinking. Nancy discovered that Jesse was actually drinking forty cups a day. Five thousand milligrams of caffeine — enough to fuel a small office — were going into one body. No wonder Jesse could hardly sleep, was jittery and confused, and asked nurses to constantly repeat instructions and information. He was too high-strung to talk about his fears and was even having more seizures, possibly exacerbated by the caffeine. Yet, in spite of this increased seizure activity, the focal point could not be located, and his surgery was delayed.

Nancy was concerned with the total picture — the patient's state of mind and body. She felt her patient needed the kind of attention that would make it tolerable for him to endure the preoperative process. She and her colleagues thus reevaluated their nursing plan and decided that what Jesse needed most was talking time. At the beginning of each shift, either she or another nurse would set aside a half an hour to meet and talk with Jesse. During these sessions there would be no interruptions, no technical care, just conversation and comfort.

These informal discussions allowed the real Jesse to emerge. One day, while Nancy sat with him in his hospital room, Jesse was disconsolately staring out of the window. Suddenly he turned to Nancy and revealed the fear and frustration he'd concealed for weeks. For all these years, he confessed, he had lived with his seizures without ever ceasing to view them as a horrible burden and source of fear. His every move toward independence was thwarted. It was as if he was tied to these helter-skelter electrical impulses in his body, to his family, and to the prospect of permanent dependence. "I'd just gotten enough nerve to move out of my parents' home," he said, "and to get my own apartment — not to mention a new job and a girlfriend — and then, wouldn't you know it, my seizures started getting worse again."

It was the human connection that helped him to become a partner in, rather than a resister against, his treatment. After that session, he seemed to retain Nancy's teaching. He followed nurses' suggestions and drank decaffeinated coffee and caffeine-free drinks. He began to sleep more. Finally, the EEG readings located the focal point of his seizures, and he was able to have the surgery.

During Jesse's recovery, Nancy and her colleagues continued to meet with him on every shift. Once again, he had to be kept quiet, his wounds had to be cleaned, and he had to be comforted. But the surgical treatment and nursing care worked. The operation was a success. After it, Jesse had some limited seizure activity that could be regulated by far less debilitating medication. He was able to finish school, get a good job, get married, and have a family. "To this day, he's okay," Nancy said with pride. "He has a life rather than a disease."

During the eight years she worked on the neuro unit, there were a number of "Jesses," patients who were clear success stories. But she also had difficult patients whom she felt she could not really reach — like another TLE patient, Jennifer Slocum.*

"She was one of my seizure patients," Nancy said, pausing to capture the painful memory. "I don't even know if I can describe how exasperating it was to take care of her. She was thirty and I was twenty-six or twenty-seven when we met."

Over the months, Nancy cared for Jennifer when the young woman came into the hospital for seizure control. The trouble was, when Jennifer was in the hospital, it was never clear which seizure was real and which was not. "Some neuro patients have pseudoseizures," Nancy explained. Long and detailed articles have been written elucidating the phenomenon of the pseudoseizure. In fact, 50 percent of TLE patients had them. These were patients, Nancy explained, who had learned to gain attention by tumbling to the floor shaking.

Just as her disease used her, Jennifer used it. "She became incredibly manipulative," Nancy recalled. "I would walk in the room and Jennifer would have a seizure."

Was it the real thing? "I decided I didn't care if the seizure was real or not. I'd treat it like it was. The problem was, treatment or not, you could never, ever give her enough time. She was never satisfied. She was bright, but she could drive you nuts," Nancy said, so many years later still struggling with her frustration.

"I never think that you should have control over a patient. But with Jennifer, the issue was the way she related. She didn't trust anyone in the world. She didn't trust me. God," Nancy said, shaking her head, "I wrote more care plans on her and thought about how to try to develop trust with her."

But she never succeeded. "It was exhausting because the bottom line is people like that make you extremely angry," she recalled.

For a nurse an open display of anger is unacceptable. "As a nurse," Nancy explained, "you're the patient's advocate. You're not supposed to get angry at the patient. So I felt I couldn't make headway."

The only way Nancy could deal with Jennifer was by talking with other nurses in an attempt to get some insight and some comic relief. She also vented her feelings in what are called "psych rounds." On every floor she has worked on, Nancy has encouraged nurses to meet with one another to discuss their feelings about their work. A psychiatric liaison nurse from the BI's psychiatric nursing department acts as a group facilitator.

In these psych rounds, Nancy could talk about her anger, guilt, and sense of responsibility. "When you're young," she said with wry nostalgia, "you think you can fix everyone and everything. You feel personally at fault when you can't. You realize these people have an awful disease. They've had surgery before. Then they have it again, and it doesn't work, and there is absolutely no recourse for them. You're with them hour after hour and you know what they feel."

Her colleagues helped her navigate those angry, resentful, and often hopeless feelings. It was during this period that she also elaborated her personal philosophy of nursing, which is encapsulated in the motto "You gotta love 'em" (her patients), no matter how challenging they are.

Over the years, Nancy has often had what many other nurses consider "difficult patients." She cringes when she hears those two words and tries never to use them herself. "It's not fair to either the patient or provider to describe a patient as difficult. For example, when I get a new patient and get a report about them from another nurse, I don't like any negative behavioral terms to be used to describe them. It colors your view of them and imposes someone else's interpretation on the patient. This then affects how you approach the person and what you listen for."

When Nancy ponders this notion of the "difficult case," she says she's reminded of the film *On Golden Pond*. Jane Fonda plays a woman whose father (played by her own father, Henry) is dying. In the movie, her cinematic mother, Katharine Hepburn, is trying to explain why the character Jane Fonda plays is having such a hard time dealing with her father. "Katharine Hepburn turns to Jane Fonda," Nancy recounts, "and says something like, he's so difficult to deal with but you have to understand, he's only trying to find his way.

"That's what's going on with the so-called difficult patient. They're people trying to find their way with terrible anxiety and suffering." Some, like Jennifer, Nancy concludes, have a harder time doing this than others. Some also have a harder time receiving the gift of caregiving — which may make them as angry at their own vulnerability as grateful for human concern and affection — than others.

Although Nancy says she appreciates all the lessons her neuro patients taught her, after seven years she felt she wanted to take on new challenges and learn about new areas in nursing and medicine. Oncology, she felt, would build on the skills she had developed while working in neurology. "In neurology," she says, "you work with people who have chronic illnesses. I have never found it difficult to deal with chronically or terminally ill patients. What you do with them is the hallmark of primary nursing — getting to know patients over time and working with them and their families. That is what I find so meaningful and what I knew I would be able to do in oncology nursing." She decided to apply for a job in the Hematology / Oncology Clinic.

Nurses in the Hematology / Oncology Clinic have more autonomy, tend to work more collaboratively, on a one-to-one basis with physicians, and often follow patients and their families for years. This, coupled with the fact that they do not have to work shifts or weekends, makes it a much sought after job that generally goes to nurses who have worked first on the Hematology / Oncology inpatient floor. When Nancy applied for the clinic position, another candidate — a nurse who had more oncology experience — was hired instead. To get more experience in oncology, Nancy worked for six months on that inpatient unit. When, in 1985, another position opened up in the clinic, she applied for it and got it. "Way back then, when I was told I had gotten the job in the clinic, it was the happiest day of my nursing career. Oncology has never disappointed me. All these years later, I still feel the same way."

Chapter 3

Not on the Charts

JEANNIE CHAISSON

It's a Monday morning in May. The day has begun with a parade of mishaps worthy of the movie *Hospital.* At 7:30 A.M., just half an hour after Jeannie Chaisson arrived at work, an alarm goes off in a patient's room. Upon hearing its steady bleating, nurses exit from patients' bedsides or leap up from behind computers in the unit's central work area. With Jeannie Chaisson among them, they sprint down one of the unit's two long corridors to find out if this emergency signal indicates a cardiac arrest or if a patient has simply hit a button by mistake.

Jeannie suspects the latter. The patient has been admitted for what is known in hospital lingo as a "rule-out" for a myocardial infarction (MI).

Translation: she's had chest pain. Has she had a real heart attack? Since the patient is demented, she can't relate her history or symptoms, so "ruling out" is a matter of observation. If this alarm signals a real emergency, she will have to be "ruled in," Jeannie explains as we trot along.

As we approach the patient's room, a number of smiling nurses are walking out the door. It's a false alarm, they tell Jeannie. All clear. Back to work.

"We get a lot of rule-out-MIs," Jeannie explains while catching her breath back at her desk. She retrieves the brown plastic notebook that holds her Kardex — the sheets of paper on which she notes information about her patients and their care plans. "Usually we rule them out. Perhaps the patient only had bad gas or stomach problems. Or it may have been stress. But sometimes, they actually have an MI. We all race down because they may be having a lethal arrhythmia."

She walks over to the unit's central work area, stops in front of the tall kiosk that holds patient charts, pulls one out, and leafs through it. In midpage she stops, rolls her eyes, and says, "What a stupid thing to say, 'rule in.' I can understand 'rule out.' But 'rule in' for an MI! God."

Six Feldberg is a forty-four-bed unit. The unit consists of two exterior corridors of patient rooms and an interior rectangle that is walled off and separated into smaller rooms or corridors comprising supply rooms, a nurses' locker room, a nurse manager's office, a patient and family kitchen, staff toilets, and a room with a huge tub and special lift to help patients being bathed get in and out. There is also a rectangular conference room, where nurses eat lunch and have their coffee breaks, and a smaller drug supply room with a locked cabinet for narcotics. At the farthest end of this central bank of offices and supply rooms, an open area is partitioned off by a chest-high wall of countertops and file cabinets. Containing a number of desks with phones and computers, it forms the unit's central work station.

The unit is painted in buff and muted blues and greens. The carpet is blue with dull green and blue polka dots. "It's done in eighties colors," Jeannie quips. "It's supposed to be calm and restful. When I came here, it was done in seventies colors — electric green and orange walls. It was great, just great. You got inured to it."

Jeri Willner, the unit coordinator, sits on a high stool next to Jeannie. Willner is a tiny woman, with a high-pitched, almost childlike voice. For years, she has been the unit's all-purpose resource person — answering phones, making sure information from the labs reaches its proper destination, filing and doing other paperwork, and, as Jeannie puts it, "haunting the interns to make sure discharge summaries and referrals actually get done."

The phone rings and Jeri answers. As she talks, her voice rises.

"No!" Jeri exclaims to the unknown caller. Jeannie looks up quizzically.

"She did what?" Jeri asks incredulously.

"But why?" she persists. "Wait a minute, I'll call you right back." Jeri hangs up and swivels to face Jeannie.

"Unbelievable," she says. One of Six Feldberg's patients was transported down to radiology about an hour and a half ago. The woman asked to go to the toilet and was escorted to the bathroom. A few minutes later, staff noticed she had not reappeared. Nurses went to check on her. The door was locked. They knocked. The woman told them she was not coming out. They pleaded. She refused. Finally, they called Six Feldberg.

That was one of the nurses outside the door, Jeri explained. She wanted to know if anyone on Six Feldberg could explain what provoked this? What should they do?

"Oh God!" says Jeannie, rolling her eyes heavenward. Then she tells Jeri she'll find the patient's primary nurse so she can go down and deal with the situation. Later, that RN returns with good news: the patient has left the bathroom. She was just anxious, the nurse reports. Rather than use words to express her feelings, she seized the bathroom to dramatize her concerns.

The unit is quiet. But not for long. About fifteen minutes later a woman wanders up to the desk. Her pale-blue-and-white johnny flaps around her. She lists slightly as she holds on to the IV pole she has wheeled along by her side.

"Can I help you?" Jeannie asks politely.

The woman launches into a diatribe against the patient who was her roommate until she was just discharged. She accuses the other woman of taking all her bras and underpants with her when she left the hospital.

"They were all new." the woman says irately. "I just bought 'em."

"I'm sorry. I don't understand," Jeannie says. "You mean she took them by mistake?"

"Oh no," the patient insists. "She stole them. I know it, she stole them all and they were all brand-new."

Rather than argue about the allegation, Jeannie promises to report the incident to Security. Someone will come up and ask her to fill out a report, she informs the patient.

"I don't want the money," the woman says vehemently. "I want my bras and underpants back."

Trying to calm her, Jeannie ushers her back to her room, promising again that she will notify Security.

Back at the desk, Jeannie turns to Jeri and remarks, "Hey, it's Filene's Basement."

She suddenly bursts into pantomime. Crooking her ear as if she had heard a phone ring, she picks up the nearest line and mimics. "Hello, this is Filene's. Ladies' Lingerie, how can I help you? Size 40D bras? No, I'm sorry, we're all out of 'em."

It's been that kind of day. And most of the ruckuses involved patients other than her own. Jeannie's patients at the moment include Mrs. Herbst,* an old Jewish woman who is here to be ruled out / ruled in. Jeannie is also responsible for Ruth Thomas,* a twenty-four-year-old African American woman admitted three days ago with a serious throat infection. Then there is another eighty-year-old Jewish patient — Mrs. Cohen,* who is demented, has had a stroke, and repeatedly comes to the Beth Israel with pneumonia. And Mr. Wilson,* a fifty-nine-year-old accountant with prostate cancer who has been admitted because of a urinary tract infection.

Before going back to check on each patient, Jeannie realizes she has left her hospital ID in her wallet. She sets off for the small, chilly room containing long rows of lockers where the nurses stow their personal gear. Spinning the combination lock to the correct number, she pulls her wallet out of a blue-and-black fannypack and rummages through its contents. An extra pair of Birkenstocks slips out of the locker. These are an integral part of Jeannie's daily uniform.

Each day, she dresses in neatly pressed chinolike slacks and an all-cotton shirt with short sleeves that buttons at the neck. The color of the pants varies, as does the shirt color (she always orders cotton, she says, because she sweats too much in synthetics).

And that is that. "I spend at least six seconds on my appearance while I'm parting my hair," she jokes. Whenever she talks about personal appearance or decoration, you get a sense that Jeannie Chaisson decided at an early age not to worry about externals. Other nurses may busily try to add an alluring detail to their work attire. They will proudly display a new coiffure, fabulous necklace, or fancy earrings. When the discussion turns to the name of the hairdresser or jewelry store where all this was purchased, Jeannie simply shrugs. "I never wear earrings," she says without passing judgment. When several nurses joke about a resident who just tried to flirt with them, she adopts a tone of mock sadness and pines, "Gee, I don't understand why those twenty-seven-year-old interns don't want to flirt with me."

With a frame that has always been tall, trim, and solid, Jeannie presents herself to the world like a Shaker woman of old — plain and proud.

Before pinning on her ID, she flashes it to me. "While my son was going through my purse the other night, he found this. He was so impressed to learn that his mother is a genuine essential service. I have to be allowed through police lines. It's great. If Boston gets nuked, I get to go to work."

Jeannie Chaisson is forty-four years old. She has been a nurse for fifteen years and throughout that entire period has combined full-time work with raising a family of three — Maddie, her daughter, is seventeen, Dan is thirteen, and Mark is eleven.

Today, as always, her work is a rapidly shifting kaleidoscope of different activities. The job of the clinical nurse specialist — an advanced practice nurse who has a master's degree — is to support the practice of bedside nurses and improve the care they provide. Nurses on the day shift generally care for four patients each. Nurses on the evening shift have six patients, and nurses on the night shift are responsible for eleven. (At night, there are fewer nurses on duty because most patients are asleep and receive far fewer tests and procedures.)

Bedside nurses are so busy simply caring for patients — and sometimes so harried — that they do not often have time to stand back and identify larger problems, reflect on or uncover solutions to them. The pressure of patient needs may also leave them with little time to study charts to discover patterns in the patients' problems and locate useful resources both inside and outside the hospital.

It is Jeannie Chaisson's job to help nurses do all this and more. At the Beth Israel, a nurse specialist like Jeannie has great latitude to structure this supportive role. Many are attached to a specific unit. Others work throughout the hospital, moving to different units as needed. For example, Marion Phipps, one of Jeannie and Ellen Kitchen's most respected colleagues, is a hospital-wide specialist in rehabilitation. Nurses who work with patients who are immobilized, fragile, or severely disabled will call on Phipps for advice — particularly when their patients suffer from skin breakdown, pressure sores, incontinence, or malnutrition. Phipps also deals with patients who don't fit into or can't use conventional hospital equipment, such as the six-hundred-pound pulmonary patient or the very frail old woman who can't sit up in a chair.

Jeannie's mission is to support nurses who are giving general medical care to a wide variety of patients with many different problems. Because nurses tend to work on general medical floors just after they graduate from nursing school, many of the nursing staff she works with are young and inexperienced. Her role thus involves teaching, mentoring, and role modeling for both nurses and physicians — many of whom are also young and inexperienced. On some days she will be available to talk with nurses one-on-one or in groups, intervene in crises, do managerial tasks, and watch for problems. Jeannie also acts as an informal career counselor. If nurses are thinking about going back to school or making a job change, they often consult with her rather than the nurse manager who is their official supervisor and in whom they would not want to confide any ambivalence about their career plans.

To teach nurses effectively, Jeannie believes it is essential for her to participate in the ongoing process of patient care. That's why she cares for patients herself two or three days a week. "If I take patients," she explains, "I can find out what nurses are up against, what systems aren't working, and what types of things are bringing patients into the hospital. Less-experienced nurses can also see how someone with greater expertise manages situations. It also helps physicians and interns when they are dealing with someone articulate and knowledgeable. If I call them about something, I already know what I want them to do, which can be very helpful."

When Jeannie is directly responsible for patients, she works all three shifts — days, evenings, and nights. "I like to work a variety of different shifts," she says blithely of her erratic schedule. "It lets me know what the issues are. People complain about different things depending on which shift they work."

When acting primarily as an educational resource, she works from 9:30 or 10 A.M. till six or seven at night. She is generally off on Thursday and Sunday. Thursdays, she says, are devoted to dealing with appointments, household chores, or just spending time with one of her three children. For half of the year, she teaches religious education at the First Unitarian Society of Newton. She is director of the Newton Schools Foundation, which awards grants to teachers in the public school system. Jeannie also directs another local program, Understanding Handicaps Inc., which has designed a curriculum on disability awareness for fourth graders in the Newton school system.

Finally, Jeannie is just completing a five-year stint as the leader of her son Mark's Cub Scout troop. "I tried to raise a lot of nontraditional Cub Scouts," she explains. And knowing Jeannie Chaisson, that's exactly what they will turn out to be.

On this particular morning, Jeannie is caring for patients herself. She begins with Mrs. Cohen,* who resides in a nearby nursing home. The elderly woman's stroke was massive and her frequent visits to the Beth Israel in the past few years have been for aspiration pneumonia, an inflammation of the lungs caused by inhalation of foreign material or vomit, which she has on this admission. A large sign placed over her bed warns staff to take Aspiration Precautions when feeding her.

Jeannie is going to feed Mrs. Cohen her breakfast. Feeding a stroke patient is extremely complicated. If not properly done, it is a risky process for the patient. While feeding Mrs. Cohen, Jeannie must constantly assess the woman's ability to swallow. Swallowing is a complex series of voluntary and automatic processes. It utilizes six nerves and twenty-five facial and oral muscles that propel food to its proper destination: the stomach. This ostensibly simple act has four distinct phases. With a stroke victim something can go wrong during any or every one of these four phases. Brain damage from the stroke can be so extensive that a patient has no muscular control of the mouth and no automatic gag reflex. In this case, anything eaten has a clear shot right into the lungs, where it can create a pneumonia.

Because some patients who seem to be in control of their swallowing may, in fact, be "silent aspirators," nurses must always evaluate each stroke patient's ability to chew and swallow. If the patient has aphasia and is thus unable to understand language, the nurse can't just tell such a patient, 'Now close your mouth. Chew. Now, swallow for me.' The patient may be unable to understand or comply with the simplest instructions, making this assessment process very difficult.

An expert nurse like Jeannie must see if such patients' gag reflex functions by slowly feeding them specially thickened food that won't go down the wrong way too easily. If a patient seems to be choking and changes color, then he or she may well be aspirating. Some patients don't choke, because they have lost that reflex. To determine whether this kind of patient is aspirating, Jeannie carefully watches for changes in color and any increased difficulty breathing or increased respiratory rate. "Patients who have no cough reflex are particularly in danger, and you have to really know what you're doing and have the time to observe closely if you're going to keep them safe."

Jeannie knows Mrs. Cohen, and thus can skip the assessment phase. She begins the process of feeding her by assembling the necessary food thickeners that will help make eating safe. "You might think a patient in this condition needs food to be more liquid," she tells me, "but that's not true. Her food needs to be thicker so that it doesn't flow into her lungs."

The old woman is lying on the bed, her eyes closed, breathing in a heavy, rasping cadence. Jeannie sits down on the bed and pats the woman's hand. "Hello, Mrs. Cohen, remember me? I'm Jeannie Chaisson. I'm going to be taking care of you today."

The woman opens her eyes and stares vacantly at Jeannie. She says nothing. Nonetheless, Jeannie continues to talk with her and explain what she is doing and why.

First, Jeannie must shift Mrs. Cohen to a more upright position so that she can eat safely. Jeannie excuses herself and returns with another nurse. The two raise the bed to a comfortable height so that they don't strain their backs. Jeannie is always cognizant of protecting her back because, on a New Year's Eve eight years ago, she hurt it while caring for a patient who fell on the floor while having a seizure. There was no room to maneuver to use proper body mechanics. The patient did well but Jeannie's back has never quite recovered. They place their hands in strategic spots under the woman's buttocks and on her back. As they explain their movements to the patient, they hoist her up toward the top of the bed and then return it to a tilted position.

Mrs. Cohen coughs vigorously and Jeannie cheers her on. "That's great, Mrs. Cohen, bring that stuff right up now. The sooner you cough it all up, the sooner you'll feel better."

Jeannie reaches behind the patient's bed and grabs a rigid tube — a Yankauer suction — similar to the kind used in dentists' offices. She then places the suction tube in the woman's mouth to draw out the secretions. "Now we're going to give you a little food and see how you do eating."

Jeannie is attentive to the smallest details. "I gave her soft food — applesauce and some custard — earlier this morning, and she chewed on it for about twenty minutes," she explains. "The fact that she took so long made me wonder about her normal diet. So I called the nursing home to double-check. Just as I suspected, they give her pureed food."

Jeannie reaches for a cup of milk. "Here's some milk," she tells her patient. "I'm just going to pour a little powder into it to thicken it so it doesn't go down too quickly and into the wrong tube." She pours powder into the milk and stirs the liquid. Mrs. Cohen takes a few sips.

"Here's your mashed potatoes." Jeannie picks up another plate and spoonful by spoonful puts the potatoes into the woman's mouth. Occasionally, the patient coughs vigorously between bites and Jeannie suctions out her mouth, applauding each rasping fit with words of encouragement. Then she thickens applesauce and spoons some of that into Mrs. Cohen's mouth. This provokes another fit of coughing, so Jeannie continues the suctioning.

"She's coughing because she has so many secretions from the pneumonia," Jeannie explains. "Some might think she's coughing because she's aspirating. But, in fact, she's just bringing up the phlegm, which I then have to suction out. Sometimes food going down stimulates her to cough. So she's somebody that I feed carefully and try not to tire too much. And if I have any doubts about the change in her respiratory status, I stop feeding her and let her rest and try again later."

She reaches behind the bed to pull out yet another device that is attached to the oxygen flow meter on the wall. She places a mask over the patient's nose and mouth so that a cool mist can be delivered into her lungs. This will loosen any phlegm and help her clear her chest.

"That's good, we're finished now," she tells Mrs. Cohen. "We'll let you sit up for twenty minutes or half an hour and then I'll be back."

"I want to change her position often," Jeannie explains once outside the room. "She's got a little red spot that I don't want to turn into a bedsore. So when I come back, I'll turn her on her side for a while to give her back a rest. When she's in an air bed, it helps distribute the weight well so that she doesn't develop bed sores. The nursing home puts her in one when her skin breaks down. But they don't have money to provide her with one all the time."

Jeannie knows that this tiny red spot can turn into a terrible bedsore, or decubitus ulcer. This is no trivial problem. In fact, a 1994 study sponsored by the federal Agency for Health Care Policy and Research estimated that the total national cost of pressure ulcer treatment was $1.355 billion per year. Thus, Jeannie's vigilant monitoring is one of the many ways in which nurses save our health care system billions.

"With a patient this prone to aspiration, some families would choose to put a permanent feeding tube directly through the abdomen into the stomach. This can help reduce the risk of aspiration. But it doesn't eliminate it. And it deprives the patient of the ability to taste and swallow food. Many families choose to attempt to continue careful feeding, and accept the increased risk of aspirations because they feel it's more humane and they hate to put a demented, elderly person through another procedure."

At the doorway, she looks fondly at the old woman. "She's demented. She only says a few words now and then, but she's my kind of gal. There's so much you can do to care for demented patients safely. You can take care of their skin, and make sure they maintain some range of motion, and see that they're turned often enough. It's good to see how well she's taken care of."

Jeannie's next patient is Ruth Thomas.* The African American woman in her mid-twenties was admitted because of an infection that made her throat so swollen she couldn't even swallow her own saliva. Her physician was afraid that the constriction would interfere with her ability to breathe and could be life-threatening. So she was admitted to the hospital to receive intravenous steroids to reduce the swelling and antibiotics to fight the infection. The treatment has proved effective and she is recovering.

When Jeannie comes in to see the patient, the woman is in the bathroom vomiting. Listening to her retching, Jeannie surmises that she probably ate more than she can tolerate at the moment. She leaves the room to get some medication. When she returns, the small, thin woman with intricately corn-rowed hair is again in her bed.

Jeannie asks how she is doing

"I was okay until I had some coffee," she replies weakly.

"Coffee is probably not a good idea for you now. How about ice chips and a cold towel? Do you think that would make you feel better?"

The patient nods limply. Jeannie goes to the kitchen and returns with a glass filled with ice chips. The intravenous line containing the patient's antibiotics isn't running well, so Jeannie checks to see if the patient has rolled over on it. This can create a clot in the line and impede the flow. Jeannie flushes it with a syringe of saline solution and checks to make sure that the medication is moving steadily.

About an hour later, Jeannie returns. The patient is still concerned about nausea. What will she do if she feels nauseous at home? she wonders. Why is this happening? she asks anxiously. Is it normal?

"You've got ten reasons to feel sick," Jeannie reassures. "And we certainly won't let you go home if you're feeling like this. Do you feel nauseated all the time?"

"The eggs went down okay," Ms. Thomas answers.

"Well, we'll see if you can keep it down next time. As long as we know that you're not dehydrated and you don't have a high fever, I'm sure you'll be fine."

After Jeannie leaves the room, I stay and talk with the patient. I ask how she feels about her hospital experience and nurses like Jeannie. Although she is exhausted and wan, she smiles enthusiastically. "They're great," she says of the nurses. "They always check up on me and see if I need anything. They know exactly what they're doing and what you need. It's very reassuring. It's like it's a group thing, taking care of you. The nurses do their thing and the doctors do theirs. That's very comforting, because you see the nurses more than the doctors."

As we walk down the corridor to see Jeannie's next patient, Mr. Wilson,* Jeannie hears a commotion inside another patient room. She stops to see if one of her colleagues can use some help. A young nurse is bending over an old Jewish woman who is rocking back and forth shrieking as if in some anguished mourning ritual. "Ai, ai, ai, I never dreamed. Leave me alone," she cries, trying to push the nurse away with a fierceness that is startling in one so frail. "I never dreamed. What are you doing to me? Leave me alone."

"I'm just trying to give you your blood pressure medicine, Mrs. Abrams,"* the nurse says quietly.

The woman is too demented and terrified to heed such rational explanations. "No, no, I don't need medicine. You can't give me that. You're not a doctor."

"I'm a nurse," the young woman explains.

The old woman gives her a skeptical look. Rearing back, she shakes her head and shouts, "No, you're not a nurse. You're not a doctor. I don't need medicine."

"Mrs. Abrams, you have high blood pressure," the nurse reminds her.

"No," the woman screams. "Leave me alone."

Jeannie offers to help. 'No, it's all right. I'll calm her down," the other nurse tells her.

Later she tracks down the young nurse to talk to her about the incident. When a patient is that agitated and you can't reach her, it's better to back off and try again later, she advises. A demented patient's mood can swing dramatically. They can be very hostile and aggressive and then, only a short time later, become quite docile. But, Jeannie adds, if you keep pushing a patient with high blood pressure to take her blood pressure medicine, she may become more and more alarmed, which is obviously not good for her blood pressure. The young nurse nods appreciatively.

Mr. Wilson's room is near Six Feldberg's long, narrow solarium. The sunlight pours through the large picture window and into the room, but the patient hardly seems to notice. He is an accountant who has prostate cancer. His tumor has blocked the flow of urine and he has to catheterize himself several times a day. This has led to an infection, which brought him to the hospital. In several weeks, after the infection has been treated, he will have prostate surgery to remove the tumor. This should help him to pass urine. Or it may have a serious side effect — he won't be able to hold urine and thus will become incontinent.

Jeannie introduces herself to Mr. Wilson. She looks at his IV and gives him some medicine. As she is talking with him, a physician enters the room on his daily rounds. Jeannie and the doctor nod amiably and Jeannie tells him how the patient is doing. "He looks good this morning and his fever is down," she says, smiling at the man in the bed, trying to include him in the conversation.

For the next ten minutes, the doctor questions the patient about his pain and other symptoms. Was the pain in his back or belly? How about his fever and chills? When did they begin? How long did they last? How does he feel now? Lifting Mr. Wilson's johnny, the doctor probes and prods. He makes sure there are no side effects from his current medication and also talks with the patient about his upcoming surgery. After reassuring the patient that things are going well, he leaves.

Jeannie, however, lingers. She pulls up one of the green Naugahyde armchairs that are standard hospital furnishing and sits down next to the bed. First she asks Mr. Wilson how the catheter affects his life. Visibly pleased to have someone that he can talk with about things he does not want most people to know, he catalogs his daily routine. For weeks, he recounts, he has had to insert a tube through his penis and into his bladder in order to evacuate urine. If he has a luncheon meeting, he goes into the bathroom to put in his catheter beforehand. If he's going out to dinner, he again makes a premeal trip to the toilet.

"I bet you do it really quickly," Jeannie predicts.

Proudly, Mr. Wilson exclaims," I'm down to about five minutes. A lot of doctors are surprised I can do it at all."

"That's because some people can't. They either can't take the idea or blockage from the tumor may prevent them."

Like two tennis players discussing the latest equipment, nurse and patient chat about the size of the catheters, their expense, how long they can be used, and how to dry them safely.

"I think you're doing a good job," Jeannie concludes. As if he'd just won a difficult match, Mr. Wilson beams. Then, just as quickly, his brow furrows.

He says he is very worried about his upcoming surgery. Can he give his own blood while he's on antibiotics? he wonders. Jeannie thinks he can but says she will find out.

Relieved, Mr. Wilson begins to relate the history of his cancer. He had an enlarged prostate, he says, and his physician felt a hard mass. After a needle biopsy detected cancer, he was given a choice — do nothing, get radiation therapy, or have surgery. Surgery was recommended, so he agreed to it.

Now he is very concerned about the outcome. "It's a bad operation," he says, no longer making any attempt to conceal his anxiety. "You pick up other problems, like incontinence."

"We have ways around that," Jeannie says. She tells him about the Beth Israel nurse who specializes in problems of incontinence and who can teach him exercises that may improve bladder control.

Mr. Wilson seems reassured to hear about this. Jeannie talks with him for a few moments longer and then tells him she'll be back soon.

Walking to see her next patient, Jeannie analyzes this exchange. She deliberately lingered in Mr. Wilson's room after his physician left because she sensed that he had not expressed all his anxieties and concerns. "With experience, you learn to anticipate the kinds of questions that people have that they haven't even been able to articulate," she explains. "You learn to recognize when somebody's worried even when they're not saying so and to know what they're likely to be worried about. A large part of what we do is calming the fears that a patient hasn't expressed or even acknowledged yet."

This important aspect of nursing work often goes undocumented and unrecorded, Jeannie says. "We don't write down in the chart, 'Well, I thought the patient was possibly worried and so I sat and talked with him for half an hour.' But, in fact, to the patient, that talk might be more important than what we do write down, which is 'I took an EKG this morning, checked his blood pressure every four hours, and gave him medication.' It's that knowledge and reassurance that allows the patient to calm down enough to get some sleep. But apart from some cryptic comment about coping, it's never going to be in the chart."

As Jeannie is leaving Mr. Wilson's room, she hears her name called. Turning around, she sees Dr. Geraldine Zagarella (or Zag, as her colleagues call her) standing in a nearby doorway. Zagarella is a fifty-two-year-old internist at the Urban Medical Group in Jamaica Plain and is also co–medical director of the Beth Israel Home Care Department, where she works closely with Ellen Kitchen.

"Would you please help me boost this patient?" Zagarella asks Jeannie.

"Of course," Jeannie replies, and the two enter the room together.

Zagarella's patient is a thirty-five-year-old woman with multiple sclerosis. She cannot move her mottled white legs and is scrunched into a pretzel-like position in her chair. To position her correctly, Jeannie and Zagarella kneel on either side of the chair. They gently manipulate each taut leg into a bent position, grab on to her torso, and, as Jeannie counts, "One, two, three," hoist her up in the chair. The woman clenches its sides as if sheer willpower will allow her to assist in this communal effort. Once she is seated comfortably, all three let out a laugh of relief. The woman thanks them and Zagarella, in turn, thanks Jeannie.

"She's very special," Jeannie comments as Zagarella goes down the corridor. "Many doctors don't get involved in making their patients comfortable. They see that as the nurse's role. When a physician does help in the hands-on care, it shows respect not only for the nurse but for the patient. If it's a simple thing like boosting a patient or fixing a pillow, why should the patient have to wait while the doctor goes off to find a nurse or the nurse goes off to get another nurse for help? Why shouldn't doctors just do it themselves?

"When Zag helps, it demonstrates that this work is not somehow unimportant for someone like a doctor to bother with. That means a lot to a patient, to know that their comfort is also important to their physician. In fact, when you think about it, many patients are reluctant to tell physicians about symptoms that 'just' involve comfort because they think that it's not important enough to bother the doctor. But those apparently trivial symptoms might be all we have to go on to determine what's causing the illness. When they see a doctor concerned about their comfort, it lets them know that they can talk about troubling symptoms, and this can give us some very good clues to the mystery of their disease."

A few moments later, Jeannie bumps into an intern she'd been looking for. The previous day, Jeannie took care of a patient who had come into the hospital with chest pain from angina. In developing the patient's treatment plan, the intern had written orders that Jeannie now questions.

Following standard Beth Israel practice, the intern had given the patient a topical nitroglycerin — nitropaste — to help control the angina. The dose of nitropaste is calibrated to the patient's blood pressure, which is checked every six hours. According to the blood pressure reading, a particular dose of nitropaste is applied to the skin and then absorbed into the body. This means that nurses must wake patients once or twice during the night to check their blood pressure and regulate their dose of the medication. In most cases, once it is determined that the patient is not having a heart attack, the topical nitropaste is discontinued and the patient is given oral nitroglycerin three times a day.

While Jeannie was with the woman, she complained about anxiety and her inability to get any uninterrupted sleep at night. Jeannie felt that waking the patient up several times a night was exacerbating this woman's fears. More to the point, the nitropaste was not controlling her chest pain. Because she had been ruled out for an MI, topical medication was no longer part of the standard protocol.

When she saw the intern, she tried to explain this to her and get her to put the patient on oral nitrates. She reassured the young doctor that this would be both safe and effective. Plus, the nurses would be able to let the patient sleep through the night.

The intern, a dark-haired young woman in a short white lab coat, seems reluctant to consider Jeannie's advice. Without making eye contact with the nurse, she insists that the patient is still having chest pain and needs the topical medication. Jeannie patiently reminds her that the nitropaste obviously isn't controlling the woman's chest pain and its administration is only aggravating her anxiety.

Faced with this argument, the intern takes another tack. "Well, she's really worried about a heart attack, or maybe cancer," the young woman asserts. "She's convinced she has something really bad. If we wake her up at night, she'll feel like we're paying attention to her."

Jeannie often expresses her astonishment at the world's foolishness by knocking on her head and prefacing her comments with a "Hello?" — a kind of extended "Is anyone home in there?" Listening to this exchange, I can imagine what Jeannie is thinking. "Hello?" she would say. "Oh, that's a good one! We wake up our patients four or five times a night so they know they're not alone. Maybe if we wake her up often enough and make her uncomfortable enough, she'll stop having angina altogether. This is obviously a voluntary activity on her part." With great self-control, the nurse refrains from ridiculing the novice doctor's notion and returns instead to her original argument. "No, I think this will only *increase* her anxiety," she repeats.

Grudgingly, the intern announces that she will "think about it" and walks off.

Jeannie looks after her. "It is not surprising that people get these ideas," she said. "Inexperienced interns often make decisions for the wrong reasons. She probably doesn't realize that when a patient is restless or frightened in the middle of the night, we nurses will find out about it and spend time with the patient. But if you wake a patient up arbitrarily, of course, they're going to be more anxious."

She hits her head with her fist and says, "For God's sake, I'd have chest pain if you woke me up in the middle of the night. Don't people know that sleep is therapeutic?"

Back in the conference room, Jeannie pours a cup of coffee, tops it amply with cream, and discusses the problem of physician-nurse relationships, or what some have called "the doctor-nurse game." The dilemma nurses often face stems from the fact that so few doctors really understand the nurse's role. Many doctors think nurses are like robots tethered by some invisible wire to a doctor's clinical judgment. Doctors write orders, and nurses follow them. If there are no orders, there is no care.

For example, Jeannie explains, you call a resident in the middle of the night because you have just taken a patient's vital signs and there is a marked change. "The resident is angry because you woke him or her up. They'll say, 'Well, why did you just check on the patient? I didn't order vital signs to be taken in the middle of the night."

Jeannie tenses the long slender fingers that are in constant motion when she talks and presses them to her forehead. "When this happens, I have to politely explain that I don't really look to doctors to tell me how to do my job. But it's generally news to them that a nurse would actually evaluate a patient who is under her care without a doctor ordering her to do it."

This is not surprising, and it certainly doesn't stem from physician hostility to nurses. It's a result of ignorance. Doctors, Jeannie says, have not been taught the fact that it is a nurse's job to evaluate patients under her care. "I explain that I try to provide certain data that the doctor has requested. But if the patient looks terrible, I'm going to use my own judgment and do an evaluation even if they haven't ordered it."

For example, Jeannie goes on to posit a typical case. A physician may write an order to call her if a patient's temperature goes up to 101.5 degrees. "But if that patient has been stable for days and suddenly goes up to 101, I'm going to call them. I'm not going to wait till it goes up another half a degree, because this in itself is a change.

I don't care what they wrote. I don't need to have their permission to call them. I can figure it out myself. If they don't want to do anything about it, that's their decision. If they want to wait till later, I'll call them again."

This fundamental misunderstanding of the nurse's role is endemic in the medical system and in the organization of the institutions that train physicians — teaching hospitals. In a teaching hospital like the BI, many of the "physicians" nurses work with are not experienced doctors, but doctors-in-training. They may be third- and fourth-year medical students, who are beginning to take on increasing levels of responsibility for patient care. Under direct supervision of an intern or resident, these responsibilities may include writing medication orders, ordering tests, seeing patients to check on their status, or talking with patients' families.

Or they may be what are known as house officers, that is, first-year residents, known as interns, who are in their first year of training after medical school graduation, and more advanced residents. Nurses also work with fellows, who have completed their residency programs and are going on for further training. For example, internal medicine residents may choose to subspecialize in oncology or cardiology, while a general surgery resident might subspecialize in orthopedics.

On a day-to-day basis, Jeannie works most intensively with these doctors-in-training. On the inpatient floors, interns rotate on and off units monthly. Because medical education and training is conducted according to an apprenticeship system sometimes referred to as "See one, do one, teach one," a medical resident will demonstrate how to place an IV in the arm for a medical student, and then will supervise as the student attempts the procedure for the first time. After the student achieves some level of mastery, he or she will be left to do the procedure alone. At some point, the student may teach less-advanced students.

The bulk of the day-to-day responsibility for patient care is left to the residents, and particularly to the interns. The resident supervises the interns, but it is the intern who spends the majority of his or her day on the medical floor. The supervising resident will come for morning rounds, to see new admissions, and if the intern calls for backup. Otherwise, residents frequently spend their time in the library or in their call room reading, studying for exams, or catching up on sleep. All are supervised by attending physicians, or "attend-ings," as they are referred to.

But the reality is that attending physicians may not spend much time on the floor or unit each day. If an attending has an office in the hospital, he or she may be seeing patients in that office or seeing patients on other floors. Many attendings who admit patients to teaching hospitals are in private practice outside the hospital and are only on the floors during a brief part of the day when they are making rounds. During the evening and night shifts, there are often few attending physicians in the hospital, and the hospital is run by nurses and house officers.

Even though a nurse may have more experience than a house officer in many aspects of patient care, it is the doctor — even the novice doctor — who is, as nursing historian Joan Lynaugh explains it, the captain of the hospital ship and who gives "orders" to the nurse — and by extension to the patient. This physician authority has been staunchly defended for over a century. And it is applied in institutions that are some of the most hierarchically and patriarchally organized in the country. In this traditional male-dominated hierarchy, nurses have been traditionally viewed as handmaidens. In the past, physician authority was so adamantly enforced on nurses that even traditional gender behavior was jettisoned. As little as thirty years ago, a nurse was supposed to stand at attention when a physician entered the room or give up her chair to a doctor if none was available for him.

Only a few decades ago, nurses were also barred from using common medical language because to do so would infringe on physician turf. "In 1956," Lynaugh recalls, "if I saw a patient on my ward who had the signs and symptoms of a myocardial infarction [MI, or heart attack], I could not write in the chart that the patient had a myocardial infarction. I could go up to a physician and tell him the patient had an MI. But to write those words in the chart would have been interpreted as exceeding my scope of practice."

An even more preposterous example of this kind of protection of turf occurs when a patient dies and it is time to pronounce death. Up until only recently, physicians were the only ones in the health care system able to pronounce a patient dead. Nurses, whose job it is to care for patients twenty-four hours a day until the patient dies, apparently could not be reliably counted on to distinguish between a dead patient and a living one. Today, in most hospitals, physicians are still the only ones who can legally pronounce death. Depending on the state, nurses in the home or in hospice care can sometimes legally decree that a dead patient is, in fact, dead.

Although a great deal has changed during the eighties and early nineties, some doctors still view nurses as replaceable subordinates, rather than valued colleagues. At the Beth Israel, as in many other hospitals, doctors are still referred to as "house officers," who give "orders" to nurses. Of course, nurses do not blindly follow those orders. If a doctor writes a prescription for a medication, the nurse must know its proper dosage and side effects and is legally obligated to raise a question if she believes it is the wrong drug or the wrong dose or if the medication is contraindicated because, owing to side effects or other concerns, the drug is not appropriate. She also needs to know about possible interactions with any other drugs the patient may be taking. If nurses neglect to play this important fail-safe role, they can be held legally liable for any adverse incident. (Nurses can and have been sued when patients suffer as a result. However, because the pockets of highly paid doctors and hospitals are so much deeper, many lawyers choose to sue the doctor and hospital rather than the nurse.)

If a dispute arises between a doctor and a nurse around medication errors or other such problems, the nurse may prevail. If, however, the dispute is around preference — the nurse prefers to give this medication rather than the one the doctor chooses, prefers to give more medication for pain, or prefers to get a patient walking at a different time than the physician stipulates, it is the physician's prerogative to win that argument.

Hopefully, such disputes do not arise too often. Doctors and nurses should work on a cohesive team. But teamwork is often an ideal rather than a reality in the health care system. That's because the groundwork for teamwork has not been laid throughout the lengthy process of medical education. Quite the contrary. Although physicians work with nurses on a daily basis, and although nurses often teach physicians a great deal about patient care, in most medical schools students learn little or nothing about nursing. In spite of the fact that they will work together in hospitals for years, medical students and nursing students rarely, if ever, learn together.

The Beth Israel does more to facilitate nurse-physician cooperation than most hospitals. Nurses from the BI often speak with medical students at Harvard Medical School on both a formal and an informal basis. Jeannie, for example, has sporadically spoken with medical students about nursing's mission. Patricia Focarelli, another nurse at the BI, is an instructor for first-year medical students in their course entitled Patient-Doctor One. Along with general surgeon Michael Cahalane, Focarelli has also organized a nurse-for-a-day program for those third-year medical students who choose to do their surgical rotation, or clerkship, at the BI. The obstetrics and gynecology clerkship has a similar program modeled on the surgical clerkship's program. These efforts are unique to the BI and are not replicated at the other Harvard teaching hospitals to which medical students are farmed out for similar rotations. (Indeed, the fact that, after two decades of promoting nursing's importance, such BI programs have not been reproduced at other Harvard teaching hospitals shows how deeply rooted physician ambivalence to nursing's role in health care remains.)

Yet, when they come to the BI as first-year residents, or interns, physicians are not given any introduction to the practice of the nurses they will work with. On Kirstein Three, Nancy Rumplik does orient new fellows to the unit and introduces them to primary nursing. In most hospitals and medical schools, however, when they enter the traditional hospital hierarchy as medical students, interns, or fellows, physicians-in-training are rarely given any orientation about how to deal with nurses or told what nurses know and do. Similarly, there are usually no explicit guidelines on particular units that help physicians to understand nursing as a profession or the individual nurses with whom they work. In hospitals, even at the BI, the constant rotation of physicians through hospital units during their years of training also discourages interprofessional connection.

In teaching hospitals like the BI, the structure of residency programs also generates increased tension between physicians-in-training and their nursing colleagues. In 1984, an eighteen-year-old girl, Libby Zion, died at New York Hospital within eight hours of being admitted. For the first time, this case brought the onerous working conditions of residents to public attention. The case led to regulations in the state of New York limiting residents' work hours and mandating increased supervision of their work. Today, medical residents are supposed to work only eighty hours a week, with sixteen-hour shifts the routine. (These regulations are, however, often flouted.) Residents in surgery and in obstetrics and gynecology, in particular, routinely work more than a hundred hours a week, sometimes spending an entire weekend on call.

At the BI, residents in internal medicine work between eighty and ninety hours a week when they rotate through the Intensive Care, Coronary Care, and Pulmonary Care Units. There they will be on-call approximately every third night and stay in the hospital for up to twenty-eight hours at a stretch. When they are rotating through other inpatient wards, they work between sixty-five and eighty hours a week and are typically on-call one out of every four nights.

Surgical residents work between eighty and a hundred hours a week, on call in the hospital thirty-six hours at a stretch approximately every third day. This is called a straight every-third schedule. There is a modified every-third schedule in which the resident will have staggered thirty-six-hour stretches but will work through an entire weekend so that she can have the following Saturday — after 11 A.M. — till Monday morning off. During that twelve-day period, the resident will be in the hospital 233 hours.

Given these spirit- and back-breaking schedules, residents' clinical judgment may not be the only thing to be impaired. Their communications skills with colleagues are profoundly strained. "The place where doctors learn to relate to nurses is during their residency or as medical students following residents and modeling their own behavior after them. But these doctors-in-training are by their situation very insecure," says physician Timothy McCall, author of *Examining Your Doctor: A Patient's Guide to Avoiding Harmful Medical Care* and a number of influential articles on the negative impact of the long hours of residency training. "They are badly stressed and suffer from chronic sleep deprivation. They don't want anyone to make more work for them. But the reality is that to do a good job, nurses often have to make more work for a resident."

Nurses like Jeannie are the ones who constantly interrupt the exhausted resident trying to take advantage of a quiet moment to read a journal article or half an hour to catch up on some sleep. "Your patient has spiked a fever, is having chest pain, has pulled out his IV, or needs to be transferred to the ICU. To the harried resident it's all bad news. Just to survive, residents will try to blow the nurse off," McCall continues. "Rather than respond to a nurse's suggestion that the resident come evaluate a patient whose clinical condition is changing, the resident may be tempted to give a thirty-second telephone order for physical restraints or suggest a patient be given Tylenol or Haldol (an antipsychotic drug given to agitated patients)."

"An undercurrent of animosity characterizes relationships between residents and nurses in teaching hospitals," says Glenn Bubley, one of the most thoughtful oncologists at the Beth Israel. He recalls his own medical training and the middle-of-the-night wake-up calls he tried to avoid. "This stems from the fact that the nurse doesn't feel her often realistic concerns about her patient are being met in a timely fashion, while the doctor feels as if he is constantly nagged by nurses. In fact, they are both right. She's right to call the doctor to get orders to help her provide care, whether during the day or at night. And the physician feels justified when he says, Hey, don't bother me in the middle of the night unless it's really an emergency."

Nurses are legally required to get doctors' orders for any change in the patient's regimen. But when doctors don't write orders in a way that gives nurses enough latitude to adjust medications when necessary, they are legally bound to call the doctor for new orders. Similarly, when doctors do not view nurses as full participants in the health care team, RNs will constantly interrupt doctors to discuss the patient's plan of care. When this happens, doctors may be tempted to dismiss the nurses' concerns as trivial and to take the easiest, least time consuming route available to deal with the problem at hand.

The result of the kind of corner cutting the system inevitably produces, McCall says, may not only jeopardize the patient's health, but may undermine relationships with the nurse. "The point is that the nurse is simply trying to do what's best for the patient," says McCall. "The resident, on the other hand, is trying to balance quality care with personal survival."

The kinds of relationships doctors begin to forge with nurses in the cauldron of their medical training have lingering effects. Once a resident escapes the militarylike rigors of the teaching hospital, he or she may thankfully leave behind the bone-weariness and nerve-jangling irritation caused by sleep deprivation and insecurity. But the newly minted physician may never overcome the by now ingrained habit of, as McCall puts it, "blowing off the nurse."

The combined legacy of gender and the socialization process of medical training produces practitioners who are "intimate strangers" — to borrow a term used by sociologist Lillian Rubin to describe male-female relationships in traditional families. Like children learning about the opposite sex from each other on the playground, most of what physicians "know" about the other health care professions is what they "pick up" along the way. "There's a kind of black box in our knowledge of what happens between the time we write orders and the time the nurses carry them out. We just don't really know what nurses do," a surgical resident at the Beth Israel explained.

"You learn not to offend the nurses, because they could hurt you if you do," another oncology fellow told me. "You'd better get along with the nurses, or they could make trouble for you," yet another echoed this negative depiction of physician-nurse relationships. Or as a fourth-year medical student recently told me, "In my experience with nurses, the nurse's role is to call the doctor when there's something wrong so the doctor can come and fix it."

According to Joan Lynaugh, "Most physicians still think that nurses are modestly educated, unambitious, and lack any commitment to their career." It's no wonder, then, that physicians respond so negatively to policy proposals that would give nurses a greater role and voice in health care delivery. Not only are they concerned about potential competition. They are also generally ignorant of the content and context of caregiving, and may genuinely believe that nurses are too uneducated and inexperienced to merit greater autonomy and responsibility.

That's what the surgical resident at the BI confided as we were talking about nursing. Adopting a conspiratorial tone, he asked, "Now honestly, can you tell me that a nurse could possibly be as smart as a doctor?" Doctors, he insisted, are some of the smartest people in the land. They've all gotten terrific grades in high school and college, spend their days poring over the latest research published in medical journals, and devote the rest of their spare time to gaining new knowledge in seminars and conferences.

He was apparently unaware that nurses might do the same — or that not all doctors graduated at the head of their class. As Thomas S. Bodenheimer and Kevin Grumbach report in their book *Understanding Health Policy: A Clinical Approach*, "between 80 to 90% of what physicians do has never been evaluated by rigorous scientific study." Moreover, "five to 15% of physicians are not fully competent to practice medicine, either because of inadequate medical skills, impairment caused by use of drugs or alcohol, or deficiencies resulting from mental illness."

In spite of this, the doctor-in-training said that he didn't know any woman from his upper-class neighborhood who wanted to be a nurse. The smart ones, he said, were trying to get into medical school. This young man acknowledged that Beth Israel's nurses were special — not, he said with a dismissive wave of the hand, like the rest of those anonymous nurses in all those other anonymous hospitals. Nonetheless, it seemed that for him Beth Israel nurses would never overcome the ultimate failing — they had not gone to medical school.

Given those widespread attitudes, it is inevitable that even at a hospital like the Beth Israel, nurses receive subtle lessons that reinforce the idea that they are inferior to doctors. These lessons in status are conveyed — either inadvertently or deliberately — in seating arrangements, body language, tone of voice, gesture, acknowledgment of effort, and lack of routine personal courtesy.

When I began observing nurses on Stoneman Four — the hospital's inpatient oncology unit — I was immediately struck by the implicit message of early morning rounds. Each day the three interns assigned to the unit sat in front of the picture window that formed the cancer ward's back wall. Leaning against the left wall, the resident faced the interns (two men and one woman) and asked them to present their cases. Behind him stood a semicircle of nurses, who were also supposed to participate in morning rounds.

But each morning, this huddle simultaneously included and excluded the nursing staff. The resident always kept his back to the nurses. He addressed the three interns, not the larger group. The nurses offered their insights about the condition of particular patients, but always from the outfield. The resident never shifted his position to look at the nurses who were speaking. Their comments were heard, but he never invited them to move into the inner circle and become full members of the group.

I watched this happen over and over again throughout the hospital. Jeannie Chaisson often confronts this subtle exclusion when she approaches a circle of doctors discussing a patient they have in common. Rather than moving out to expand the circle so that she can enter it, they often continue their discussion with each other and force her to stand outside, straining to catch the drift. Jeannie is not a woman who tolerates much nonsense or disrespect. She simply moves into the circle and the discussion.

But on Stoneman Four, day after day, the semicircular formation at morning rounds remained impermeable. I kept hoping that one or two of the nurses would just go up and sit down next to the interns, thus disrupting this daily pattern of exclusion and relegation to a secondary role. But during the weeks I was on the unit, the nurses abided by this "doctors only" seating arrangement.

Some feminists might have hoped that an influx of women into medicine would alter relationships between doctors and nurses. Female doctors, some perhaps thought, would evince more sisterly solidarity toward their female nursing colleagues. The fact that more women are in medicine today than ever before has not transformed traditional relationships between physicians and nurses — particularly at the doctor-in-training level. Female physicians and medical students are socialized into a system that does not foster collegiality between the two disciplines. The legacy of nursing as the female career in health care also exacerbates this tendency. Male doctors don't have to be concerned about being mistaken for a nurse when they enter a patient's room. Women do. Many female physicians who — understandably — want to be acknowledged for their education and skill complain that patients are constantly confusing them with nurses. And not all have learned to distinguish between themselves and their nursing colleagues in a way that doesn't denigrate the latter.

Recently, I was invited to speak at a conference sponsored by a nursing school and a female medical students association. When I arrived at the dinner after giving a speech to the two groups, several female medical students gathered round me. They knew I was a longtime feminist and were eager to discuss their trials and tribulations as women in medicine. One third-year student angrily complained that patients often mistook her for a nurse when she went in to examine them or take a history.

I asked her how she responded when someone mistook her for an RN. "Well, I tell them I'm not a nurse and I'm not a manicurist, either," she said defiantly.

My heart sank. "It's a shame you can't think of a way to distinguish yourself from nursing without putting nurses down," I suggested.

In many accounts, both in the media and in talking with individuals, female physicians often measure their success in elite terms — as how far they have moved away from nurses. Thus, some female surgeons complain vociferously because they feel it is demeaning when they are asked to share the same locker rooms as operating room nurses. One sign of their arrival in the higher ranks of medicine seems to be their own female-doctors-only locker room. Thus it is that women in medicine may reproduce the same gender-based hierarchies that have inhibited their own professional ambitions.

The tragedy is that disciplines that should recognize their interdependence and complementarity are pitted against each other. This creates higher and higher barriers that well-intentioned doctors and nurses who, in fact, want to work together, have a difficult time scaling. Today, for example, when some nurses try to distinguish their work from that of medicine, they may paint the missions of the two professions in stark blacks and whites. Nurses, they insist, are patient advocates. Nurses, they may say, care, while doctors cure.

This depiction often infuriates physicians. When nurses claim the role of patient advocate, many doctors feel that this is a direct repudiation of their own caregiving mission. "What does that make me, the patient's enemy?" retorts BI general surgeon Leon Goldman, who is a strong supporter of nursing. The dichotomy between caring and curing also serves to paint nurses right out of the health care picture. When nurses stake out caring as their exclusive territory, it obscures the fact that nurses — not just doctors — help patients to be cured.

This century-long antagonism makes building bridges between medicine and nursing an arduous endeavor. At Columbia University's College of Physicians and Surgeons, internist Rita Charon tried to bring medical and nursing students together for lectures and discussions about their professional roles and the health care functions that they share. "The attempt has failed every time. The professional suspicions already implanted in the young students and the deep hostilities no doubt cultivated by their teachers and the wider culture complicate what should be a normal part of professional maturing."

Similarly, when a nurse like Jeannie Chaisson offers her hand to doctors, she is often rebuffed. "The notion that doctors learn from nurses is not acknowledged in this system," Jeannie admits sadly. "But in fact, what physicians learn about symptom management, skin care, and functional issues — how patients get along on their own, what their lives are like, how they adjust to their illness — they learn from nurses.

"You often have to teach inexperienced doctors on a unit like this. When they're new in a field, it can be very frightening. We have very sick patients, with many failing systems. We don't always know what's going on, why they're doing so poorly, or which failing system is causing the problem. So we're sometimes crash-diving."

Because they have little hands-on experience and clinical judgment to rely on, many interns and residents may seek security in tests and technological fixes. "They want to generate a lot of numbers and lab values. They want to know blood pressure, potassium levels, and oxygen saturation levels, and check the pulse, and listen to the lungs so they have something solid to hold on to. The problem is that this is not a substitute for clinical assessment, for really going over what's happening."

What the doctor needs to do, she believes, is take a thorough history to find out what happened to the patient and how he or she looks right now. It's not good enough, Jeannie explains, to count how many respirations the patient is having a minute. The doctor needs to know how the person is actually breathing. Similarly, it's not enough to say that a patient is confused. Clinicians need to listen to what the patient is saying and pay attention to his or her perceptions.

"All of this," Jeannie says sympathetically, "is very hard and requires an ability to integrate information and knowledge at a level that some young doctors and nurses don't have yet. Because of this, doctors-in-training may do things that don't always have a clinical effect on the patient. But it makes the inexperienced doctor — or nurse — feel like they're doing something."

It takes a lot of work to help people understand what patients are going through, Jeannie comments. What makes this work even harder is the fact that many novice physicians and nurses have not had enough life experience to understand the kinds of things that are frightening to sick and vulnerable human beings.

"Most of the people you see here — particularly doctors-in-training — are very young," Jeannie explains. "They've been in school forever. They've probably had a fair amount of external control over their own lives. Few of them have been sick themselves or have dealt with the loss of a loved one. For them, the big issues have been academic ones — like getting into medical school and finding enough money to pay their tuition or loans."

"You can't offer a seminar on how to know what your patient is going through," Jeannie says. "What you as a nurse can offer them is your own experience and knowledge."

The two professions ought to work closely together, Jeannie voices her ideal, pooling their strengths so that practitioners utilize the correct procedures and medications, the correct symptom management and rehab methods, and anything else the patient requires. "This kind of collaboration allows you to treat the whole patient. So the patient is not only getting the right drugs to treat the infection, but is getting everything else they need to get better."

No matter what the obstacles are, Jeannie tries to refashion traditional nurse-physician relationships. But then Jeannie is used to bucking traditional ideas of authority in both medicine and nursing and has been doing just that ever since she entered nursing school. In fact, her path to nursing was as atypical as Nancy Rumplik's was traditional. Jeannie Chaisson was raised a Catholic, one of eleven children. She was the first girl after two boys, to be followed by two more boys, four more girls, and two other boys.

Her father is an engineer who runs a family-owned heating, ventilation, and air-conditioning company. Much to her grandparents' chagrin, Jeannie's mother dropped out of high school to marry her father. She had the children and then — when the youngest was in kindergarten — began to take courses so she could return to school. She passed her high school equivalency test, went on to college at the University of Massachusetts at Boston, and then to law school. "She was the only grandmother in her law school class," Jeannie exclaims proudly. Now she is an attorney in private practice in Auburndale, where she often handles appeals for people who have been denied disability benefits after an illness or accident. When she works on those cases, she frequently uses Jeannie as a consultant.

Jeannie grew up in the Auburndale section of Newton, about ten miles outside Boston. Behind her parents' red wooden house is the house her grandparents lived in. All through her childhood, Jeannie's extended family was only a walk across the garden away. As a teenager, when her grandparents became ill — her grandmother with a stroke that left her weak and demented for several years, her grandfather with cancer that killed him in a matter of months — she often helped her mother care for them.

Today, her parents still live in the same house and she and her husband live in her grandparents' home. Her father's brother lives in an apartment in Jeannie's basement. Jeannie's house was originally a summer cottage that overlooked the lake and a huge expanse of forest and meadow. Now, the stillness is gone. On a summer afternoon, when she's sitting in the comfortably cluttered living room telling me about her decision to become a nurse, we can hear the steady hum of traffic on Route 128 — the major artery that leads north to Maine and New Hampshire and south to Cape Cod, Rhode Island, and Connecticut. She gazes across the small family enclave and concludes, "We've been on this hill, in one place or another, since the turn of the century."

The house matches the temperament of its owner. Jeannie laughs when she describes all the renovation projects she and her husband have planned since they moved in fourteen years ago. But the couple has never had either the time or the money — and certainly not the inclination to devote their lives to getting it — to do all the renovations. So the house, with its comfortable disarray, is a long-term work in progress.

Unlike Nancy, Jeannie was not one of those nurses who recognized her calling at an early age. "I never wanted to be a nurse. Even in nursing school, I didn't want to be a nurse," she states candidly.

Like many members of her generation, Jeannie didn't go directly from high school to college. The summer after she graduated from high school, she worked in a sheltered workshop for the mentally retarded in Needham. Then, during what would have been her first year in college, she worked part-time at a bookstore and part-time in the Boston public schools as a school volunteer. "That," she remembers, "was tremendously depressing. We were supposed to be teaching English as a second language. But we had no expertise, no resources, and no help. The principal of the school was a one hundred percent angry Irish biddy. In fact, I later learned it was the school Jonathan Kozol had taught in and written about in *Death at an Early Age*. It's since been closed."

Jeannie soon resigned that position. "I had a big problem with allowing the system to pretend it was dealing with a problem when it wasn't. I didn't want to be part of that pretense."

Jeannie then enrolled at the University of Massachusetts at Boston and spent three-quarters of a year taking courses in anthropology, Chinese history, Russian, and French literature. But halfway through the spring semester, the U.S. mined Haiphong Harbor and the students went on strike. She was among them. Rather than return to school the next year, she went to Maine to live on a farm with some other acquaintances. For the next two years, she returned to Boston part of the time to earn enough money to continue living in Maine. It was her experience on the commune that led her to nursing. When one of her housemates became pregnant, the woman decided to have a home birth. In the traditionally staid medical community in Maine there were few childbirth options. A woman in labor went to the hospital and was sent into a twilight sleep until the baby was born. Meanwhile, the baby's father paced the floor in the visitors' lounge outside.

Through the burgeoning women's health movement, Jeannie and her friend found a midwife. The midwife delivered her friend's baby without any incident. But Jeannie decided that if she was going to have a baby herself, she would want a midwife who had more medical knowledge. In other words, a nurse midwife — which is exactly what Jeannie decided to be. Nurse midwifery, she felt, combined her political passions, intellectual interests, and her earlier experiences of caring for both younger siblings and ailing grandparents. Jeannie decided she would get a basic nursing degree and then a master's in midwifery.

For the basics, she went to Boston University (BU). At that time, BU had a well-known school of nursing, since closed — over faculty objections — by the university's controversial president, John Silber, and his trustees.

"Overall, I hated nursing school at BU," Jeannie recalls. She loved the courses in the standard arts and sciences curriculum but was troubled by the quality of teaching in the nursing school itself. "A couple of the instructors were good, but at the particular time I was there a lot of the instructors were even younger than I was. They had academic experience but really no on-the-job nursing experience. And it showed."

Outspoken and self-confident, Jeannie was the kind of student who challenged professional dogma and her instructors' sometimes disparaging attitudes toward patients.

For example, she remembers a course at BU in which the lecturer advised students to bring a section of newspaper along with their black bag of nursing paraphernalia on any home visit to a poor patient.

Why the newspaper?

"So that you could put your bag down on it and keep it clean when you went into their homes," Jeannie explains, shaking her head in disbelief at the memory. "I told her, 'I don't really see how it's going to be helpful to me as a student nurse to insult the people whose homes I'm going into. Do I wrap newspaper around the patient's arm before I put the cuff on?' I asked."

In those days, nursing instructors were also promoting a very formal definition of nurse-patient relationships. "One day I was working in the labor and delivery unit and was talking to a woman in labor. She actually asked if I had any children. By this time, I had had my first child, and I told the patient I'd also been through labor. She asked me what my labor was like. That's obviously what everybody wants to know — how bad it's going to be.

"So I told her that mine was actually very easy. Then I asked her how her labor was going."

When Jeannie told her instructor about this conversation, she was horrified. "Oh no!" the instructor exclaimed, "you should never give any personal information to a patient. Nursing is a professional relationship."

Jeannie did not agree and said so. "I told her that this is crazy. Obviously I wouldn't go on and on for three hours about my labor. But I do have a personal life. And there is a personal relationship between a nurse and patient. A real helping relationship can't be purely professional. There's got to be some sharing, and that's okay. My feeling is that as long as you don't dwell on me, but concentrate on her, you answer people's questions."

She lowers her voice and draws out the syllables as she repeats her instructor's response. "'Oh, no!' the instructor said. 'That's totally unprofessional.'"

Jeannie pauses in her nursing school recollections, sighs, and then sums up. "So, basically, there was just all this bullshit. I had a few excellent nursing instructors and a few who should not have been invited back for a repeat performance. But then," she allows with a chuckle, "some of my teachers probably felt the same about me."

When she was in nursing school, Jeannie had the first of her three children — Maddie. "That's short for Madeleine. That's Madeleine — M-A-D-E-L-E-I-N-E — like the famous church in Paris," she jokes. "Not Madeline — for the house in Paris that is covered with vines and has the twelve little girls in two straight lines." Bob Persons, whom Jeannie later married and who is the father of her two sons, Mark and Daniel, adopted Maddie soon after their marriage. "Maddie's birth father and I did not want to get married," she states with typical candor.

Although Jeannie didn't want to be with Maddie's father, she did want the child. "I'm totally pro-choice," she explains staunchly. "But my choice was not to have an abortion. I was twenty-four, almost twenty-five years old, and I figured I could manage a baby and I did."

Managing a baby, going to school, and working part-time was, however, an effort. Her tests, for example, were usually scheduled in three-hour blocks and were invariably slated for Fridays — the one day when she had no babysitter. With Maddie on her hip, she would arrive precisely an hour and fifteen minutes after the exam began. Mother and infant waited for someone to emerge early from the room. Jeannie would then ask this fellow student to watch Maddie while she took the test. "They were all multiple choice and I could do them in twenty minutes.

"I aced all of the tests," she recounts. "I'm good at tests," she says without a hint of boasting. "But," she adds, "I didn't get good grades in the clinical courses. The problem was that I would argue with them all the time."

During her final year in nursing school, she met Bob, her husband of fifteen years. He's a mechanical engineer who designs heating systems.

"One day, Bob was with a friend at work," Jeannie recounts with a smile. "I liked how he looked and I told his friend to bring him over for dinner. That's how I snagged him."

She finished nursing school in December 1979, when she was twenty-seven. "I didn't go to my graduation. I'm sure they probably invited me, but I didn't want to go," she says irreverently. "I don't have my diploma. It's probably in an office or a landfill somewhere."

Jeannie Chaisson was twenty-seven when she got her Bachelor of Science in Nursing degree. Her first job was at the Mount Auburn Hospital in Cambridge, where she worked for two and a half years. During this period, she abandoned the notion of becoming a nurse midwife. "I investigated getting a job in labor and delivery or postpartum care and decided I couldn't do it. I couldn't put up with obstetricians and deal with policies that were ridiculous."

She says she also recognized that she would not have been able to deal with women who did not take good care of themselves while they were pregnant. Indeed, impatience fills her voice when she talks about women who smoke, drink, or take drugs during a pregnancy. Jeannie knew that she would not be able to disguise those feelings of disapproval if she felt a woman was compromising the health of an unborn child. Besides, she says, she found working with the elderly more enjoyable. "I'd been doing that for a long time with my family members before I ever became a nurse, and I was good at it."

Her two years at Mount Auburn were an invaluable learning experience. As a new nurse, you learn, she says, what someone looks like when heart failure causes fluid to back up into the lungs; when a patient develops a high fever or is having a seizure. "What nurses do after this initial period," Jeannie explains, "is to develop the ability to put these individual episodes into the broader context of a patient's life."

Jeannie also learned to value patients and families. "We were very understaffed at the Mount Auburn. Things were very chaotic. But we had great patients. On the medical floor most patients were old Armenian, Greek, or Italian ladies. Their daughters-in-law, granddaughters, or daughters would come in and take care of them. These family caregivers knew we nurses were very busy. Instead of being resentful and demanding, they would help care for their family member. It was a lot of fun to see families and patients working together in that way."

Dealing with the nursing hierarchy in the hospital was not fun, however. "It was the old system with a 'charge nurse' running an assembly line of care," says Jeannie, describing the team nursing model. "The nursing role was splintered by task. Someone took all the vital signs. Someone did dressing changes or breathing exercises. The charge nurse was the overseer. It was her job to take all the doctors' orders and communicate with the physician. There were nurses there who were trying to institute primary nursing, but there was no institutional support for it."

It was this lack of institutional support that led her to leave Mount Auburn. Her decision about where to work next was deeply influenced by a personal crisis. Her husband, Bob, who was thirty-one, developed a serious case of rheumatoid arthritis. "It was hard for him. He was a young guy and he was very, very sore, and he was dealing with a disease that he knew would impact his whole life. The experience," she reflects, "was one very quick way to develop the empathy that can be so helpful in establishing relationships with patients."

Bob's condition was so bad that he couldn't even manipulate the pins for a diaper, which made it difficult for him to help care for the couple's two young children — Dan, the baby, and Maddie, who was five years old. Jeannie planned to stay home until her husband's medication began to alleviate his pain and disability and then return to work by the winter of 1982. But by late October of that year, she was pregnant again with her younger son, Mark, and horribly nauseous from morning sickness. When the nausea passed, she resumed interviewing for jobs at other hospitals. But prospective employers took one look at her protruding stomach and suddenly the jobs that were vacant before the interview had been mysteriously filled.

Her only alternative was to work in home care. Week after week, Jeannie would go into patients' homes, and assess their need for care. Finally, in 1983, when her son Mark was three months old, she got a job at a suburban hospital. In order to determine where she wanted to work within the hospital, she worked as a float nurse — a nurse who is not attached to any particular unit but who floats between units when needed. As she moved around the hospital, she was, however, disturbed by the quality of its nursing care.

"The general orientation of the nursing staff was 'Don't do it if it wasn't ordered by a doctor.' And if it was ordered by a doctor — even if it was inappropriate — they would do it," she recalls with disgust.

For example, one of the patients she was "floated" to care for was a woman who had developed a decubitus pressure ulcer — or bedsore — on her heel while she was in the hospital. It seemed that nobody had anticipated the obvious: that the skin over any bony protrusion continually pressing against the patient's bed — the heel of a foot, or the edge of a hip bone or pelvis — will begin to break down because of lack of blood flow until it ulcerates. It is, of course, the nurse's responsibility to recognize this common side effect of being bedridden.

"But, in this case," Jeannie remembers, "they just thought that their job was to follow physicians' orders. If the doctor had ordered the nurses to put sheepskin under the heels or to turn and position the patient more frequently, they would have done it. But they couldn't use their own knowledge to initiate basic nursing care."

Jeannie also found, much to her chagrin, that nurses were too quick to use restraints for their personal convenience. Restraints are only supposed to be used in extreme cases, when patients present a danger to themselves. For example, when someone might pull out an IV line necessary to his or her survival. Restraints, she pointed out to her coworkers, are not supposed to be used because a patient will pull off a catheter and pee in the bed, creating a mess for nurses to clean up.

Tired of swimming against the tide, Jeannie decided to look for work elsewhere. By that time, the Beth Israel Hospital was already developing its reputation as the Mecca for nursing in Boston. Jeannie had, in fact, spent a few months there during nursing school. She applied and interviewed with Karen Dick, nurse manager of a general medical unit.

Karen Dick still remembers that 1984 interview. Most of the other candidates she talked with were in their early twenties, just out of school and with a fairly traditional outlook. As Dick recalls, "These young women all seemed to have taken the same course in how to dress for an employment interview. They arrived in low-heeled pumps, well-tailored suits, and silk blouses. Each one had exactly the same string of pearls."

Jeannie was thirty-one, with several years of nursing experience. She was also the mother of three children and was herself most definitely a child of the sixties. She came to the interview wearing a pair of plain flat shoes, neatly pressed chinos, and a short-sleeved, all-cotton knit shirt, and she carried a fringed suede handbag. Dick was surprised, but not at all put off, by Jeannie's attire. In fact, she was intrigued. By that stage in her career, Karen Dick says, she had mastered the art of the interview. She could tell within ten minutes whether she liked a candidate or not. Always on the alert during an interview session, her staff had learned to recognize the subtle signals of a hiring decision. If Karen came out and gave the applicant a tour of the unit, there was a good chance the person would be offered a job. If Karen shook hands with her at the door and said she would be in touch, that was it. She had made her mind up — no.

Jeannie Chaisson got the tour.

After four years on the job, in 1987 Jeannie began studying for an advanced practice degree. When she enrolled at the University of Massachusetts at Worcester, she had two options — becoming a nurse practitioner or a clinical specialist (moving into nursing education or administration was too far removed from direct patient care to appeal to her). She chose the clinical specialist track because of her own firsthand experience of how such nursing specialists improved the quality of care at the Beth Israel. She also felt that this kind of education would allow her to address the kinds of systemic challenges she wanted to tackle. "I wanted to support and improve practice for a lot of practitioners. I felt that being a clinical specialist improves quality of care throughout the whole setting."

When Jeannie graduated, a nurse specialist position opened up on her unit and she got it.

The patients Jeannie likes to care for the most are those that many would consider to be the most difficult: elderly, sometimes demented patients who cannot voice their wishes, complaints, or needs. Several days after she cared for Mr. Wilson, she is trying to bathe and groom one of these "difficult" patients. Mrs. White* is demented — perennially confused and sometimes aggressive. On this particular day, Jeannie enters the old woman's room with a basin of water and a number of towels slung over her arm. From her bed, the old woman — gray hair disheveled, eyes wrathful — looks at Jeannie scathingly. As Jeannie steps closer, she spits out, "If you come near me with that, I'll scratch your eyes out."

Unruffled, Jeannie approaches the side of the bed. She smiles at Mrs. White and says, ' I know you don't want this bath, but we have to do it. So listen, let's make a deal. If you let me give you a bath today," she ventures, " I promise I won't try to comb your hair."

The old woman looks at her dubiously. But the rage of the cornered bull seems to fade from her eyes and she reflects. After a few moments, she gives in. "All right," she allows and Jeannie begins the bath.

Afterward, as we are walking down the corridor, Jeannie is far

more cheerful than one might expect her to be after such an encounter. She beams. "I just love patients like that," she says. I ask her
if she is being serious or sarcastic.

"No," she says emphatically. "I'm not being sarcastic at all. I just
love spunky old patients who still stick to their guns. It's such a challenge to try to figure out how to take care of them without hurting
them or compromising their autonomy."

"But," she adds, "you'll notice I gave her that bath really quickly so
she didn't have a chance to scratch my eyes out."

Chapter 4

A Special Visitor

ELLEN KITCHEN

In 1987, when he was eighty-three years old, Albert "Mac" McKay* left his apartment near Symphony Hall to do his weekly grocery shopping. A 190-pound, five-foot-ten-inch former bus driver, with florid skin and a bulbous nose, he had until that morning been suffering from the more minor ailments of the aged. A touch of arthritis in his knees bothered him occasionally, and he had an enlarged prostate. But none of this was troublesome enough to cause Mac to see a physician.

Mac took his time in the market, carefully checking the price of toilet paper, cereal, and frozen dinners before making his selections. He stood in line, paid his bill, and was only a block away from home when he suddenly collapsed. Mac was rushed to the Beth Israel Emergency Unit. The doctors discovered a benign tumor on his back. Pressure from the tumor on the spinal cord had caused his collapse.

The surgery to remove the tumor went well, but it was obvious that Mac would need follow-up. The Home Care Department was called and he was referred to one of its medical directors — John Jainchill. Ellen met him shortly thereafter and began to follow his case in the home.

Mac was a typical elderly postoperative home care patient. He now had complex medical problems, some confusion and memory loss, and great difficulty getting out and navigating the activities of daily living. "By the time I met him, he had a lot of cognitive problems and was functioning at about the age of a twelve-year-old. He needed a lot of help, not just with physical activity, but with basic problem-solving," Ellen recalls.

"The main reason people go to home care," Ellen explains, "is that it is difficult for them to get to the physician. They are essentially homebound. They need to be seen frequently and are able to stay at home because they have constant monitoring. If they are able to maintain their independence, it's only because they have someone to coordinate their many physical problems and emotional and social needs."

Ellen has been providing that kind of monitoring and coordination since her initial encounter with Mac. She has a vivid memory of her first visit with him. After studying his chart at the hospital, she rode her bicycle from the Beth Israel up Boylston Street and then turned right on Massachusetts Avenue toward Symphony Hall. To more-affluent Boston residents and out-of-town visitors, the area is best known for its cultural and architectural monuments — among them the rectangular brick building that is home to the city's major orchestra. Across the street, the world headquarters of the Christian Science Church takes up a full square block with a beautiful domed cathedral and long reflecting pool.

This neighborhood is, however, also home to a large number of poor and elderly Bostonians. Directly across from Symphony Hall, two white high-rises flank the south and northeast corners of Massachusetts Avenue. These apartment buildings are subsidized by the city and provide shelter for elderly people and those with disabilities. Behind Symphony Hall is Morville House, another building for the elderly, owned by the Episcopal City Missions. And then there are other — often shabbily maintained — apartments that line the warren of streets near the BSO's home. Mac lived in one of these, in an apartment four floors up without an elevator.

When she learned where he lived, Ellen immediately wondered how someone in his condition could now manage to haul himself up so many flights. Then she saw his apartment — several truly horrible rooms that reeked of age and neglect (Mac at the time had a dog). The dun-colored walls hadn't been painted in years. The plaster on the ceiling was pockmarked and crumbling. The carpet was thread-bare, the sink stained from countless unrepaired leaks.

The moment she walked in the door, Ellen understood her mission. The apartment needed a thorough cleaning. Its occupant clearly required assistance doing his laundry, cleaning, cooking, and shopping. He also needed help with bathing and dressing. His use of medications would need to be managed and follow-up visits with physicians arranged. All of this would be possible. But little would happen if Ellen was unable to win Mac's trust.

That was the hard part. Mac was a classic loner. Somewhere, far in his past, there had been a brief marriage followed by a precipitous divorce. He had one son whom he hadn't seen for decades, and a brother who had simply drifted out of Mac's life. Forging relationships and relying on other people had not been a big part of Mac's experience. Indeed, his adult life seemed to revolve around a series of relational close calls and escapes.

But Ellen Kitchen is exceptionally adept at penetrating the cracks in her patients' relational armor. "What you do is go slowly and try to show people that you're on their side" is how she describes her goal. Soon after Mac's first hospitalization, Ellen and her colleagues had a chance to do just that. "Mac had a fire in his apartment and was forced to move out of it," Ellen recounts. "We were then able to get him into a building with an elevator. So he saw that we were helpful to him because we found him a new and better place to live."

Gradually, Mac also accepted Ellen's offers to help bathe him. After he became used to the process, she arranged for a Beth Israel home health aide, Bea McIntyre, to come and take over that aspect of his care.

The home care staff's ministrations became even more invaluable later on when Mac had prostate surgery. Ellen visited him frequently in the hospital. When he got home, his wound needed to be kept clean, which would not have been possible without Bea's services. Equally important to Mac was Bea's help walking his dog when he was in the hospital and recovering at home. "Over time," says Ellen, "he realized that we really were here to help him, not to take over his life."

Over the next few years, Ellen continued to work with Mac as he developed other problems that required regular attention. He began having periods of confusion, what might have been transient ischemic attacks (TIAs), or warning signs of a stroke. A small clot or piece of atherosclerotic plaque breaks off from a bigger blood vessel — for example, the carotid artery in the neck — and lodges in a smaller blood vessel. This occlusion cuts off oxygen supply to the brain. In his case, Mac developed slurred speech and some difficulty walking and even more difficulty getting through the day.

Because of Mac's history of falls, the team could not prescribe Coumadin, a strong blood thinner that affects clotting. If Mac were taking Coumadin and fell, he would be at serious risk for a hemorrhage. He was put on one aspirin a day, which would serve as a milder blood thinner. And Ellen increased the services of his home health aide.

During one particularly severe winter, Mac slipped and fell while he was out grocery shopping. He didn't hurt himself seriously, but when Ellen next visited, she found an empty refrigerator and bare shelves in his kitchen. Ellen discovered that Mac was afraid to go out to replenish his dwindling stocks of food. Although he resisted the idea initially, Ellen was able to persuade him to get a homemaker, who would help with various chores. For several years, the homemaker's services were paid for by a state agency. But then, one day, an agency caseworker arrived at Mac's door to evaluate his condition. Because he was still able to get out by himself and was not totally housebound, the agency terminated his homemaker services. Ellen pleaded with them to reverse their decision. She explained that, although Mac was capable of going shopping, he really couldn't be relied upon to do all the chores of life unassisted. The agency would not reverse its decision, and Mac had to start paying $25 a week for homemaker services, which was, for him, a significant expense.

Mac still lives in the apartment Ellen helped him find. Since Ellen met him, his dog disappeared and he acquired a cat. He briefly befriended a student at Simmons College, Emily,* who lived in his building, but who later moved to California. He also bumped into an irascible old-timer — Harry* — who is ten years younger than Mac. He had known Mac years ago but lost touch with him. They discovered they live in the same neighborhood. When Harry realized how much Mac's health had deteriorated, they became friends again. "Harry comes over quite a bit now," Ellen comments. "He drives Mac crazy sometimes. But he's glad to have the company and stimulation."

Over the years, Ellen has tried unsuccessfully to get Mac to walk the short distance to Morville House, check out the bulletin board there, and take part in some of the many activities offered to seniors in the area. A self-proclaimed "eternal optimist," she won't stop encouraging him to get out more and do things with other people, even though she knows that a lifetime habit of social isolation is hard to change — especially when someone is old and sick. During a period of seven years, Ellen has visited Mac on a weekly and sometimes biweekly basis. He has become increasingly weak and more infirm with each year. He needs more and more help with every aspect of his daily life.

I first heard about Ellen Kitchen when I was at a conference for nurse executives in Florida. I was talking with Mary Brunell — at that time a nurse executive from Yale New Haven Hospital who had been a nursing administrator at the Beth Israel — about my longtime interest in covering nursing. "You're lucky," she said. "One of the best nurses I ever encountered is right there in Boston. You should do a story on her."

She proceeded to tell me about Ellen Kitchen, a geriatric nurse practitioner in Beth Israel's Home Care Department. "You should see her," Brunell prodded. "Each morning she leaves Brookline Avenue on her bicycle and bikes around Boston to see her patients."

It was the image of the bicycle that captured my attention. The image was so wonderful, so marvelously against the grain of everything associated with modern medicine — all the high-tech equipment, the screeching ambulances, and the doctors and nurses racing around in emergency rooms shouting frantic commands like "Type and cross four units of packed red cells stat." Instead she was offering me a nurse on a bicycle. In a major American city. In the 1990s. The offer was too good to resist. After the conference, I called Ellen and asked if I might observe her work. That inevitably led to her inclusion in this book.

Ellen is one of the "new nurses" much publicized of late. In the mid-nineties, both the media and organized nursing have advertised "advanced practice nurses" — like nurse practitioners (NPs), nurse midwives, certified registered nurse anesthetists, and clinical nurse specialists — as one solution to a serious component of America's health care crisis. The United States has become noted among industrialized nations for its dramatic imbalance between physicians in general practice and those in medical subspecialties such as orthopedics or oncology. Most nations have a fifty-fifty or even a forty-sixty split between generalists and specialists. Their systems focus more on primary and preventive health services and, as a result, they spend less on health care overall — with far better health care outcomes — than we do. Although this has recently begun to change, in the U.S. health care system about 70 percent of all physicians are specialists, while only 30 percent are engaged in primary care. As recently as 1993, only 15 percent of medical school students said they would choose to go into general or family practice after graduation.

Nursing has for years offered an alternative solution to the problem of primary care: nurse practitioners, they say, can provide such needed services. Nurse practitioners are trained to do routine primary and preventive care. That has always been their mission. Working in collaboration with physicians, getting a physician's advice when a problem goes beyond the scope of their expertise, they take care of patients in the home, in some hospitals, and in clinics. Nurse practitioners, moreover, have been particularly attuned to the needs of those patients that the medical establishment has long neglected — like rural populations, poor people, minorities, the homeless, high-risk mothers and their babies, and the elderly.

As a nurse practitioner, Ellen Kitchen is one of America's hundred thousand advanced practice nurses. These nurses work in several areas. About forty thousand are clinical nurse specialists like Jeannie Chaisson. Another five thousand are certified nurse midwives, who generally have eighteen months of graduate education beyond the baccalaureate. Nurse midwives provide prenatal and gynecological care, deliver babies at home, in hospitals, or in birthing centers, and care for mothers after they have had their babies. Advanced practice nurses also include certified registered nurse anesthetists (CRNAs), who were the forerunners of the advanced practice nursing specialists. CRNAs have two to three years of post–nursing school education and they administer more than 65 percent of all anesthesia given to patients in this country each year. They are often the only anesthetists working in 85 percent of rural hospitals.

Finally, there are about thirty thousand nurse practitioners (NPs) like Ellen Kitchen. These nurse practitioners are products of programs that generally offer a master's degree. Most specialize in a particular field. Thus there are pediatric NPs, adult, family, women's health NPs, and a growing number of geriatric nurse practitioners. They work in doctors' offices, nursing homes, hospitals, clinics, or in their own offices. They deal with a variety of basic and routine health problems and perform activities we have come to associate exclusively with physicians — such as evaluating patients, diagnosing their problems, prescribing medications, and suggesting treatment plans.

As the American Academy of Nurse Practitioners defines the profession, "Nurse practitioners are primary health care providers . . . they provide nursing and medical services to individuals, families, and groups. . . . Emphasis is placed on health promotion and disease prevention as well as diagnosis and management of acute and chronic diseases. Teaching and counseling individuals, families and groups are a major part of nurse practitioners' activities."

Nurse practitioners appeared on the health care scene in 1965. The original nurse practitioner model was developed by nurse Loretta Ford and physician Henry Silver at the University of Colorado. Ford and Silver were trying to fill the gap in access and ability to pay for primary health care for children and their families. Because so many physicians were in specialty practice and so few nonspecialists were willing to care for low-income and rural individuals, the time was ripe for nursing to move into what had been considered exclusively physician terrain. Ford and Silver were trying to educate nurses to work with physicians in their private offices, as well as in clinics in the inner city and rural areas.

The nurse practitioner movement was greatly enhanced by the social agitation of the late sixties and seventies. Health care activists in the patients' rights movements of that era — like those in the family physician movement — felt that every American should have access to basic health services. Since there were not enough physicians willing to help realize this goal for children and the poor, activists successfully sought resources to fund programs that would educate nurses to provide primary care services. The United States government's Public Health Service, some state agencies, and some private foundations such as R. W. Johnson, Kellogg, and Commonwealth made resources available to schools of public health as well as to nursing schools, and academic health centers.

Since nursing's fate has always been intimately connected to the position of women in society, this attempt to broaden nursing practice also gained energy from the women's movement. Many early nurse practitioners certainly rejected the traditional view of nurse as physician handmaiden and wanted even more autonomy from physicians than the initial Ford / Silver model of the NP gave them.

Congressional passage of Medicare and Medicaid in 1964 and 1965 also created a climate hospitable to nurse practitioners. As a result of this legislation, there was an enormous influx of patients flowing into the health care system. Someone had to care for them. Again, because of the scarcity of primary care physicians, in many instances that someone was a nurse practitioner. Initially, organized medicine fully supported this professional nursing development. During this brief period, some in the AMA encouraged those nurses who believed health care should serve a broad public. Since that time, however, organized medicine has tried to constrain the scope of practice of these nurses — limiting their ability to prescribe medications, refusing to share vital information with nurse practitioner colleagues, restricting access to hospitals, and insisting that nurse practitioners practice under the supervision of a physician.

In an excellent article entitled "Revisiting 'A Nurse for All Settings': The Nurse Practitioner Movement, 1965–1995," Barbara L. Brush and Elizabeth A. Capezuti discuss the considerable barriers physicians and their allies in state legislatures, the hospitals, and the insurance industry have raised to nurse practitioners. In the mid-eighties, insurers who had been selling malpractice insurance to NPs suddenly decided not to continue to provide them such coverage. When nurses protested, insurers reinstated coverage, but at prohibitive rates. To successfully regain affordable coverage, NP organizations argued that such insurance company denials constituted unfair restraint of trade.

Physicians have long fought to keep NPs from being reimbursed by private insurers, and every advance in reimbursement has involved costly and protracted battles. And physicians have opposed moves to give NPs caring for patients the ability to prescribe medication for those patients. State governments can choose to give prescriptive authority to NPs. The fact that some do and some don't has to do with the power of the physician lobby in a particular state — not with nurse practitioners' qualifications. "NPs working in areas with a limited supply of physicians or in areas unattractive to physicians have apparently been deemed more capable of prescribing medications. How is it, for example, that NPs in Oregon are more competent to independently write prescriptions than are NPs in Pennsylvania? . . . Why is prescriptive authority associated with NP practice in Arizona, but considered to be the domain of the physician in Oklahoma?" Brush and Capezuti ask, highlighting the almost ludicrous state-by-state discrepancies.

Defenders of nurse practitioners have countered these attacks by publicizing studies and analyses that document the high quality of the care delivered by nurse practitioners. Barbara J. Safriet, a non-nurse who is associate dean and lecturer on law at the Yale Law School, prepared a lengthy review of this material entitled "Health Care Dollars and Regulatory Sense: The Role of Advanced Practice Nursing." It cites the many research studies that affirm nurse practitioners' ability to give high-quality care and analyzes the barriers to practice these nurses constantly confront.

Safriet's article discusses the most far-reaching study of NP effectiveness done so far. It was issued by the U.S. government's Office of Technology Assessment in 1986. Called "Nurse Practitioners, Physician Assistants and Certified Nurse Mid-Wives: A Policy Analysis," the report concluded that "within their areas of competence, N.P.s and C.N.M.s provide care whose quality is equivalent to that of care provided by physicians." Safriet writes, "The OTA also reviewed 14 studies whose results demonstrated a *difference* in the quality of care provided by NPs and M.D.s. Of these, 12 showed that the relative quality of care given by NP's was *better* than that given by M.D.s." Several studies indicated that patients are more satisfied with NP than with MD care because of the amount of information conveyed, the reduction of professional mystique, and the costs of care.

Safriet concludes her article by citing survey results that explain why so many members of the public say they would actually prefer to go to a nurse practitioner rather than a physician. In 1991, Jerry Avorn and his colleagues at Harvard Medical School interviewed a random sample of 501 internists, family practitioners, and general practitioners as well as 298 nurse practitioners. Over the telephone, investigators asked each one to tell them what they would do in the following case.

"'A man you have never seen before comes to your office seeking help for intermittent sharp epigastric [stomach] pains that are relieved by meals but are worse on an empty stomach. The patient has just moved from out of state and brings along a report of an endoscopy performed a month ago showing diffuse gastritis of moderate severity, but no ulcer. Is there a particular therapy you would choose at this point, or would you need additional information?'"

Twice as many physicians as NPs would have initiated treatment without seeking that information. Sixty-three percent of the physicians would have reached for a prescription pad. Had they asked for additional information, they would have learned that medications currently used were two aspirin tablets four times daily for stomach pain; that the patient's son was killed in a car accident six weeks earlier, that he drank five cups of coffee per day, had only one large meal daily at lunch, smoked two packs of cigarettes per day and had two cocktails with lunch and two glasses of wine at night.

Eighty percent of the NPs sought this information — which is why most recommended a change in diet, counseling, and trying to deal with the patient's heavy use of aspirin, coffee, cigarettes, and alcohol.

The Avorn study concluded that "far more nurses than physicians elicited the basic historical information necessary to make an intelligent treatment plan for the patients presented." This, Safriet said, "has inescapable implications for both the quality of care and its cost." "Many have argued that the health care system must find a way to provide reimbursement for the time spent in history taking and patient counseling. While this is probably true, it is interesting to note that in this instance, nurse practitioners, who are reimbursed at a lower level, appear to have performed these tasks more completely," Avorn and his colleagues added.

On a Monday in May of 1993, when I go along with Ellen to see Mac, she parks her bicycle and walks across the street to Mac's brick apartment building. At the sound of the buzzer, Mac, who expects her visit, buzzes her in. The elevator takes us to the fifth floor, and we go down a barren corridor to a door that is ajar. Ellen walks directly into a cramped studio whose one room serves as living room, bedroom, and dining area.

A single bed hugs the left-hand wall; on a table next to it, there's a lamp with a badly stained shade and a clock radio. A tattered overstuffed chair occupies the corner of a bay window, alongside a small desk with a TV on top. To the right of the front door is a second-hand 1950s-style aluminum and Formica table with two chairs. Beyond it is an archway separating the main room and a long, narrow kitchen. To the left of the front door, Mac stores his cane, an umbrella, and a shopping cart. The bathroom and one closet are set back behind another doorway near the foot of his bed.

The apartment's drab cream-colored walls have few decorations. There is a poster of the basketball player Larry Bird in his Boston Celtics uniform. Above the table, Mac has hung a small American flag, a real estate calendar, and a red plastic wall clock. Taped to the front door is a sign Ellen has left that says Take Pills Every Morning.

Mac sits passively on the edge of his bed. His thick white hair is neatly combed and he wears bedroom slippers, a pair of old corduroy pants, and a loose-fitting flannel shirt over an undershirt.

Mac's face lights up when Ellen walks through the door. Before she can inquire about his health, he thrusts out his hand and presents her with his gift of the week, a shopping handout from Toys R Us. Perhaps she might find something in it for her three-year-old son, he says hopefully.

"Oh, thanks, Mac. I missed the Sunday *Globe* and I was going shopping with my son tomorrow," she says.

Then he hands her another newspaper clipping from one of his favorite commentators, Paul Harvey. Again, Ellen's gratitude is genuine. She knows how paltry Mac's resources are and that this gesture, like the other, is his attempt at reciprocity.

Without any further preliminaries, Mac then launches into a recitation of everything that's happened to him since she saw him last. He's been getting odd phone calls in the middle of the night. Sometimes two or three times a night. The calls wake him up and alarm him. His cat has also been jumping on his bed and interrupting his sleep. Though seemingly small, both problems have defied his attempts to find a solution to them.

"Do you have any idea who could be on the phone?" Ellen inquires.

"Nope."

"How long has this been going on?"

Since she saw him last.

"Well, you go to bed pretty early," Ellen reflects, suggesting that he just turn the phone off. "Whoever is calling will probably get frustrated and give up."

Mac hadn't thought of this and nods heartily. "It's a good plan," he agrees.

As for the cat, Ellen points out that Mac can put the large plywood board that's stored behind his bed in the doorway between the living room and bathroom to keep the cat confined at night. It won't hurt the cat, and he'd finally be able to get some sleep. Hearing this, Mac again seems greatly relieved.

Ellen asks if Mac has heard from Emily, the former Simmons student who was his neighbor and friend.

Yes, indeed, Mac reports with delight. He received a letter just the other day. He sighs and says, "I wish she'd come back."

"Yes," Ellen agrees. "She was a good friend."

Ellen then turns to the subject of Mac's health. First she wants to know if he has been getting out much.

Mac looks at her sheepishly. Not much, he says.

Why? Ellen asks.

At first he claims that it's because he's too tired.

Suspecting there is more to this than just fatigue — understandable in anyone over eighty and in his physical condition — she probes further. "Is that all?" she asks. "What about those accidents you were having? Are they still bothering you?" Blushing slightly, he confesses that when he goes out, he sometimes has a terrible urge to pee. No sooner has he turned the corner than he has to hurry back to the apartment to avoid having an embarrassing accident right there on the street.

Ellen is not surprised. This has been an ongoing problem and it has been hard for Mac to deal with. For the umpteenth time, but without a trace of impatience, Ellen reviews the situation for him.

"Because of your congestive heart failure, Mac, you have to take that water pill [diuretic] every day — remember, it's the one shaped like a football. Because your heart isn't pumping that well, your kidneys are also having trouble working, so this helps you get rid of any excess water. But if you take the pill before you go out, it will make you urinate when you're out for a walk."

Confused, Mac frowns and says, "You mean I should take it before I go out?"

"No, no," Ellen quickly counters. "It takes about four hours to get rid of the water pill. If you take the pill at ten in the morning, it's effect will be finished by two P.M. But if you take it at ten, and then go out at eleven, you'll have to pee. What time do you like to go for your walk, Mac?"

"Oh, about eleven," he replies. "I'm usually back by twelve or twelve-thirty."

"Then if you take your water pill at twelve or twelve-thirty, it will be much better," Ellen says. "Just don't take it at ten if you're going out right after. I keep going over and over this with you, Mac, because it's important for you to walk. It's good for your heart, and the more you do, the more you'll build up your endurance."

Once they've discussed his daily exercise, Ellen takes out her stethoscope and blood pressure cuff. She takes his blood pressure sitting and standing. "It's up a little bit since last week," she notes and then walks over to check a small plastic box on the desk next to the television. The box is a daily medication reminder. It is divided into a number of rows that she can mark so she can arrange a patient's pills in a way that helps him utilize them correctly. Ellen uses this device to lay out Mac's pills so that he can take them on schedule.

Like most elderly patients, Mac is on multiple medications. In his case, there's a daily vitamin pill, an aspirin once a day to thin his blood and prevent any more TIAs, and Lasix, the diuretic prescribed for his congestive heart failure. Many elderly patients can't remember the names of these pills, or even their purpose. Arranging them thus not only reduces their considerable confusion about which pill to take when, it also enables Ellen to determine if all the pills were used, and to ascertain if a patient is failing to maintain a medication regimen.

A quick glance at Mac's plastic box tells Ellen that Mac has indeed missed several blood pressure pills. She doesn't want to scold or embarrass her patient, but the issue of missed medicine is of grave concern to her.

"What happened, Mac?" she asks, turning from the kit to her patient. "It seems you miss medicine every couple of weeks. I just hate to see you miss it, because your blood pressure is so well controlled, and you've been doing a good job taking off weight."

She once again goes over the medication schedule. Then she scans Mac's body, palpates his ankles, runs through the rest of his personal medical checklist of major and minor aches and pains. In an impressive show of memory, she scans the list of his afflictions. How's the ankle that was bothering him? Did he have to take any Tylenol for his arthritis? What about his back, has it been acting up? Has he been troubled by the ringing in his ears that he complained about several weeks ago?

She goes into the bathroom to get Mac's scale to weigh him, and after noting his weight in the chart turns to his other needs. She notices the dirty linen on his bed and asks Mac to get up so that she can change it. Then she strips the bed, places the sheets in his laundry bag, and tells him to ask his homemaker to wash them when she comes next.

As she's about to make the bed, she realizes that the mattress is slightly soiled. "When did we flip this bed last?" she asks, as if to herself, and suggests that it be turned over again. The old man manages to lift a corner of the mattress and, together, the two of them turn it over. Then she makes the bed. Next comes the kitchen. Ellen whisks the dirty dishes off the table, quickly washes them, and looks in the cabinets and fridge to make sure Mac has enough food.

Hearing all the kitchen noise, Mac tells Ellen that his friend Harry has come by several times to cook dinner.

Great, Ellen says.

Finally, she checks the calendar to find out when Mac has his next scheduled appointment with his urologist. How will he get there, she wonders, by cab or public transportation? Cab, he says.

To make sure he can find the doctor's office once he gets to the hospital, Ellen calls to confirm Mac's appointment and get detailed directions for him.

"You register on the first floor, when you walk into the Kirstein Building. Then you go up to the fourth floor. We'll talk about what the doctor said when I see you next Thursday," she says, packing up her bag to leave.

Before she does, Mac thrusts another flyer, from CVS, into her hands.

"What's this about, Mac?" she asks.

"I want to give a razor to Emily. I saw this ad in the paper. But do you think it's all right? I asked Harry about it and he says girls don't use these."

Ellen carefully studies the ad. She smiles and hands it back to him.

"Oh no, Mac," she says, "that's not true. This is top of the line, the Cadillac of razors. I'm sure she'll love it."

"Home care," Ellen says, "means taking the time to get to know patients and their families so you can understand their medical and social history very well." It demands the patience and expertise of an experienced nurse who willingly enters the world that the patient — rather than the health care professional — inhabits. And it requires a willingness to engage enthusiastically with the most banal details and dilemmas of a patient's life as it is actually lived.

As Ellen practices it, home care involves relationship-building and detective work. It is essentially "case management" — but a far different kind from that so widely promoted by the owners and managers of today's market-driven health care institutions, who often turn "case managers" into "case messengers." In the business environment, case management is defined as analyzing the case histories of thousands of patients and arriving at statistical norms of illness that are then superimposed on each new individual case and clinician.

As determined by this process, an elderly male with congestive heart failure and diabetes might be entitled to only a few visits from a nurse, some from a home health aide, and some from a homemaker. Each visit, the nurse is then told, should take precisely twenty minutes, and, during that time, nurses should not be guided by their own experience and clinical judgment, but by road maps compiled by MBAs. No matter how much an individual patient may deviate from the statistical norm applied to his or her case, the square peg of case management must still be squeezed into the round hole of the patient's actual needs — with the result being less than satisfactory care. In the corporate model of case management, nurse practitioners are often asked to manage care from afar: they may never even deliver the care they manage. Rather, they supervise the direct care given by less-skilled, and thus less-costly, personnel or spend their time pushing other professionals — nutritionists, social workers, physical or occupational therapists — across the patient care chessboard.

To Ellen, managing her "cases" means something very different. It involves carefully studying each individual patient's living situation and understanding who the patients are and what care is appropriate for them. She delivers much of this care as well as coordinating all the help her patients are receiving so everyone works as a team on both medical and social problems.

"Elderly housebound patients are often confused or inarticulate about their problems," she points out. "But when you go into their homes, there it is in front of you. You can see exactly how they are responding to treatment and care. You can see if it is safe and then do things to make the environment safer. You'd be amazed," she exclaims, "what you learn by just walking into a bathroom, bedroom, or kitchen."

According to the American Academy of Home Care Physicians, on any one day in 1996, nurses make more visits to patients' homes than doctors did in the entire year of 1995. When Ellen goes into a patient's kitchen to wash the dishes or quickly scramble an egg, she is doing a lot more than simple housework. She is discovering if the house is clean, if it conceals health hazards, if the patient has enough clean linen and food, and if the food is the kind the patient should be eating. This kind of health care and personal safety detective work could easily be conducted like — and perceived as — a total assault on an individual's privacy and autonomy. No matter how needy, frail, or confused many of Ellen's elderly patients may be, they don't necessarily welcome with open arms the succession of well-intentioned helpers — nurses, social workers, home health aides, and homemakers — who come their way. For many elderly people, it's bad enough that they must spend so much of their final years in hospitals, pharmacies, and doctors' offices. To have the health care and social service systems invade their homes as well adds insult to injury. Ellen is acutely aware of this tension. "What I've found, for the most part, is that so-called 'difficult patients' are either terrified that you're going to place them in a nursing home or that you're going to come in and try to make tremendous changes in their lives. A lot of times, these patients are just trying to hang on to their independence."

Ellen recalls, for example, the trials of one nursing student she supervised who was supposed to care for an elderly woman who suffered from confusion and memory loss. The woman repeatedly forgot to take her hypertension medication, and her house was in terrible disarray that cried out for a homemaker's help. The young nurse went to Boston's South End three or four times to see her, struggling each time to find a parking space, only to be refused entry to the apartment. The woman would come to the door and say, "No, I'm not going to let you in."

Ellen herself recently had to cope with another troublesome case, a seventy-eight-year-old woman with emphysema who was angry about the fact that she was hospitalized to begin with (because she didn't believe she had the disease) and then felt she was discharged too soon. Forced to use oxygen at home and severely limited in her movements, she knew that she couldn't make it alone anymore and had to have people coming in to help. "On the other hand," recounts Ellen, "every time you were there to help, she launched into tirades. You just couldn't get around her anger. It was difficult to examine her, talk to her about her meds, and find out how she was doing. She just vented all the time. It was bad enough for me, but the poor aide was ready to jump out of a window."

Although Ellen has encountered many patients like this in her career, she views each one as a special challenge. Her approach is to go slowly. You enter patients' houses as a guest, she explains, not as a general imposing martial law. At first you make little suggestions that will change things for the better and produce immediate, perceptible benefits. Perhaps you order a commode for their bedroom, or a toilet seat extender, the installation of rails that help them safely enter or exit the bath, or someone to help them do their laundry. Gradually, she says, most patients come to appreciate the help and feel less threatened by it.

There are, of course, exceptions; people who say, "I'm sorry, I don't want this anymore." If patients are adamant in their refusal of home care services, the burden will inevitably fall on family members, if they have any. Patients who are isolated and alone will fend for themselves until their next medical emergency. "The longer you're a nurse," Ellen says, "the better understanding you have of human nature. So you do your best to get them to see that you're only trying to help. Sometimes, it just doesn't work."

Like Nancy and Jeannie, Ellen was raised as a Roman Catholic and comes from a large family. This is no coincidence. Although none of these three nurses went to Catholic nursing schools, a large percentage of the hospital schools in the forties and fifties and sixties were in Roman Catholic hospitals. Because nursing tends to faithfully reflect the upper-working-class and middle-class composition of the wider population, in the Northeast, with its large Catholic population, nursing continues to be a popular occupational choice for young, white, female Catholics. (Nationwide, nursing is still an overwhelmingly white profession, with only 8 percent minority representation.)

Although Ellen says she never intended to be a nurse, caregiving was obviously a part of her growing up. As the third of seven children — three girls and four boys — she helped care for her younger siblings. As a child whose grandparents lived nearby she was, like Jeannie Chaisson, used to being around, being cared for by, and finally helping to care for elderly relatives. For expert nurses, caregiving does not come "naturally" but is a skill they learned first in their families and communities, and later, in school and on the job. Ellen, like Nancy and Jeannie, initially learned about caregiving at home and then built on this foundation in nursing school and the professional work that followed it.

Despite her traditional upbringing, Ellen Kitchen's path toward nursing also reflected the modern woman's desire for greater independence. After finishing high school in the Long Island suburbs of New York City, where she grew up, she briefly attended community college but quit when she was nineteen. She took several odd jobs on Long Island. She then followed a boyfriend to Boston. After they broke up, she recalls becoming homesick in Boston. She returned to Long Island, took a waitressing job, worked as a secretary, and then decided to go back to Boston two years later. During her second stint in Massachusetts, she decided to take a few college courses at what was then Boston State College, an institution that has since merged into the University of Massachusetts. She enjoyed biology and, in her spare time, served as a volunteer in a nursing home in her neighborhood.

It was a very posh place, she recalls, geared toward helping the elderly maintain their independence. Although most residents got out a lot, they were still frail and needed help from staff or volunteers like Ellen when they shaved, bathed, and went for walks. At that time Ellen also had a paying job at the Magic Pan — a crêperie on Boston's Newbury Street. She was still taking courses at Boston State, concentrating in the humanities — English, psychology, philosophy. But it was the experience in the nursing home that defined her future. "One of the nurses there was a young, vivacious recent graduate who was full of enthusiasm and ideas," she says of that first encounter.

The nurse's excitement was contagious. "What made me finally decide on nursing was working with older people. I always liked working with older people. I loved my grandparents. There were also a lot of older people that lived in the Back Bay section of Boston, where I was living. I wanted to have an impact on improving the quality of their lives."

At Boston State, she began to focus on the courses needed to gain entry to nursing school. As soon as she was able, she transferred to Boston University's School of Nursing.

Just before she graduated, a sympathetic professor urged Ellen not to specialize too quickly but to find a first job on a medical-surgical floor that would give her a solid grounding in the basics of nursing. Like Jeannie Chaisson, Ellen had been introduced to the Beth Israel during a rotation in nursing school. She had been assigned to a medical floor managed by Peg Reilly, who is now the Beth Israel's associate vice president of nursing. Having experienced firsthand the Beth Israel's commitment to nursing, she interviewed with Reilly.

Ellen found Reilly was very encouraging, to say the least. "I had finished nursing school in August, and I wanted to travel to Europe before I started work. I told Peg about this. Peg thought that was a terrific idea. She was unbelievable. She asked me when I wanted to start. 'When you get back and want to start work, just drop me a postcard,' she told me. I have never encountered anyone who was so flexible. It was a great way to start."

While she was working on the medical floor, Ellen finally decided to devote her career to geriatrics. Again, the mentor factor was critical to her decision. Both Peg Reilly and Mary Brunell — who was at that time a unit-based clinical specialist — encouraged Ellen to advance professionally and expand the borders of her knowledge. "They were very instrumental in encouraging me to take classes and go to workshops and work with the geriatric team at the hospital. So, with the support of these wonderful nurturing mentoring relationships, I spent a lot of time developing professionally.

"Mary and Peggy and [clinical nurse specialist] Marion Phipps were professional colleagues and personal friends," she continues. "They were doing a grant on function in the elderly and asked me if I wanted to help.

"I swore that I'd never go back to nursing school after undergraduate work. I worked all through school." Ellen laughs at her failed resolve. "Since I was taking all these courses, I decided it was ridiculous not to enroll in BU to get a master's degree."

When she entered graduate school, Ellen had no intention of going into home care. Although she liked working with elderly patients in the hospital, her undergraduate experience with home care was disappointing to her. During her initial stint in nursing school, she had done a rotation in the community. It was an experience in sheer frustration. Like a young litigator eager to leap into a case containing the most challenging legal technicalities, Ellen wanted to apply her newfound knowledge and skills to her patients. She wanted to go out and *do something*.

When she was assigned to see patients in a senior housing project in Roxbury, one of Boston's poorer, African American neighborhoods, she embraced the opportunity to apply her knowledge of complex medical and nursing problems like hypertension, diabetes, and chronic lung disease and to devise intricate care strategies for her patients. She would leave school loaded down with pamphlets about low-salt diets and managing hypertension that she planned to give to patients with cardiac problems, or brochures about nutrition and diet for her diabetic patients. What she encountered was an unexpected obstacle — her patients.

Instead of attending dutifully to her educational curricula, her patients' eyes would hurriedly glance at the materials, and then they would get down to what really mattered to them. "They would confess their fears about being alone," she recounts. "They would tell me what their daughter-in-law said to them when she came to call over the past weekend, or complain about how a son had forgotten to stop by for a visit. They didn't have anyone to talk to all day. I would come back the next week hoping that this time they would have looked at the written material and get down to *my* business, and all they would do was gab and gab and gab. The pamphlets had just collected dust, because for most of these people mine was in great part a social visit. And I would get incredibly frustrated," she says, laughing at her youthful illusions.

That's it, Ellen thought, I will never do home care. Absolutely, I will never do this.

By the time Ellen finished her nurse practitioner training, she had matured as a person and as a nurse. She had also benefited from the encouragement of another mentor — a home care instructor who had worked in the field for five or six years and was deeply committed to the kinds of chronically ill, housebound patients home care nurses care for. Ellen says it soon became clear to her that home care represents an extraordinary and little-appreciated challenge. "There is no one else going out there and caring for these patients but us."

Ellen also found that home care was a respite from some of the obstacles to the care of patients in the hospital created by growing insurance company interference in health care decisions. What she valued in home care was precisely what she felt she was losing in the hospital — the chance to develop relationships with patients. As a young nurse, she might have put the attainment of technical prowess above the development of relational skills. As an older and more experienced one, she discovered that her technical expertise allowed her to do what she found to be initially frustrating. "As I became more expert in my nursing skills, what I realized I liked about the practice was really working with the patients, talking with them, and getting to know them." She also valued giving patients the time they needed to recover from the immediate effects of a procedure or acute episode and to regain a sense of confidence in their bodies and their ability to cope before they went home.

In the early eighties, she could devote time to her patients — time to reach beyond their illnesses and into their lives. But then, in 1983, Diagnostic Related Groups (DRGs) appeared, and that time became a luxury. Patients' complaints were categorized according to statistical averages, and length of hospital stay was dictated by insurers and seemed to decrease year by year. With DRGs, the race was on to get people out the door. "Toward the end of my work in the hospital, patients got discharged if they were ambulatory and relatively continent and relatively safe. That's it, they went home."

This was not only hard on patients, but difficult for nurses. "As a nurse, your time got really contracted. You were trying to teach people things and get people ready functionally a lot faster. And it was not always possible to do the teaching and caring that needed to get done."

In this climate home care became far more appealing. "By the time I left the inpatient setting, insurance companies were forcing us to discharge patients so quickly, with so many problems, that I became frustrated at having to subordinate nursing decisions to insurance company mandates." In home care, she points out, you have far more autonomy and more time to get to know, work with, and educate patients.

Far from being a professional backwater, home care had turned into a haven for nurses who wanted to practice and care for patients free from the kind of interference they often faced in the hospital.

For those patients who are able to make full use of the benefits of home care, Ellen becomes the hub of the wheel around which all the patient's other services revolve. She typically sees six patients in an eight-hour day; when she works a ten-hour shift, her caseload may include as many as eight. If patients are stable, like Mac, or Mr. Cousins, a patient with prostate cancer, she will probably visit them once a week. If they have a more serious problem, or have just returned from the hospital, she may see them daily or even twice a day. One of her patients, for example, had a huge abdominal wound that needed to be dressed. Ellen attended to her on a daily basis for a year. When Mrs. Gloria Beauchamp,* one of Ellen's oldest and dearest patients, developed an ulcer on her toe, she dressed it once a day, then every other day, and then every three days.

Ellen generally sets aside at least an hour for each patient. After seeing Mac, for instance, she may walk across the street for a routine check on Mr. Cousins and then around the corner to see Mrs. Henry* and Mr. James.* One of her colleagues may ask her to check on a patient of hers. Then she may bicycle to Brookline to see Mrs. Beauchamp, and she may finish the day with one of her most challenging patients, eighty-eight-year-old Mr. Fitch.*

On any given day, Ellen runs the gamut of the experience of aging in America — with every possible ethnic, class, and racial variation. Mrs. Henry, for example, is an enormous, cheerful black woman who has had serious angina. She has been plagued by severe chest pain but has improved dramatically since Christmas. Although she is fiercely independent and tries to get out as much as possible, her weight makes it difficult for her to get to the doctor's office for the extensive monitoring and follow-up care her heart problems require. Like Mr. Cousins, she lives alone, and her appearance and apartment are neat as a pin.

Only two floors down, in the same building, Ellen enters a different world when she helps out a colleague by visiting a patient who is not part of her caseload. The woman needs to have a blood sample taken, and Ellen's colleague was not able to see her in time to do it. So Ellen fills in. The patient in question turns out to be a heavy-set African American woman in her late fifties who lives with and is responsible for her own daughter and her daughter's three young children. In the squalid living room, the wood floor is scored with ugly black slashes. A faded gray carpet barely conceals the deep marks. The patient sits on a torn fake-leather chair, and a cockroach roams freely across the battered coffee table on which her feet rest.

As the woman stretches out her arm for the needle stick, one of her grandchildren scrambles across the living room floor.

Mr. James is another variation on the theme of race and poverty. A former alcoholic, he has just come back from the hospital after having had major surgery on a dissecting aneurysm. He has many complex social and physical problems that need a great deal attention.

"The reason I'm following up on Mr. James," Ellen explains, "is that he was seen over the weekend, and I'm concerned about his hydration and nutrition. I want to draw labs on him, check his vital signs, both sitting and standing, to see if he's still dropping his pressure precipitously."

She's also worried about his smoking. Only a few days out of the hospital, he's already back to ten cigarettes a day. And then there is his financial situation. Although he's reluctant to confide such embarrassing matters to his white, middle-class nurse, he has told his homemaker that his son cleaned out his bank account the last time he came for a visit. If this can be confirmed, Ellen will talk to his social worker about finding a way to prevent further financial abuse of the old man — a not uncommon problem in some families, no matter what their income level or race.

After stopping at a local bagel shop for lunch, Ellen gets back on her bike for the fifteen-minute trek to Brookline to see Mrs. Gloria Beauchamp, whom she calls "Mrs. B." Mrs. B.'s apartment is located in a well-tended low brick building on a pleasant tree-lined street. Ellen hitches her bike to a tree and walks up the two floors to the apartment. The door is open, and as Ellen enters a wide central hall, Mrs. B.'s two small white poodles yelp at her feet. Mrs. B. found her cherished pets at an animal shelter. Their previous owner never walked them, and they became accustomed to relieving themselves on papers indoors. Although someone now walks the dogs, they've never been completely broken of their former habit. The hallway is thus covered with newspapers intended to catch their mistakes. Familiar with this system, Ellen immediately spots a wet section of paper, scoops it up, walks back into the kitchen, and deposits it in the garbage. Then she finds another piece of newspaper and re-covers the wood floor and Oriental carpet.

Her ninety-two-year-old patient is perched in a comfortable armchair. Mrs. B. seems remarkably trim for a woman of her age. She greets Ellen with a broad smile and stands up briefly to display a bright-red-and-white dotted sundress that her homemaker sewed for her. Mrs. B.'s home could not be more different than the apartments of the elderly patients Ellen visited earlier in the day. She has lived in this sunny, spacious two-bedroom apartment for thirty-seven years. Its walls and hallways are a museum of mementos. Old photographs of a trim, twirling dancer swathed in satin or gauze, draped Ginger Rogers–like over the arm of a tuxedoed partner, adorn her living room walls. Dance trophies sit on window ledges and fill the mantel above the fireplace.

Mrs. Beauchamp was an amateur painter of some ability. Soft watercolors of flowers and sunscapes fill every other available wall space. The living room and dining room are crowded with lovely old oak furniture — small armchairs and rockers whose worn backs and arms are concealed under brightly colored shawls or lace doilies. The tops of tables are cluttered with dainty Dresden figurines and other assorted bric-a-brac.

The gracious old woman, who has been Ellen's patient for four years, had a stroke ten years ago and now has difficulty making herself understood. But Ellen is as comfortable translating her slurred speech as she is keeping track of her myriad physical complaints — arthritis, congestive heart failure, peripheral vascular disease, and dental problems. Ellen sits nimbly on the edge of a small Eastlake chair with a scalloped wooden border and asks Mrs. B. about the arthritis in her knee. "Oh, honey, this morning I could barely move," she drawls as she tucks a stray hair into the bun at the base of her neck. "I had so much trouble sleeping last night."

"Are you thinking about anything?" Ellen asks.

Mrs. B. smiles knowingly. "About old times."

"Good times, I hope. I know you like to doze in the afternoon. But don't sleep for more than an hour, or you won't be able to sleep at night," Ellen advises.

Next Ellen inquires about the woman's friends, her homemaker, and her homemaker's son, who's had his own health problems. Her son was knocked down and injured at school and has had a hard time recovering. Ellen knows that if the homemaker can't resolve her own family health problems, she won't be able to take care of Mrs. B. Situations like these arise frequently, and Ellen is often involved in sorting out the personal difficulties of a patient's other caregivers. In this case, she learns that the child is fortunately on the mend and such intervention won't be necessary.

When Ellen asks about her other health problems, Mrs. B. lets out a cheerful guffaw. "Honey, I'm just falling to pieces — piece by piece."

To emphasize the extent of her afflictions, the old woman raises her legs and points her toes. The slender and muscular limbs are covered with protruding veins. Her toes are gnarled. One toe has an intractable ulcer. "It keeps looking like it will heal, and then it doesn't, but we've managed to keep it from getting infected," Ellen says.

Tenderly, she removes the woman's stocking and bathes her foot. As Mrs. B. submits to these ministrations, one of her poodles jumps into her lap. The old woman cradles the dog and coos softly in its ear. "She's thirteen years old," she tells Ellen as she draws her long, elegant — albeit crooked — fingers through its coat. "I'm worried about her. She has terrible feet, they're almost as bad as mine."

After Ellen wipes and rebandages the ulcer, she examines Mrs. B.'s medicine box. "Have the pink pills helped the cramping in your legs that you were complaining about?" she asks.

Ellen takes the woman's blood pressure, listens to her heart, and compliments Mrs. B. for all the progress she has made since her last hospitalization four years ago for congestive heart failure.

But Mrs. B. complains about difficulty eating. Ellen asks her to describe the symptoms. The old woman opens and closes her mouth repeatedly. "Each time I chew, I bite myself," she says. Ellen reaches into her backpack, removes a small flashlight, and peers into her patient's mouth to see if there are any sores. She can't find anything noticeably wrong and advises a visit to the dentist anyway, which she immediately calls to arrange, along with the necessary transportation.

As the two continue talking, Mrs. B. reminisces about better days. "Imagine," she says in her difficult-to-decipher slur, "I used to teach square dancing and dancing to people with cerebral palsy. I used to take the dogs out two or three times a day and painted and danced all night, and now I can barely walk around."

It's so ironic, she mutters, even the people who used to take care of her are gone. "There was that doctor, you remember, Ellen." She turns to her nurse for help.

"Yes," Ellen says. "His son died while he was quite young, and he was so upset he stopped practicing and Mrs. B. had to switch to see Dr. Zagarella [co–medical director of Home Care]."

"Sometimes it's hard, Ellen dear," she says matter-of-factly. "Nearly all my friends are gone."

Ellen squats at her side, one hand resting gently on the old woman's arm. "I don't know why the Lord is keeping me here. He must have some reason," Mrs. B. says, looking down at the younger woman with a wry smile.

The many physicians Ellen Kitchen has worked with have come to understand the benefits nurse practitioners can bring their patients. Sadly, however, organized medicine has been unable to make this conceptual and professional leap. It remains wedded to its prejudices about nurses in general and nurse practitioners in particular.

In the spring of 1994, at the height of the debate about government-initiated health care reform, the political arm of the state medical societies in Florida, California, and Texas — all affiliates of the AMA — sent out a fund-raising brochure that reportedly raised $9 million in six weeks. "Don't Let Reform Fowl Up Health Care," the brochure warned in bold letters next to a picture of geese taking flight. According to the text, "flocks of non-physician practitioner groups" were "using the call for health care reform as a decoy to lower licensing requirements and broaden their scopes of practice." The doctors' mailing claimed that making any changes in licensing requirements and expanding autonomy for "providers who did not attend medical school is a serious and dangerous threat to the health of the United States."

What prompted this thinly veiled attack on nursing was the fact that two major health reform proposals that year — the Clinton administration's managed competition plan and the Wellstone-McDermott single-payer bill — sought to expand the functions of advanced practice nurses. Drafters of this legislation were responding to polls in which ordinary Americans said that they viewed nurses as more trustworthy and far less self-interested than physicians.

A survey conducted by the Clinton administration, for example, found that encouraging patients to see a nurse practitioner instead of a physician was one of the health care cost-containment measures most widely supported among the general public. Removing legal barriers to advanced practice nurses' ability to serve the American public would allow nurses greater prescription-writing authority and more control over their own licensing requirements and encourage physicians to collaborate more productively with their nurse practitioner colleagues in patient care decisions.

The alarmist response of the state medical associations cited above was designed to rally physician opposition to these reforms. The AMA quickly followed this attack with a less sensationalistic report of its own on what are called "non-physician providers" that it distributed to the media, Congress, and state legislators. The bottom line was the same: physicians should oppose efforts to expand the scope of practice of nurse practitioners. And, even after the Clinton health reform proposal had clearly stalled and died in Congress, the AMA, at its 1995 convention, reaffirmed its opposition to giving advanced practice nurses a broader role and voice in health care.

Those physicians who work closely with nurses and who have discovered the benefits of such collaboration are dismayed and distressed by the organization's persistent efforts to drive a wedge between the two professions. They know that physicians cannot serve their patients as isolated individuals; that the health and well-being of patients hinges on the quality of the collaborative relationships between two professions, which are intrinsically interdependent.

As Geraldine Zagarella, co–medical director of the Home Care Department, states: "A better working relationship among all health care professionals will result inevitably in better patient care. Any attempt to destroy such relationships weakens our health care system."

"If the AMA asked the majority of physicians who work closely with nurse practitioners how they feel, I think they would find them very supportive of this nursing role," Ellen comments. "Nurse practitioners deal with the episodic illnesses patients have in a way that saves patients problems and also saves money. Things get much better managed."

The idea — voiced by some physicians — that nurse practitioners are dissatisfied women who are trying to find a back door into medicine is, to Ellen, ludicrous. "This is a total misperception of the nursing role," she says. "Obviously, there is some medical management in what we do. But what many physicians don't understand is the science of nursing. They don't understand all the teaching we do, how we help patients alter their lifestyle, and, particularly in the home, how we help people organize their lives so they can maintain their independence.

"If people haven't worked with nurse practitioners," she concludes sadly, "they won't understand the whole gamut of things we do."

What nurse practitioners do, Ellen explains to me as we walk out of Mrs. B.'s apartment, is erase the invidious dichotomy so often drawn today between the "medical problem" lodged in the patient's body and the so-called "social problem" divorced from the physical complaint and conveniently abstracted from payer or provider responsibility.

How can we separate the two, she wonders? If a patient can't sleep because she can't get into bed; if a person doesn't bathe because he can't afford to have rails installed in the tub; if she develops a urinary tract infection because she doesn't know how to access a device to raise her toilet seat — all of this, Ellen knows from vast experience, will soon impact people's health — perhaps seriously — and by extension escalate costs in our health care system. Bridging those two worlds, she insists, is what health care should be all about. "And why would the AMA want to oppose that?" she asks.

Chapter 5

The Meaning of Illness

NANCY RUMPLIK

When Nancy Rumplik first heard about the spousal abuse, she was not surprised. Deborah Celli, her breast cancer patient who had survived Hodgkins' disease in her teens, was used to being a victim. Just as she was reaching adulthood, she was given what she thought would be a terminal sentence. She recovered, but the worry never really ended and seemed to become an inalterable fact of her life. "I want to know it's not going to happen again," she once begged Nancy. "If someone could only promise it won't happen again, but I know they can't. I dreaded this. I swore I'd never go through it again. It makes me so scared. If it happened a second time, it could happen a third time."

After her first course of treatment for cancer, she went to a community college for a year. She dreamed of becoming a teacher. Although she did well in school, she ran out of money and quit. She then married, had two kids, and got cancer again. Luck was clearly not on her side. Her self-esteem had been badly battered over the years — by cancer, by her other setbacks, and now by her husband as well.

Over the course of her weekly chemo sessions, details of Deborah's troubled life emerged — first in tentative hints, then in clear, unambiguous accounts. Initial glimpses came in discussions about her self-doubt and about her children. How could she handle them? Was she a fit parent now that she was so sick? What would happen to them? Would they get sick, too?

In responses to such questions, Nancy tried to get a clearer picture of her daily life at home. How was she taking care of her two girls? Did she have help? Did they go to preschool? Was there respite care? The answer was an across-the-board no — no help, no preschool, no respite. The obvious next question was, what about her husband? What was he doing to help in all this?

At first Deborah was taciturn, uncomfortable talking about Richie, as she called him. She preferred to focus on the girls. How could she manage? she asked repeatedly. She was so tired each day. It was hard enough for her to drag herself out of bed just to go to the bathroom, wash, and force herself to eat and drink. And yet, she also had to care for two rambunctious preschoolers, aged one and five. It was a big enough job when she was healthy. Now that she was sick, it seemed overwhelming.

In one session, she broke down because she had hit one of her kids. "I just hit her on the side of the head, I didn't really hurt her," she moaned, guiltily. "It's so hard to control her. She keeps getting into things. She is so lively," she explained, pouring out the frustration that is common to every parent. "But I feel like I'm abusing her. I'm so afraid she's going to grow up insecure and thinking badly of herself."

Nancy asked if Deborah had ever gone to a parents' counseling group.

No, she replied, that had not occurred to her. In fact, she didn't know such groups existed. Nancy explained that she could call one of the social workers on the unit, Judy Bieber, who would help arrange it. Nancy left the room and, within only a few moments, reappeared with an elegantly dressed woman. Judy pulled up a chair and listened as Deborah and Nancy explained the problem. The solution, Judy suggested, was to get a team into the home to evaluate the kids and then get further assistance.

Turning to Deborah, Judy asked, "How would you feel about that?"

Deborah brightened visibly at the prospect of getting help and agreed instantly. "That would be so great," she said, as if unable to believe that such a gift were possible.

"I'll call right away," Judy promised. She left the room and returned a short time later to announce, "We've gotten the ball rolling."

With social work assistance, Deborah eventually enrolled her older child in a Head Start program, which allowed her to give more attention to the other girl.

Gradually, during the treatment sessions, as her life became more manageable and she felt less isolated, Deborah began to trust Nancy more and more. There seemed to be few people in her life who were on her side, but it became clear that her nurse and other caregivers were among them. This encouraged her to reveal more about her domestic problems — the biggest one being her husband.

It was not simply that he did not understand her illness and despair or that he quickly tired of her complaints about her nausea and fatigue. Or that he did little to help her cope with the girls. He was an active source of disruption and pain. Thus, one day she revealed that Richie had a drinking problem. On another she said, "Rich was arrested for drunk-driving the other day. That wasn't the first time. This time, he lost his license. I really know how to pick them, don't I?"

In yet another chemotherapy session, she described more bouts of drinking and shouting and told Nancy that her husband threw tantrums worse than those of his young children.

She soon admitted that the abuse was not just verbal. No wonder the girls were out of control, she confessed. Her husband was out of control, too. "He doesn't just shout and get drunk. He lashes out physically, at me, at the kids. He even once hit his own sister during a fight. Can you imagine that?" Deborah asked. "Hitting your own sister?"

After weeks of such discussions with Nancy, Deborah makes a desperate plea for help. Nancy is sitting in her office. It is a small, rectangular space painted teal blue and crammed with five desks for the five nurses who share it. Each has a telephone and a lockable shelf above, where they can store their purses and valuables. A bookshelf contains essential texts on nursing and oncology. Nancy is going over charts when the phone rings. As she sits listening, her normally placid expression shows distress and then outrage. She talks calmly to

Deborah, asking her not to make any swift decisions, to wait until she and Deborah's physician can talk about it, and then hangs up. She walks quickly out of the room and down the hall to Hester Hill's office.

"You won't believe what's happened," Nancy tells Hester. "Her husband isn't just hitting her anymore, he's pulling her hair out."

To anyone dealing with cancer patients, this form of abuse seems particularly cruel. Here is a woman fighting to save her life. That struggle is causing her to lose a fundamental part of her identity — her hair. Rather than helping Deborah cope with this side effect, her husband has joined the disease in attempting to strip her of all self-esteem.

To both women, this may portend much worse to come. Over the past summer, local newspaper headlines have reported a series of violent incidents in which husbands who used to batter their wives were now murdering them. Both the nurse and the social worker feel they must act immediately to prevent this worst-case scenario from materializing. "The good news is we'll cure her cancer, but the bad news is her husband will really hurt her," Nancy says to the slim social worker, whose black hair is peppered with gray and cut in a fashionable bob. Hill has spent her career counseling cancer patients, and she nods in agreement. Nancy also tells Hester that Deborah is so overwhelmed she is threatening to stop her treatment altogether.

Hester says she will try to come up with some options for Deborah. Throughout the day, Nancy does the same. At lunch, Nancy and her colleagues Paddy Connelly and Mary Whitley devote their entire lunch in the large, bustling BI cafeteria to a discussion of Deborah's latest revelation. Over the hour, several possibilities are considered. Perhaps Deborah should go with her children to a shelter. Perhaps Deborah should move in with her mother, who has been supportive during both her experiences with cancer.

Nancy also reports that Deborah says she is upset because she can't deal with her husband and children as well as the nausea from her chemotherapy. Nancy tells her colleagues that she wants to talk with the oncologist about giving Deborah Cytoxan by a different method to reduce the side effects of the treatment. Nancy explains to me later that if Deborah takes the Cytoxan intravenously, she'll be nauseated for twenty-four hours, but then the nausea will fade. With the pills, the nausea lingers for the entire fourteen-day cycle of oral medication.

By balking at her treatment, Deborah is clearly trying to draw attention to her nightmarish situation at home. That is a shrewd — albeit probably subconscious — move. She has been talking about spousal abuse in increasingly detailed terms. Her caregivers have tried to help her deal with her husband and family. But threatening to stop the treatment brings the issue to a head. A family problem her caregivers regarded as chronic, but perhaps less critical than her cancer, has now erupted into a medical emergency. In our health care system, medical emergencies take precedence over emotional ones.

Nancy knows that if Deborah is going to remain in treatment, her doctor, a dedicated clinician, must join their intervention in the ongoing saga of her home life. Although she has paged him several times, she is unable to locate the doctor until the late afternoon. As the clinic quiets down, she leaves the main treatment area and catches him in the corridor outside her office.

"Let's go over to my office," she suggests, explaining that she needs to talk with him about Deborah Celli. Once inside, the doctor slumps in a chair and stretches out his legs. As the late afternoon light deflects off the Formica-topped desks and bookshelves and is absorbed by the deep blues of the carpet and walls, he listens to Nancy's account. He winces and seems to blanch, drawing a hand across his face in pain, when she gets to the part about Deborah's husband pulling out her hair. He is jarred by the desperation so apparent in his patient's refusal to continue with part of her treatment.

Yet, he expresses his caring by focusing on efforts to deal with Deborah's cancer. Each time Nancy refers to Deborah's domestic troubles, he interrupts with questions, not about her emotional state, but about her treatment schedule.

"She says she can't handle the Cytoxan and cope with her kids," Nancy explains. Before she can continue, he interjects, "When did you say she had her last cycle? When is she due for another?"

He listens as Nancy mentions suggestions of temporary shelter for Deborah and her children. The nurse asks for his advice about enlisting Deborah's mother in their attempts to resolve this crisis. He agrees that her mother has been helpful in the past and then comments, "You know we can't change her life. These problems have been going on for so long. How many pills did you say she has taken?

"We can't change her life," he keeps insisting. "We have to keep her safe," he adds, and agrees that her mother should be consulted. But he does not voice the same kind of urgency in this conversation that Nancy, Hester, and the other nurses had displayed, and he continues to argue that this has been a long-standing dilemma.

They agree that Deborah should be given some immediate relief from her nausea. No more oral Cytoxan for a while. The doctor says he will call the patient to discuss this with her. But clearly the job of continuing to provide the kind of emotional support necessary for Deborah to complete her arduous treatment will largely be left to the nurse and social worker.

In yet another session, this division of labor is highlighted. Again, the doctor joins the patient and the nurse. He asks Deborah how she is doing now that she is back on the Cytoxan pills after her brief reprieve. Sheepishly she looks up at him, blushes, and confesses that she has skipped a pill or two. "But I'll make it up next week," she hastens to assure him.

Startled, the doctor says with great intensity. "No, you can't do that. You can't just skip pills and make it up later by taking more medication."

Clearly upset, he stops talking for a moment, collects himself, and then adds, "It really shakes me up that I come in here and just by accident find out you've blown off some pills. Have you done this before? Have you blown off any pills before?" he asks with grave concern.

Visibly affected by her physician's urgent tone, Deborah stammers that no, this is the first time, honestly, it's never happened before.

He shakes his head and frowns. "I want to believe you. But it really scares me. What if I hadn't asked and you hadn't taken the pills? Or worse, if you'd taken an extra week's worth and you screwed up all your white counts and they went down?"

He tells Deborah that he needs to put her on IV Cytoxan "so at least we'll know that we've gotten it into you. Then you can take the pills again the next cycle. I want you to stay well," he says, his voice full of emotion. "I don't want you to do anything foolish and then, if you're not well in a year, ask yourself, 'Did I hurt myself?'"

As the doctor speaks, Deborah's guilt and embarrassment seem to give way to an appreciation of his deep concern for her. But just as he stands up from the bed preparing to leave the room, he adds, "So I'm sentencing you to IV Cytoxan today."

Deborah pales. The doctor continues explaining the details of the treatment to Deborah. He then leaves with Nancy behind him.

When he is well away from the doorway, the doctor turns to Nancy and sighs. "It's a little disconcerting to learn this like that. I always assume my patients are highly motivated and take their pills. But who knows how many of them get thrown out." He again shakes his head in frustration and he walks away.

Nancy remains there thinking about the situation for a moment. Then she walks over to another colleague at the nurses' station to ask if she will switch her lunch hour with Nancy. "I have to stay and talk with a patient," she explains.

Walking back to Deborah's room, she stops and turns to me. "She's going to feel that she disappointed the doctor, the parent. She's going to feel she disappointed me. She walks around with enough guilt all the time for anyone." She says that she just can't leave Deborah with the feeling that she is being punished.

"We've got to talk this through, because what she did is understandable," she comments. "What these people go through is so difficult, and sometimes they just do things like this to maintain some control."

Nancy opens the door and sits down on a stool next to Deborah. Leaning close to her, she puts a hand on the woman's arm and asks gently, "Was it hard for you to tell him?"

Deborah looks shattered. "I didn't want him to be mad at me. When I got the prescription, I didn't get it filled right away. Then, when I wanted to get it filled, I didn't have any way to get to the pharmacy." She lowers her head in a characteristic gesture of shame.

"This isn't a punishment, you know," Nancy reminds her.

"Yes, it is," Deborah counters.

"It may feel that way. But the important thing is for us to support you so you can get through this. But you have to understand that if you took the pills the way you were going to, your counts would have bottomed out entirely. You would be in the hospital with an infection and really sick. You can't make up medication. That's the thing about chemo."

"I want to do it right," Deborah wails. "You know, I want to do it right. I don't want to be sick again," she insists.

"I know," Nancy says softly. "It's hard for you to look to the future when you feel so rotten you just want it to end. It doesn't escape us how hard it is for you to do this. It doesn't surprise us that you didn't take the pills. I don't blame you. It's an easy way to cope and fix it. But we have to look to the future and what's most important. Your long-term health is most important."

Deborah looks up at Nancy and smiles faintly. "You're so good to me, Nancy," she says. "I just wish I could take you home with me."

It is inevitable, when you talk about nursing, that comparisons are made with the work of physicians. Many have observed that doctors focus on diseases, while nurses focus on illness — what patients experience when they get sick.

Physicians, of course, try to help their patients cope with the experience of illness. But in our society, the practice of medicine has moved inexorably toward the disease-fighting model, with its concentration on the technology of research and cure. Everything in our health care system — from medical education to reimbursement mechanisms — so compellingly draws the doctor's attention to sick cells, organs, tissues, and limbs that some may forget the care of the soul.

Some physicians reproach the medical system for just this tendency to confront a patient's disease while hardly relating at all to the patient. Eric J. Cassell, M.D., clinical professor of public health at Cornell Medical School, observes in *The Nature of Suffering and the Goals of Medicine:* "The relief of suffering, it would appear, is considered one of the primary ends of medicine by patients and the general public, but not by the medical profession, judging by medical education and the responses of students and colleagues."

Arthur Kleinman, in his book *The Illness Narratives: Suffering, Healing and the Human Condition,* similarly analyzes medicine's failure to understand that "illness has psychological and social meanings." According to Kleinman, "one unintended outcome of the modern transformation of the medical care system is that it does just about everything to drive the practitioner's attention away from the experience of illness. The system therefore contributes importantly to the alienation of the chronically ill from their professional caregivers and paradoxically, to the relinquishment by the practitioner of that aspect of the healer's art that is most ancient, most powerful, and most existentially rewarding."

This is nowhere more evident than in the cancer ward. Cancer treatment can be one of the most technological and dehumanized areas of health care. Since 1971, when President Nixon signed the National Cancer Act and the nation "declared war on cancer," it has been almost impossible to escape military metaphors and the individual treatment modes they reflect. While people die after merely "having" heart disease or diabetes, obituaries of people who have died of cancer invariably depict them as having "battled against," "fought against," or "waged war against" cancer for a number of years. Popular media accounts and even more technical discussions of cancer research and "cures" are replete with references to "armies of invading cells," "mutinous cells" — as if cancer cells themselves had a conscious malevolent intent — and "cell-kill ratios." Even some critics of the cancer research establishment use the same terminology, claiming that its current priorities are causing us to "lose the war" against the disease.

Kirstein Three is one of the front lines in this "war." In the oncology clinic's waiting room, material advertizes the many advances in research and the programs available to cancer patients. Annual walks to raise money to fight cancer are announced. When I first visited the clinic, its bulletin board displayed an article by Paul Tsongas about his experience with cancer. This oft-told success story, involving a painful and expensive bone marrow transplant, has inspired many other cancer victims and mirrors the professional optimism of medicine's own leading "cancer-fighters." For his personal service in the "war against cancer," Tsongas became, for a time, a medical "medal of honor" winner.

But the public eventually learned that there was more to his story. As the former Massachusetts senator was running unsuccessfully for the Democratic nomination for President in 1992, it was revealed that he had a recurrence of cancer during his campaign, and had also failed to disclose a 1987 recurrence of the disease when he released information to the press about his medical condition. News of these setbacks did not, of course, change the dominant view of cancer; rather, it merely confirmed how difficult an "enemy" it is to "defeat."

In our "don't just sit there, do something" culture, when we get sick we are supposed to become characters in a heroic medical narrative that conceals the remorselessness of pathology, the intractable fact of human vulnerability, and the inevitable inadequacies of medicine. To many of the participants in the medical drama, aggressive treatment — even when it fails — represents a quasi-religious quest for immortality and meaning. As the medical sociologists Renee Fox and Judith Swazey have described it, the medical system is permeated with the idea that one must have the "courage to fail," that is, to pursue cure at all cost — even at the cost of an agonizing death for the patient.

This courage to fail is embraced not only by physicians, some nurses, and other medical professionals, but by patients and their families and friends. Family members, for example, often say they want "everything" done for their loved one — meaning all the advanced technology available. They do this not only because they believe this will help a loved one defeat illness and death, but because our society teaches us to equate the search for cure with the best care. Some relatives or friends feel that the only way they can demonstrate concern, affection, and caring for a patient is through the gift of high-tech treatment.

In many journalistic accounts of cancer fights, the patient's gruesome death — which may be as much a result of the treatment as of the disease itself — is imbued with greater meaning because it occurred in the course of "fighting back." Consider Madeline Marget's 1992 book *Life's Blood*. The subject of Marget's book is her own sister, whose demise, after a bone marrow transplant, was truly horrific. In spite of this fact, the author argues, "before the advent of modern chemotherapy, in all its gross imperfection, people with leukemia *always died* of it. If they were lucky, they had the companionship of decent people . . . and the solace of a spiritual life — assets still available to anyone who can find them — but their dying was physically ugly and unenlightening. They were not part of a continuum of cure . . . They were stricken: that was all."

"In bone marrow transplantation," Marget continues, "a terrible trade-off always exists. The person may be cured, but he may die. If he does, his dying is likely to be more painful and protracted than it would be with less aggressive treatment. If he lives, he may be left disabled, perhaps disastrously so." Marget goes on to affirm that no matter what their fate, these patients will have contributed to the advancement of science and that the mechanisms of disease "will be at least a little better known" because of their treatments. "Whatever bone marrow transplantation's inadequacies, however, it isn't necessarily a failure."

When hope is so firmly tied to cure, it becomes very difficult for health care professionals, patients, and families to abandon that pursuit under any circumstances. Doctors, patients, or their families idealize the quest for cure, and the consequences for patients are usually downplayed.

As I watched doctors in the clinic and on the floors, it almost appeared that some were engaged in a massive exercise in denial, as well as flight from the sad fact that more than 50 percent of all cancer patients will die of the disease.

Consider, for example, some typical medical language. One afternoon, I was standing in the cramped kitchen at the back of the clinic pouring myself a cup of coffee when a second-year fellow came in and stopped to chat. I asked him about his day, and he launched into a discussion of one of his patients. The man, he said, had been "free of cancer," but it had recurred after six months. I almost choked on my coffee. "Wait a minute," I interjected, "how could the patient be 'disease free' and the cancer 'just recur'? Obviously he wasn't disease free, was he?" I asked incredulously. The young man seemed surprised. Pondering my question, he replied, "Of course, he wasn't really 'disease free.' I guess we just use funny language, don't we?" He sipped the rest of his coffee and then went back to work.

In this case, there seemed nothing particularly amusing about the mystification this language produces in both patients and physicians. Imagine how stunned this patient would have been had he been told he was "disease free" and then learned he now had cancer again. Where did it come from? he would have wondered. Was it new? Old? How did it happen? he would have desperately asked his doctor.

Sometimes the avoidance implicit in medical jargon is simply outrageous. When discussing cases that are not going well, doctors in every area of the hospital talk about how their patient, not the treatment they propose, has "failed." In oncology, when a patient is given several cycles of highly toxic chemotherapy and the tumor does not shrink, it's often said that she's "failed X number of cycles of CMF." In an ICU, it may be said that "the patient failed a trial of multiple antiarrhythmics and died after a V-Fib arrest."

To say that a patient "failed" a therapy is to make a revealing statement. In what can be interpreted as a classic case of projection, practitioners may use this expression to allay feelings of guilt or failure when a treatment flops. Although doctors and nurses don't intentionally want to hurt their patients, with this turn of phrase, blame is conveniently shifted from the practitioner and placed squarely on the shoulders of the patient. The sick person is now responsible for the fact that he or she has not been cured, has not recovered, and may, in fact, be deteriorating. After all, to say that someone has "failed" suggests not merely that something has gone awry, but that the patient — the victim of illness — has actively participated in this outcome.

Nancy Rumplik objects strenuously to anything she perceives to be a put-down of her patients. Which is precisely how she views this metaphor. "This type of comment lays blame on the patient. It contributes to their feeling that it's their fault that they got sick, and now it's their fault if they don't get better. This places more stress and adds more guilt onto people who are already struggling for answers."

She pauses to clarify her thoughts and then continues. "I can't tell you how many patients — perhaps more than thirty or forty percent, especially if they're men — will make some comment like, 'If I just hadn't been so stressed, if I hadn't smoked, if I'd only exercised more, I wouldn't have gotten sick.' Our job is to tell them that no, it's not their fault. Our job is to make them feel better, not worse." When you say they've failed the therapy, Nancy says, you're not helping them, you're just adding to the burden of insecurity and vulnerability that is crushing them.

Nurses and doctors, Nancy insists, must always attend to patients' suffering. That is the essence of their job — to share a patient's dramatic, often overwhelming confrontation with illness. That is what her career is all about.

"I'll never forget as long as I live, when I was an LPN," Nancy recounts one afternoon before she rushes off to attend a class in her master's program in nursing administration and family nursing after work. "I was in school and one of our instructors said, 'You will hear things from patients that no one else will ever tell you in your life. They will tell you things that they wouldn't tell anyone else.'"

She pauses as if struck once again by the power of this statement. "It's really true. It's part of the privilege of being a nurse."

When I ask Nancy if she feels comfortable sharing some of those secrets, she replies, "Well, I had a patient once who told me something she'd never told anyone before she died." She hesitates. "I guess it's all right to tell you, because she's dead, although she made me promise I would never tell anyone. She told me that once when her daughter was away and left her grandson with her, she baptized him with water. She was Catholic and was afraid her grandson wouldn't go to heaven because her daughter refused to have him baptized.

"People often tell you these things to get rid of their guilt. Another patient I remember came in every three months with his wife, and I used to talk to her. She was taking care of her husband while he was dying of cancer, and she told me she hated him. She took care of him because she felt it was her duty."

Nancy does not receive these kinds of confidences passively. She actively solicits them by creating an atmosphere in which people can feel comfortable talking to her. Nancy sits with patients while delivering their chemotherapy and talks with them about issues that are both related and unrelated to their conditions. With a thirty-two-year-old woman suffering from terminal leukemia, she steers the conversation to how her children and husband are faring. She helps a fifty-year-old woman who has advanced metastatic breast cancer deal with the discovery that the tumor has now moved into her eyes. The woman reveals her terror of going blind and speaks with frustration of her visit to an eye specialist, who unfortunately seemed himself blind to her concerns.

"How was your weekend at the Cape?" Nancy asks a man with Kaposi's sarcoma and listens intently to the reply. Had her kids been home for Thanksgiving she queries a sixty-eight-year-old woman with lung cancer and spends another fifteen minutes on a recitation of the family meal. "Where did you find that wonderful turban?" she exclaims to a woman with breast cancer, and again, the search for just the right disguise for baldness seems to fascinate her.

As casual as these exchanges appear, they enable Nancy to establish the kind of rapport and connection with patients necessary to uncover problems that patients will not readily acknowledge or reveal. Nancy knows that you can't get the facts if you don't know how to interpret the patient's responses and probe into them. For example, you can give a patient a questionnaire to fill out. One question might be, "Do you have help with the shopping?" The patient might answer, "Yes. My son helps me." The nurse might think, Oh great, there's no problem here. But in a face-to-face conversation, the patient's hesitancy in answering a question or his body language might convey hints that he really has difficulty getting his son to do his shopping. The son may do it only occasionally. He may have to call his son six or seven times in order to get the young man to go to the market. That's why you have to talk to patients in person. You can't just ask them to fill out pieces of paper and expect to learn anything definitive about their lives.

By her attentiveness to the mundane aspects of a patient's daily existence outside the hospital, Nancy also confirms that patients have lives whose meaning is not completely altered by disease. When Nancy engages in what some would consider trivial chitchat, she is actually helping to create a semblance of normalcy in the extremely alien and abnormal environment of the modern hospital. Hospitals today have become the quintessential "total institution" described by sociologist Erving Goffman in his work *Asylums*. Goffman defined these "total institutions" as "part residential community, part formal organization." They are, he said, "forcing houses for changing persons; each is a natural experiment on what can be done to the self." In hospitals, sick patients are confronted with the prospect of losing not only their lives, but their identities as well.

Nancy reassures her patients that they can survive the experience of hospitalization and illness; they can find in this foreign land someone who speaks their language and tries to understand the culture they came from, who will act as their guide and companion.

Nancy's guidance is not just a pleasant luxury. Without Nancy Rumplik and their other nurses, patients would not be able to survive some of the most arduous medical treatments, such as bone marrow transplants.

Take Carol Benoit.* While Deborah Celli is dejected and often depressed — so overburdened that she seems to live life in slow motion — Carol is a cascade of loud, splattering eruptions.

Married, with three young children, Carol has had Hodgkin's disease with involvement of her liver since she was in her early thirties. She had chemotherapy but did not respond well to it. During her initial treatments, a Hickman catheter was inserted into a vein in her chest. Such devices are used for the administration of chemotherapy that cannot be delivered directly into the smaller veins of the arm. This becomes necessary when repeated chemotherapy and blood sampling have hardened the peripheral veins and made them inaccessible. Thus, via a surgical procedure, a small tube is placed into a large central vein — usually in the neck or shoulder. The tube protrudes from the point of insertion and allows blood to be drawn or drugs to be administered directly into the large venous system. The patient has to flush the line out daily to keep it clean and prevent infection. Even if that is carefully done, the line may become infected. During her treatment, Carol contracted an infection in her Hickman. It had to be removed and another inserted.

Nancy and her oncologist, Steve Come, cared for her through all this. But in spite of their efforts, the cancer resisted remission. The physician felt Carol's only hope was a bone marrow transplant. After months of hesitation and debate, Carol agreed.

A bone marrow transplant is perhaps one of the most difficult procedures imaginable. Unlike kidney or heart transplants, most bone marrow transplants aren't really transplants in the conventional sense. They are bone marrow rescues. These procedures are performed when other chemotherapeutic protocols have been unsuccessful over either the long or short term.

The excruciating "transplant" process has a number of steps and stages. After leaving her children with her husband, Carol entered the hospital. First she went down to surgery and was put to sleep. Over the course of one to two hours, one of the attending physicians on the Beth Israel / Dana-Farber Cancer Institute transplant team pushed a large needle into both sides of her pelvic bone in ten to fifteen different spots. A syringe was attached to the needle and with each pull about 20 to 25 cc of blood — about five tablespoons — with its blood cell–producing marrow was drawn out. Once cleaned of any extraneous noncellular material, such as little pieces of bone, and with a preservative added, the blood was frozen and sealed in plastic bags and saved to be infused back into the patient.

Carol then went home and a week later was readmitted to the hospital. She was sequestered in a special room reserved for transplant patients on Stoneman Four, where she spent the next three weeks. There she endured high-dose chemotherapy. The doses were so high that they would wipe out her capacity to regenerate her own blood — with its infection-fighting and blood-clotting components — and thus make it impossible for her to survive. That is why the patient's healthy marrow has to be harvested — to rescue the patient from the chemotherapeutic assault. The harvested marrow is reinfused into the patient one or two days after chemotherapy is completed.

Carol, like all transplant patients, had to remain in one of the special rooms dedicated to use by patients with compromised immune systems. Because the biggest risk to such patients is infection, these rooms have what is called laminar flow, with negative air exchange. When the door opens, a special mechanism prevents germs from the outside hallway entering. The rooms are carefully cleaned out between patients, and before the patient's arrival are filled with their own sterile supply of medicine, tubing, syringes, and equipment. Anyone entering the room usually has to don gloves, a mask, and a gown. Everything — every pen, book, glass — that goes into the room must be cleaned before it is brought in. Anyone with a cold or other illness is barred from patient contact. This period of risk lasts until the reinfused bone marrow "engrafts," or starts producing more cells. The process of engraftment can take up to three weeks.

Patients who go through these operations are so weak they have trouble even sitting up in bed and are subject to numerous complications that must be rigorously monitored. They often develop terrible mucositis — that is, mouth sores — and esophagitis — sores along the lining of the esophagus. They have diarrhea and vomiting and sometimes skin reactions. The chemotherapy drugs' toxicity may make them vulnerable to potentially lethal bleeding from the bladder wall, and they are at risk for complications in almost every major organ system. Because preservatives have been added to their marrow, allergic reactions to the preservative can occur when the marrow is reinfused into their bodies. Similarly, they can develop an allergic or immune reaction to the blood products — platelets and red blood cells — that they receive. The smallest sign of a complication must be immediately noticed and acted upon, because it may signal a life-threatening catastrophe or a routine complication that must be addressed.

Transplant patients are, furthermore, subject to wild mood swings and acute depression because of their isolation and the kind of physical assault they undergo. Many of the drugs they take — steroids, antinausea medication, and others — may severely affect not only the body but the psyche. Many patients are given antidepressants or anti-anxiety medication.

The kind of nursing care these patients require is extraordinarily intense. While Carol was in the hospital, her primary nurse on the inpatient oncology unit, Stoneman Four, checked on her perhaps every fifteen minutes, or sometimes even more frequently.

She would wash off her pen, or anything else she was carrying into the room, don her gloves and mask, and enter. The room seemed to engulf her. Even when one is outside the hospital's main buildings, the medicinal smell of chemicals and disinfectants can seem over-powering. The smell becomes more intense on the hospital floors. But Carol Benoit's room seemed a humidor of affliction. Inside, the fumes from its peculiar mixture of blood products, stale vomit, and disinfectant penetrated every pore. People are terribly sick and can feel very alone in the other rooms on Stoneman Four, but the trans-plant rooms seem to reduce this illness and solitude to its very essence.

A picture of Carol taken before the transplant was pinned to a small bulletin board opposite her bed. Nurses often ask patients to bring in pictures that were taken before they began their treatment. Because the person undergoing treatment is so deeply altered, care-givers and patients alike appreciate reminders of an existence free of disease as well as the possibility of returning to that state. In this case, Carol's smiling, ruddy face was surrounded by a halo of curly red hair.

The woman in the bed could not be more different from this pho-tograph. Her head was totally bald. Her eyebrows and eyelashes had disappeared. Her face, arms, and legs were as hairless as a baby's. When her hospital johnny flapped open, you could see that she no longer had pubic hair. The chemicals had acted like sandpaper, smoothing down every surface, eradicating every identifiable trace that was uniquely Carol Benoit. What was left was a head that looked like every other head sheared by chemotherapy. Carol looked like the kind of small primitive Grecian figure exhibited in museums. The ancient sculptures are formed of a series of balls, like a miniature stone snowman, with stublike arms jutting out at the sides. The surface is pale, like Carol's skin, and finely sanded. The figures look like a child's attempt to sculpt an adult reduced to everyman. Which is what the drugs have done to Carol Benoit.

The disease and transplant process have narrowed her life. "It's like they're going to hell and back," her nurse says. "It's the combination of the intensity of the chemo, the side effects, and the experience of isolation. She's hooked up to so many machines. There's a Foley catheter irrigating her bladder because the chemo is so toxic it could burn it out. She has an IV pumping a liter of fluid into her each hour and then draining through the three-way Foley. The IV also gives her antibiotics, and blood products."

Everything and anything can go wrong, she adds. "The chemo made her incredibly nauseous. Yesterday the drug gave her severe chest pain. Her blood pressure dropped. She had projectile vomiting for six hours plus copious amounts of diarrhea. She was incontinent of stool. I have to be very careful when we infuse the platelets, because earlier she got platelets and had rigors [intense shaking]. Sometimes she's so tired she can't even tell you what's wrong. You have to use all your experience to ask, 'Is it this? Is it that?' They're always on the edge of something about to happen. You always have to be prepared."

For the patient, the ordeal seemed interminable. When no family member was present, the door shut behind the nurse and Carol was utterly alone. When her family was not there, the nurse's comings and goings and Nancy's visits represented some of the only human contact in a world overwhelmed by technology.

"You have to coach these patients through the whole thing," Carol's inpatient primary nurse explains. "You have to talk to them about what they're going through, about what's happening right at that moment. You have to tell them that we're here to relieve their symptoms, and try to reassure them that this will pass. And then you have to support the family, because the patients look so scary. They have no hair. They look so sick. They *are* so sick."

Lying in her bed exhausted after an episode of vomiting, Carol Benoit talked to me about her nurse's care and the experience of transplant. "When you discuss the procedure with your doctor, they tell you you're going to be really sick." So, Carol thought sick, like when she had chemotherapy before. But she says, "There is no way you could ever imagine being this sick. No way you can imagine it at all. You see the doctor so rarely through all of this. I don't think I could have survived it if it weren't for Nancy and my other nurses."

Difficult as the ordeal was, when Nancy visited her on the floor, she was chafing at the bit to go home early and was discharged more quickly than was originally projected. Now she is in the clinic for one of her many follow-up visits. Posttransplant patients like Carol visit the clinic three times a week to be monitored and perhaps to receive further blood transfusions.

Again, it is Nancy who is central to communication, evaluation, and education in this postprocedure phase. Weakened by her ordeal, Carol lies on a hospital bed in the small treatment room at the far right-hand corner of the main treatment area. Her curly red wig has been replaced with a pale peach turban, which she wears to conceal her baldness. Her face is as transparent as parchment. The upper part of the bed has been ratcheted to an upright position, and Carol is leaning against it for support. Nancy pulls up a rolling stool and perches beside her. Carol reaches out her hand and grasps Nancy's hand tightly. To Nancy's first question, "Carol, how are you?" her eyes well with tears.

"I'm so worried about getting an infection, Nancy. I feel awful. I keep having the chills and feeling nauseous. What's happening to me?" she asks in a panic. "I swing up and down, through such highs and lows. Is this what happens after a transplant?"

"I don't know anyone who feels good posttransplant, Carol," Nancy says, trying to calm her.

"Yes, but this!" Carol exclaims. "I was so weepy this weekend. I don't understand. I did so well in the hospital. I couldn't believe it. You remember, Nancy." She appeals to her nurse as the chronicler of her medical history.

Knowing how easily Carol panics, Nancy delves more deeply into the subject of her anxiety, asking Carol to talk more about her feelings.

"I guess I thought all the anxiety would disappear after the transplant," Carol says as her fingers clench and unclench over the thin blue cotton blanket that covers her. "The whole period for those months before it, when we were debating whether I needed the transplant, was so bad. It felt like such a relief when they told me I did need it, because then I could do something about all this. I guess I expected to get out of the hospital and be perfect."

Nancy strokes Carol's hand as she listens. She has heard this story countless times. What is to Carol a complete break in the pattern of her life is to Nancy normal for such patients. When she talks to patients, however, she never trivializes their experience. "Carol," she says slowly, emphasizing each word, "you are going to be fine. You're going to get through this like you got through the hospital. But you have to understand that this is a major transition. Going home from the hospital seems like it's going to solve your problems. But it just adds different problems. That's because for three weeks nurses took care of you for twenty-four hours a day. They met all your needs. Going home is harder than you imagined. It is for everybody. It's a major ordeal. Your body has to build both physically and emotionally."

Carol tries to assimilate the information, but she is fixed on the conundrum of her emotional roller-coaster ride during and after transplant. "It's so hard to understand why I get so emotional now, when for three weeks I was like the Rock of Gibraltar," Carol repeats.

Understanding that her patient will have to sift through her concerns over and over until she can make some sense of her feelings, Nancy does not interrupt. She continues to try to reiterate that Carol's responses are normal. At the same time, she is careful to get across crucial information. "Now remember, this is a major transition. You have to be careful. You have to watch yourself and come in here if you have a temp that goes up to a hundred and one. You have to come right in to the EU. If you're home alone and your husband is working, you'll have to call an ambulance."

Carol tries to listen attentively. Unfortunately, the possibility of serious complications is not a subject that is foreign to her. "Yes, I know," Carol says. "But remember what happened when my Hickman line got infected two years ago." She reminds Nancy that none of the doctors would listen to her when she insisted that there was something wrong with the line.

"I'll never forget how sick I felt. And I was right. It was infected," she says almost triumphantly. She asserts with pride the knowledge of one's own body that is so often preempted by medical personnel. Patients may be told that there is nothing wrong with a body that they live with daily because "objective indicators" have not yet registered the presence of an infection or other complication. But in this case as in so many others, the patient often knows best.

"Remember, Nancy, I was right," she says almost defiantly.

"Carol, yes, I remember. You know just what it's like when you have a blood infection, and you have to act on it if it happens."

Nancy sits with Carol for a few more minutes before leaving. But this is only round one.

Several days later Carol calls frantically from home. Again it's a busy day in the clinic, but Nancy takes time to talk. Carol tells Nancy that she is starting to spike a fever. When she began to feel ill, she took her temperature and it was 100.2. A few hours later she took it again: 100.5. Now it's the magic number — 101. More, in fact. It's actually 101.2.

Carol is getting increasingly nervous. Should she come in to the hospital? she asks Nancy. Will the attending physician want to admit her? Should she just come into the clinic? Can she get an answer? And soon?

Her husband, Phil,* is about to leave for work. The couple live an hour from the hospital. Since she can't drive herself and hates to come to the hospital in an ambulance, she wants Phil to drive her in. If she has to be readmitted through the EU (the route through which patients are admitted to the hospital for an emergency condition or other crisis), she would rather Phil take her before he goes to work. But what does the physician want?

Nancy tells Carol that she will page her doctor and find out. Once she manages to track down the physician, it's confirmed — Carol should indeed come in to see if she has an infection.

When Nancy informs Carol of this, the patient is beside herself. This running back and forth to and from the hospital is putting an enormous strain on her and her marriage. Last week, she says, she came into the emergency room with low blood counts, feeling terrible. Rather than being admitted to the hospital, she was sent home. Then she ran into more trouble the next day and was finally admitted. Again, the line was infected and had to be pulled and replaced. Before she left the hospital, Carol was told she would need blood. Why did she have to come in to the clinic for blood only a few days after she left the hospital, when she could have gotten the blood in the hospital and avoided another difficult two-hour round trip?

After listening to this litany of justifiable complaints, Nancy tries to calm Carol and encourage her to come in to the clinic. Then she goes off to find Frank McCaffrey, another of the social workers on the oncology unit, who has worked with Carol's team for years. A small, slim man with close-trimmed hair who dresses in neat casual pants, muted shirts, and colorful ties, McCaffrey tells Nancy that just the other day, after Carol's emergency room snafu, Phil approached him in the clinic. Phil seemed to be at his wit's end. Almost in tears, he told Frank that his boss had been riding him about taking too much time off work. He works from three in the afternoon to eleven at night. He is free to help Carol and chauffeur her in the morning but must be at work in the afternoon. When his wife is passed like a football from the EU to home, then to the hospital for a few days, then home, then back to the hospital, it is a nightmare for him. Each hour he is away from work adds to the risk that he will lose his job. If he loses his job, the family loses more than his income. It loses his health care insurance as well. How could they survive without that?

"I certainly understand what he's going through," Nancy commiserates. "I don't understand why they didn't just admit her when she was in the EU."

The two surmise that it was because her counts were borderline, and the hospital wanted to avoid an unnecessary hospitalization that Carol's insurance would refuse to pay for.

"I think Carol went home probably a little too early after transplant," Nancy confides to Frank. "She wanted to go home and didn't realize how hard it would be." Nancy shakes her head sadly at decisions that are not in her hands and that she might have handled differently. "There isn't a lot of confidence-building going on here."

The social worker agrees. His beeper sounds and he looks for a phone. Before he leaves, Nancy touches his shoulder with warmth and gratitude. "Thanks so much for helping with Phil," she says. When Frank can deal with his concerns, she says, it makes the job of dealing with Carol easier.

To care most effectively for their patients, Nancy and other nurses in the clinic try to encourage as much collaboration with physicians as is possible. Every July, when the new crop of first-year fellows arrives on the unit, Nancy conducts an hour-and-a-half informal orientation to introduce them to primary nursing, discuss how the two disciplines can work together, and describe the unit's systems and flow. "Our focus," she says, "is on getting primary nurses involved early on in the process of patient care. For example, if there is a new patient, we want to meet them as soon as possible. We want to be alerted to what a person needs sooner rather than later. For example, if a fellow knows a patient needs Neupogen — a very expensive drug that costs a hundred and fifty dollars a day — tell us right away so we can get preapproval from their insurance company. If someone needs hospice, tell us."

The message, she underlines, is, "We're involved, we're part of the team."

She believes that physicians need to understand the long-term role a primary nurse plays in a chronic disease like cancer because a primary nurse like Nancy will care for many patients for years. If they have a cancer like breast cancer or lymphoma and are in active treatment, patients like Carol Benoit will be coming in regularly for chemotherapy or other treatments. Patients with leukemia are in the clinic once or twice a week. Similarly, patients who have had bone marrow transplants require significant follow-up care and monitoring.

Many patients come in for follow-up visits for years. For example, when Deborah is through with her period of intense treatment, she will visit the clinic every two months for a year, every three months the second year, and perhaps only once every six months the third. If things are going well on those visits, patients tend to check in with their nurses but require little more than a hello.

Nancy is frequently on the phone with patients who have questions or problems. When patients come in for treatment the first time, Nancy always tries to call back a day or two later to make sure they are doing well. If a patient is having intense side effects, if he or she is having trouble coping with treatment or is developing a complication, Nancy will either deal with the problem herself or consult with the patient's physician. Nancy manages many patients' side effects, such as pain, nausea, vomiting, diarrhea, and mouth sores, either on her own or in consultation with the physician team. If drugs are recommended for these problems, an experienced nurse like Nancy may suggest the specific drug and discuss her ideas with the physician, who will either agree or disagree. If she has worked with that physician for a long time and is familiar with particular drugs, the physician may do little more than rubber-stamp her decision. Smart fellows know that much of the practical side of medicine is learned from nurses.

Nancy also follows her patients when they are admitted to the hospital or are in the Emergency Unit because of a crisis. Many of her patients bounce in and out of Stoneman Four, the oncology ward, or other general medical floors as well as the ICU. They may be receiving anticancer drugs that require close monitoring. They may suffer from infections and need IV antibiotics or other treatment following chemotherapy. They may be in severe pain or they may be dying.

Nancy's concern is not just with her patients but also with their families or close friends. On any given day, she will spend a great deal of time in her office or in the clinic on the phone talking not only with patients, but with family members. In attending to her patients' lives and relationships, Nancy also functions as coordinator of the care provided by other members of the health care team. When Deborah Celli breaks down in tears and confesses that she needs help with her life; when she doesn't understand how to get her medical bills paid, Nancy is the one who calls in the social worker or talks to the pharmacist. When a patient needs care at home, Nancy arranges for and maintains contact with the visiting nurse and home health aide.

Nancy is also one of her patients' primary educators and will go over explanations about treatments and their physical and emotional impact. Physicians, of course, explain the terms of their patients' treatment when they meet with them initially and in follow-up visits. But nurses reinforce their lessons and add many of their own.

This is not an easy business. Nancy knows from long experience that people who have serious illnesses are hardly in the best state of mind to absorb complex information. They come to the hospital frightened, anxious, often in terror. What seems to be the simplest of messages — take one pill in the morning with breakfast and another at night with dinner — may elude their capacity to retain information. Going beyond this to informing them about an aggressive chemotherapeutic protocol or the impact of bone marrow transplants is a daunting endeavor. Reading a multipage consent form for a chemotherapy regimen or bone marrow transplant makes it clear that patients with serious illnesses inhabit an entirely different psychological space than those who are healthy. The bone marrow transplant consent form catalogs the treatment's potential threats to every organ system in the body; explaining the high risk of irreversible damage, and even death.

A healthy person reading this form would be astonished that anyone could contemplate risks of such magnitude. But people who are sick are not "rational choice-makers." They are desperately trying to fight off death — often at any price. Both physicians and nurses speak of patients with whom they have spent hours discussing diagnosis, prognosis, and treatment options, who nonetheless retain little or nothing of what they have been told. Or patients may mobilize the impressive human capacity for denial to deal with their illness. Again, Nancy often recognizes and deals with their denial, fear, and anxiety.

In order to help educate her patients, Nancy must understand how to convey information and *when* to convey it. If a patient is in tears because she has just learned that she has a recurrence of cancer, this is obviously not the time to discuss the latest details of how the cancer will be fought. If a patient has just heard the physician tell him there is "nothing more to be done," talking about what it means to be dying of a terminal disease may be out of the question at that particular moment. If a patient is suffering from intense nausea and vomiting, it may be necessary to educate the family rather than the patient so someone can take charge of the patient's care at home.

In an example of the long and arduous process of making sure patients really understand what physicians have told them, Nancy comes to work one morning and walks into an exam room to begin administering chemotherapy to a new patient. The patient is an old man who sits in a wheelchair. His squat, pumpkinlike head is covered with gray curly hair that recedes slightly at the forehead. His hands — with stubs of fingers that seem to have been worn down to squared-off tips by years of manual labor — grip the arms of the chair, polishing the steel with silent sweeps of apprehension. His son — who is in his late thirties — is next to him. He seems to be planted there, a dull, inert lump fixed to his seat.

The old man is seventy-four and had colorectal cancer. He's had surgery and will now have chemotherapy ordered by his attending physician. The more mature physician, however, has assigned the daily supervision of the case to a first-year fellow — young, kind, but by definition inexperienced.

This is Nancy's first meeting with the patient. She introduces herself, and expecting that the fellow has explained the treatment process, she quickly goes over the routine. The old man nods absently.

Pulling out a tourniquet, she wraps it tightly around the man's forearm. The tray on the cabinet next to her prominently displays several syringes and small vials. Saline solution hangs from the IV pole just behind her right shoulder.

All is ready. She begins to probe the veins in the crook of the man's arm to insert the finely honed needle. The old man averts his face. It is a typical gesture. She has seen this happen thousands of times. Like a Geiger counter measuring the surface of emotions and sensing what is percolating under the most commonplace gesture, she detects in this movement a signal that there is more going on than fear of a needle stick. She pauses and asks, "What is it?" and removes her hand from his arm. "Is something wrong?"

The old man begins to speak and out flows a torrent of heavily Greek-accented speech, almost a parody were it not so anxiety-filled.

"All my friends who've had chemotherapy have died. It's going to kill me," he announces with total certainty.

"Why? Why you do this?" he continues. "I've had a good life. I don't want to die like this. God gave me a fine life. I've lived it. My wife died like this, with this cancer. The medicine was supposed to make her live. But she died."

Nancy looks surprised. "Didn't the doctor explain this to you?" she asks. "You may get a bit nauseous, but we have drugs that can help you."

He doesn't seem to hear. "My friend, last year, he had chemotherapy," he repeats, as if counting each medical failure like a bead on his rosary. "He's dead." The old man stares at Nancy, defying her to contradict this logical conclusion.

"Did you talk to the doctor about this?" Nancy interrupts. Turning to the son, she tries to elicit information from him. "Didn't the doctor talk to you about this?"

Sitting stolidly in his chair, the son simply shrugs. His uninterested gaze speaks of frustration.

The old man continues his litany of dread. Nancy tries to reassure him. Finally, he sticks out his arm in a gesture of capitulation.

"Here," he says, thrusting his arm in her face. "You gotta die, you gotta die."

Nancy does not say a word. She looks at his arm and its defiant challenge. Then she stands up.

"No," she pronounces. "I am not going to give you chemotherapy if you feel this way about it. Please excuse me a moment." She leaves the small room and closes the door behind her.

Outside, she shakes her head. She walks down the corridor and sees the fellow in charge of the old man's case. Walking up to him, she briefly describes the situation. "He thinks we're going to kill him. Right now. On the spot. We cannot give him chemotherapy under these circumstances. We have to talk to him together."

The doctor agrees and follows her back into the room. Very solicitous of the patient, he reviews the drug regimen and explains its potential side effects.

The old man clearly does not take it all in. But the doctor is here. The doctor is authority. Even a young doctor who has just begun his career must be obeyed.

"I don't mean to bother you, Doctor," he says apologetically and smiles deferentially. "Anything you say, Doctor."

Nancy does not seem surprised. It has happened so many times — this dance between authority and intimacy. This "I don't want to bother you, Doctor, anything you say, Doctor," followed by the confession — "Nurse, help me, I am terrified, I've had a good life, why are they doing this?"

The doctor remains there for a few more moments. Whether resigned or reassured, the old man is ready. When the doctor leaves, the old man sticks out his arm again, and the first round begins.

When I was in the hospital, I asked Nancy's patients how they felt about the nursing care she gave them. Invariably, these patients responded emphatically: Nancy and their other nurses were crucial to their curing, recovery, or coping.

Why? I asked. What made the difference?

Again, they responded, "The nurses really care. They are really there for their patients."

But what, I probed, does the word "caring" mean to you? Two of Nancy's gay patients explained what it means for a nurse to care and what it means to a patient to be cared for.

Dave Andrews* has had HIV / AIDS for a number of years. He has seen many friends die, cared for many others, and been active in the AIDS community for a long time. He has Kaposi's sarcoma (KS), an AIDS-related cancer. As he sits in the clinic getting his chemo, we talk. "The nurses, doctors, and receptionists here are really exceptional," he says. "The attitude is simple friendliness, which is so reassuring. I was admitted here twice, and I've visited friends. I'm just overwhelmed by the nursing staff here. If I've had to be here overnight, they let my significant other stay overnight. They let friends stay till midnight. They don't adhere to all sorts of strict rules."

Dave says he appreciates the fact that his caregivers acknowledge that gay lovers or friends are part of the informal system of caregiving that HIV patients depend on. "In a lot of hospitals, they usually say only family members. Then they turn to you and say, 'You're not a family member.' But for many of us our significant other is more important than a family member."

Dave says he values the consistency of having one nurse, someone whom he knows, over time, who can act as a barometer for his physical and emotional state. This consistency, he says, is important because living with cancer and AIDS is a "double whammy." What he finds so important, he continues, is the matter-of-factness, openness, and honesty of Nancy and the other nurses. "The nurses here realize that, in many cases, they're the first ones who validate that a person has AIDS. This is particularly important to many of us because, for example, my family would not talk about it. No one would bring it up.

"It wasn't until I was hospitalized that anyone acknowledged the problem. And it was the nurses who did that. They just said, 'Yeah, with PCP [*Pneumocystis carinii* pneumonia], it's AIDS related.' They talked about it matter-of-factly. This validated the fact that I had it. They did it without being brisk or cold, and it was very comforting."

Healthy people may not understand that many sick people find it unbearable when their friends pretend that all is well and try to bury the fact of illness beneath a barrage of good cheer. "It's good to hear people talk about it realistically," Dave continues, "like, you're here, you're sick, let's do something about it."

Several hours later, Nancy is delivering chemo to another gay man with KS. Jack McDonald* is, like Dave, in his late thirties, trim and dark-haired. He is struggling with the same kinds of issues that so many of her Kaposi's patients confront. What he values, he says, is nurses' competence and their acceptance.

In this case, Jack not only has AIDS but is the lover of a man who has a far more serious case of AIDS than he. "Here, they not only care for me, but accept me as Bill's* mate. I've been with Bill for thirteen years. You are like husband and wife. But it's extremely difficult being a gay man and being with someone for a long time, because many people can't accept our relationship." To illustrate, he tells me stories about hospitals that would not allow him even to come into the emergency room with his partner.

"Caring, to me, is including me in the decisions," Jack says. "It's not being judgmental, treating me as someone who has a significant part in someone else's life. Even though we're not a traditional legal family, the nurses still recognize me as someone who's involved with that other person. When you come to a place like this, they treat you with open arms. When you don't get treated that way," he says, "it hurts. It really does."

In the literature of nursing, caring is often said to be the core of nurses' work. Indeed, the public often believes in a neat dichotomy between the work of physicians and that of nurses: Doctors cure and nurses care. In hospitals, one realizes that this is a false division of labor. Many doctors are extremely caring, and nurses also play a big role in curing. There is, however, a cultural paradox that clouds most people's ability to perceive this reality. We may be able to accept that doctors can be caring, but we have trouble understanding that nurses also help us heal and cure.

While I was researching this book, I told a friend about an incident between Nancy and Deborah that occurred while Nancy was administering Deborah's chemotherapy. My friend's reaction was illuminating. She had no trouble accepting my description of Nancy's caring relationships with her patients. But she balked at the "medical" function of the nurse.

I must have gotten it wrong, she said of my description of Nancy's initial session with Deborah. After all, it must be the doctor, not the nurse, who administers chemotherapy. And all this business about the nurse managing the patient's nausea. That, too, is the doctor's job, isn't it?

My friend had never been in the hospital and certainly had never spent any extended time in an outpatient oncology clinic. But she had watched TV and read her daily newspapers. She had learned her lessons well. My account of nursing contradicted the message that doctors *are* health care.

I had to laugh at the idea that the average medical specialist would spend hour after hour sitting at a patient's side administering chemotherapy, track down a drug at local pharmacies, and / or listen to the patient unravel the tangles in her conjugal life. Of course doctors care about their patients. But what Nancy does is not the doctor's job, but the nurse's.

Ironically, the propaganda about the physician's role in health care has been so pervasive and effective that even many of Nancy's patients attribute her accomplishments to either physician expertise or effective hospital administration. When I was talking to Jack, he concluded his ode to Nancy's nursing care with the following: "I don't know if the doctors give them a special course on patient relationships or if they just choose them [the nurses] well." Similarly, another of Nancy's patients gave physicians the credit for nursing education. "The doctors here really train them well, don't they?" she commented.

But, of course, when both curing and caring, Nancy, not her physician colleagues, is responsible for her own work. That work — the work of nursing — said Florence Nightingale in her classic volume *Notes on Nursing*, is to "put the patient in the best condition for nature to act upon him." Or as the distinguished nursing scholar Virginia Henderson defines it, "The unique function of the nurse is to assist the individual, sick or well, in the performance of those activities contributing to health or its recovery (or to peaceful death) that he would perform unaided if he had the necessary strength, will or knowledge. And to do this in such a way as to help him gain independence as rapidly as possible. This aspect of her work, that part of her function, she initiates and controls; of this she is master."

Chapter 6

A Mentor of Their Own

JEANNIE CHAISSON

On the Friday before Mother's Day, Jeannie Chaisson is sitting at the high counter at the central work station, going over charts. A young nurse with reddish curly hair wearing blue scrubs and a worried look approaches her. Can I talk with you for a moment, she interrupts.

Jeannie sets aside her work, swivels in her chair, and says of course. The young nurse then launches into a long story about a patient for whom she is caring. The woman is in her seventies and has just had a massive stroke. As a result she also has a severe pneumonia and is dying.

"Do you have a particular question?" Jeannie asks.

The nurse seems to hesitate. No, there's nothing in particular, just . . . She mumbles and her voice trails off.

Aware that there is, in fact, a problem the nurse wants to raise, Jeannie probes. "Are you sure?"

The nurse then says: Well, today is Friday and Sunday is Mother's Day. The woman has a daughter in her forties and two granddaughters. It would be so hard for her family if she died on Mother's Day, the nurse elaborates. No one wants to do anything heroic to try to prolong the patient's life, she adds, but imagine how her daughter and granddaughters will feel for the rest of their lives if Mother's Day is associated with the patient's death. But what do you do in a case like this?

Jeannie sympathizes with the nurse's concerns and suggests they go and see the patient together. They walk down the corridor and enter a single room. The woman is lying on the bed, her wispy gray hair spread out on the pillow. Her mouth is open, and she is taking loud, rasping, gurgling breaths. After checking the monitor of the IV infusion pump that is delivering morphine to make the patient more comfortable, Jeannie walks over to the bed, bends over the woman lying in it, and gently strokes her hair. Because she is always careful to speak to patients even if they are comatose, Jeannie introduces herself and explains the purpose of her visit.

"I'm Jeannie Chaisson, a nurse on this unit, Mrs. Jones.* I've just come in to see if you're comfortable. We want to make sure you're not in pain."

Inert and unresponsive, the woman continues to expel her excruciatingly labored breaths.

"You have to make sure that the dose is okay for someone who is not used to morphine," Jeannie explains. "Even though she can't speak, you can try to tell if she's comfortable just by the way she moves and breathes."

Hearing the patient rattle again, Jeannie turns to me and describes the physiology of the patient's breathing. "She's Cheyne-Stoking. When someone is dying, they start up breathing, breathe more deeply for a few breaths, then stop and pick up again. It's a breathing pattern that usually indicates near coma. The brain stem controls basic functions like breathing. When patients are near death their ability to keep oxygen and CO_2 levels balanced is decreased. So the oxygen levels go down and the carbon dioxide levels go up, and then the brain picks that up and tries to normalize it. People who are severely compromised can stop breathing for up to a minute or even longer. It's called Cheyne-Stokes respiration. It was named after two physicians."

After leaving the room, Jeannie and the young nurse sit down in the nurses' conference room. As a clinical educator, Jeannie looks upon this room as her favorite classroom. In it, she can engage in what she calls "situational teaching." "Some nurse specialists will conduct in-services on particular medical problems. They'll gather a group of nurses together to discuss an abstract case of renal failure.

'This is what renal failure looks like,' they explain. Rather than tell people what renal failure is in the abstract, I like to work with a nurse caring for someone with renal failure. Then you can show a nurse what a particular symptom of renal failure looks like and demonstrate how to care for a person with that problem.

"Some people think of the word 'teacher' and conjure up an image of a classroom, where you sit people down in front of you, face a sheaf of notes, and say, 'All right, congestive heart failure is characterized by these symptoms. It's treated by these drugs. Now repeat after me.' But people tend to forget that information."

Jeannie likens her process of situational teaching to storytelling. She and a nurse go in and see a patient together. The nurse tells Jeannie her version of the patient's story. Then Jeannie adds important details she feels will make the account more cogent and accurate. Then, most important, if the patient is able, he or she adds others.

"I'm augmenting their story." Jeannie sums up the process. "It's not taking over. It's just adding a chapter."

These chapters are best added, she feels, in the moments when nurses process their day, raise their concerns, and vent their emotions. This provides an opportunity to help nurses learn from one another. As Jeannie talks to the younger nurse, a group of their colleagues are gathered around the long rectangular table having lunch. Orange trays brought up from the hospital cafeteria contain an assortment of sandwiches and salads. Jeannie pours herself a cup of coffee, sits down next to the young nurse, and urges the young woman to share her dilemma with her colleagues.

The nurse eagerly relates her fear that the woman might die on Mother's Day and talks about the woman's family. The nurses around the table understand her concerns immediately. Had Jeannie not been present, the conversation might have ended there. Rather than allowing the other nurses to turn from this reflection, Jeannie, the storyteller, augments the nurse's account. "She's got a lot of secretions in the back of her throat. It becomes a question, doesn't it, of whether it will make her uncomfortable to suction them or whether it will make her more comfortable."

"It's so hard to figure out which is better or worse," the nurse agrees.

"It's a very long wait for the family," Jeannie comments. "At this point, all she's getting is fluids. And it's hard for them to see her not eating, and hard for us. People tend to want to be more aggressive. But that doesn't make sense."

In a case like this, when a patient is not aware of what's going on, she continues, it's a matter of figuring out what will make the family feel better. "The issue," she suggests, "is how much explanation does the family want? What do they feel they need to know? What do they feel they should be doing in order to believe they're doing the right thing for their loved one? We need to ask them if they feel they want the dying patient to have some hydration or if they're comfortable withdrawing that as well. The language we use is very important because most often it's done wrong so that families feel pressured to make a particular decision. But there's more than one correct decision."

Later she discusses the value of such interactions. "These nurses are seeing a tremendous amount of pain and suffering. They are constantly dealing with families who are under stress. There is no automatic way for them to get support for what they do. So if they can talk about what they are doing and why, just the act of putting words to their actions and feelings helps them plan. You have to do this informally, over lunch or coffee, while it is happening. If we said, 'We're going to set aside an hour at ten o'clock next Wednesday to talk about all this,' no one would come. This way, they're all here, all thinking about it."

Jeannie's mission is not only to allow nurses to talk, but to allow them to question. How can they navigate the system? How can they find the resources they need? Who has the resources they need? "I'm the person people seek out for information because I've been a nurse for a long time. I have a great memory for all sorts of bizarre trivia. So if a patient is coming in with a strange condition that we've never seen before, I'm the one who's likely to know what it is and what causes it. And if I don't know, I know how to find out."

"It's rather self-effacing," Jeannie says of her job. "In my estimation, if I'm doing my job well, then it doesn't look like I'm doing anything."

When it looks like Jeannie "isn't doing anything," she is, in fact, attending to the things that make a difference in the lives of patients and the life of her unit. This involves the art and science of noticing and decoding the smallest signs and most elusive signals. Whether they are staff nurses working at a patient's bedside, clinical nurse specialists surveying the daily life of an inpatient unit, or nurse practitioners working in a patient's home, nurses constantly register the subtlest changes in a patient's status. In so doing, they find meaning in what many of us would find meaningless and focus attention on problems that most of us would dismiss as trivial.

But for a patient whose life has been disrupted by illness, it is often the minute and mundane that matter most. That's because illness disrupts the routine activities of everyday life. When you are sick, the molehills of life quite literally become mountains. Eating, sleeping, walking, breathing, these are some of the mountains that nurses have charted and help patients scale.

While I was watching Jeannie feed Mrs. Cohen, the old woman with a stroke, I suddenly understood the import of Virginia Henderson's definition of nursing. And I also understood why so few people share this understanding. The average American knows he can't perform an operation, conduct research that will discover a cure for cancer, or develop some new biomedical device. But most people think it's easy to feed a sick person, empty a bedpan, or help someone walk down the hall. What's the big deal? Anyone could do it, most of us imagine.

Lacking much familiarity with illness, we superimpose "healthy thinking" on the experience of caring for the sick. But this obscures our ability to understand the complexity of caregiving.

Even though I've spent years listening to and observing nurses, it was only when I watched Jeannie feeding the old woman who had had a stroke that I finally "got it."

Before this encounter, I thought I knew all I needed to know about strokes. I knew people often became paralyzed, and that they had trouble talking and eating. I hoped it would never happen to me. Before I observed Jeannie and her colleagues, if someone had said that it takes an experienced nurse to feed a stroke patient, I would have thought, But, that's nonsense. Anyone with a little sense and sensitivity can feed a sick person. Why do we need to pay a nurse to do that?

Now I know better.

This aspect of nurses' work is as challenging as the more dramatic, life-saving activities they engage in. The medical system is awash in drama. But if the meaning of illness also lies in the disruption of the everyday, who, other than nurses, has the knowledge and experience necessary to attend so intelligently to this aspect of the human condition?

Several days after the Mother's Day discussion, Jeannie informs me that we are off to the first meeting of the swallowing group. The what? I ask. The swallowing group, she repeats. Okay, I say, let's go.

We march to the elevators and go up to the tenth-floor surgical conference room located at the end of a warren of staff surgeons' offices. Six other nurses sit around a long table. They are Marion Phipps, Jeannie McHale, a clinical nurse specialist in the pulmonary intensive care unit; Linda Grant, a clinical nurse on a large medical floor; Ann Connor, a stroke nurse specialist; and Ann Howard and Kristin Russell, staff nurses in the Medical Intensive Care Unit (MICU).

Marion Phipps and Jeannie McHale have initiated a research project on swallowing. Phipps explains that her long experience caring for stroke patients with swallowing problems had led her — along with other Beth Israel nurses — to try to find out why so many of these patients were getting aspiration pneumonias and to learn what could be done to prevent it. Phipps was also on a panel set up by the federal government's Agency for Health Care Policy and Research to establish guidelines for poststroke rehabilitation patients. She thus began to search the nursing literature for insight and guidance on the subject of swallowing.

What she found was little of either. Phipps then met with clinical specialist Adele Pike, who worked at that time on Seven North, a special medical surgical floor that was also set up to study and encourage nurse-physician collaboration. Pike agreed that this was a fruitful area for exploration and the two recruited Jeannie McHale, a clinical nurse specialist on the MICU. McHale was interested in the nutrition problems of patients after their breathing tubes had been removed. How were decisions made to feed such patients, McHale wanted to know.

Pike, Phipps, and McHale held informal discussions, and Phipps also decided to look at the Beth Israel's nursing procedures manual to see what advice nurses were given as they tried to assess swallowing. What she found was both insufficient and disturbing. "All nurses were told was how to assess a gag reflex," Phipps recounted. "But, in fact, the problem of eating and swallowing is far more complex."

The three clinical specialists agreed that the hospital needed an accurate tool to help nurses assess their patients' difficulties with swallowing. At that point, Kathy Horvath, the hospital's director of the Center for the Advancement of Nursing Practice, suggested that Phipps, McHale, and Pike meet with Barbara Munro, a prominent nurse researcher and dean of the Boston College School of Nursing, and Mary Duffy, director of the school's Center for Nursing Research.

Although most people are familiar only with medical research, nursing research is one of the foundations of nursing care. Indeed, careful investigation and observation — the first steps in any research — go back to the origins of modern nursing. Florence Nightingale was one of the first health statisticians and an extremely well-known one. She also argued for nursing based on knowledge and careful inquiry. "If you cannot get the habit of observation one way or another," she wrote, "you had better give up being a nurse, for it is not your calling, however kind and anxious you may be.

"In dwelling upon the vital importance of sound observation, it must never be lost sight of what observation is for. It is not for the sake of piling up miscellaneous information or curious facts, but for the sake of saving life and increasing health and comfort."

The nineteenth-century definition of investigation and scholarship certainly differs from the late twentieth-century version. But Nightingale clearly outlined a vision of nursing grounded in research rather than in "woman's intuition." Although it took nursing decades to follow up on Nightingale's vision, her ideas have provided some of the building blocks of contemporary nursing research. (Observation, after all, is the first step in any research.) Today, every major nursing school and most major hospitals and medical centers conduct nursing research. Moreover, students at most four-year nursing schools take courses in statistics, experimental design, and survey research. Masters' students take advanced courses in research design, while doctoral and postdoctoral students work with nurse researchers on major studies.

Nursing research — funded by the National Institute for Nursing Research (NINR), which is a part of the National Institutes of Health, and by other sources — builds on basic science to explore how patients experience and respond to disease and dysfunction and how they weather complex medical procedures and treatments.

Nurse researchers investigate how RNs at the bedside can better ad-minister and monitor treatments so that they will be most effective in curing or abating symptoms. They challenge conventional wisdom about caregiving activities and techniques. This research often re-veals how patients' understanding of their medical problems and treatments can be enhanced and their emotional concerns more fully addressed.

Nursing research differs from medical research in important re-spects. Nursing research focuses less on survival itself and more on the quality of a patient's life after treatment or procedures or while on medication. Nursing research asks how patients live — what their quality of life is — after they survive. It also asks how the family care-givers upon whom many patients depend handle the burden of caring for a sick or dying relative.

The importance of nursing research is increasingly recognized by such prominent research bodies as the federal Agency for Health Care Policy and Research. Established in 1989, this agency's mandate is to "enhance the quality, appropriateness, and effectiveness of health care services and access to these services." The agency has cre-ated a series of clinical practice guidelines panels in which experts come together to review data on a specific condition — heart failure, acute pain management, cataracts — and to make recommendations about treatment. Unlike many other research bodies that are led ex-clusively by physicians, the agency's panels are often cochaired by a nurse researcher precisely because of nursing's focus on quality of life and burden on families. It was participation on such a panel that led Marion Phipps to her search for better information on swallowing problems.

Munro and Duffy encouraged Phipps and her colleagues to con-duct a full-fledged research study on this problem. To develop their assessment tool, Phipps, Horvath, and McHale decided to survey current knowledge of the hospital's nurses. Under the auspices of the Center for the Advancement of Nursing Practice, hospital nurse managers identified twelve nurses considered to be expert in caring for patients with swallowing problems. The nurses were then broken into two groups, and Phipps met with each three times for two hours a session. Patty Lydon, Jeannie Chaisson's nurse manager, nominated Jeannie to participate in one of those two groups.

A blond woman in her early fifties, Phipps speaks so quietly that the nurses around the table have to lean in to catch her words as she explains her goals. "We don't understand what nurses do in their everyday practice around the issue of eating and swallowing. The problem with what we do as nurses is that so much of it is silent. So often, observation and interpretation is not documented. So we're here to look at the silent knowledge you have."

To make that knowledge speak, Phipps had asked each nurse to prepare and present a narrative account of a patient or patients she cared for. Marion passes out the narrative Jeannie wrote for the group. It is called "N.P.O." (*non per os*), that is, nothing by mouth, and describes her experiences with two patients she has called Lena and Hal.

Hal is an elderly man who has suffered a major disabling stroke. He can no longer use the right side of his body and can no longer swallow safely. Small bits of any food or drink that he attempts to eat slide right down into his lungs. A feeding tube placed in his stomach now provides the nutrition that he needs to live. The problem is that calories and protein are not enough for Hal. Periodically he is admitted from home to our hospital unit with pneumonia caused by food in the lungs. "Hal," his nurses always ask, "what did you eat this time?" He is unable to speak to answer us, but we find out from his family sooner or later. Take-out Mexican food, Girl Scout cookies — some temptations could not be passed up.

Hal's indiscretions are a topic of discussion with his doctors and his nurses. Those who don't know him are annoyed. "Why does he keep doing this? He should know that he's going to get pneumonia again. This is such a waste." Those who have been through this a few times have a glimmer of understanding — for Hal, there are times when it is too much to ask that he never eat or drink anything; there are times that it seems worth it to suffer the consequences. There are always a few anxious days and nights when breathing is painful and difficult, times when Hal's caretakers have to suction thick secretions out of his airways so that oxygen can enter, times when his high fevers cause him to toss and moan.

This time, Hal's need to taste, to eat like the rest of us, has been his undoing: despite our efforts to treat the pneumonia, he dies.

Lena is an elderly woman who comes in to our medical unit because of a fever. She is very lethargic when she arrives, and intravenous fluids are used to provide hydration and some calories while antibiotics treat her infection. But after her fever leaves and her infection clears, she remains lethargic. She opens her eyes at times but never speaks, sits up, or seems aware of what is happening around her. Her son and daughter visit daily and don't understand why we do not feed her. "How can she get better when she is starving?" her daughter asks. She is certain that after a few meals her mother would perk up, recognize her, converse with her as she used to. But the nurses' cautious attempts to see if Lena can swallow in her sleepy state have shown that the answer is no. In the face of Lena's children's anger and insistence that inadequate nutrition is what is causing the lethargy, a trial of intravenous nutrition is started, but this does not wake Lena up.

There is growing desperation in the faces of Lena's children as she fails to get better. One day her daughter is found spooning soup into Lena's mouth; most of it dribbles out and down her chin. The nurse is concerned and orders the daughter to stop, explaining that Lena cannot swallow and that this attempt to feed her is harmful. That night, Lena starts to cough and her temperature rises, signs of pneumonia.

Some nurses and doctors are angry with Lena's children, seeing their force-feeding as abusive. But her children never intentionally harm her. They see the withholding of food as the harmful thing. The gap between the viewpoints of the doctors and nurses cannot be bridged. One side sees the futility of wishing for what can no longer be; the other knows only the sorrow of seeing the mother who struggled to see that they were always fed go hungry herself.

What Jeannie conveys in these two stories is her knowledge that the problems of eating and swallowing are not simply medical conundrums. They are not just part of "The Riddle" — the medical mystery of ferreting out disease, treatment, and cure — that Sherwin B. Nuland describes so well in his bestselling book *How We Die*. It is their human and social meaning that is paramount to her.

Perhaps she feels this because eating is such an important part of her own life. Her conversation is full of anecdotes about her cherished breakfasts at the Knotty Pine — an Auburndale coffee shop that serves, she says, the best home fries in the area. The small restaurant is an artifact of the fifties that has managed to cling to survival in the chic, Yuppie era of the nineties. Across from a long, open griddle area where short-order chefs cook up eggs of every variety, bacon, sausage, and muffins dripping with butter, customers sit at worn red-leather booths amid a decor of fifties-style knotty-pine paneling. Jeannie, a vegetarian who skips the meat, savors her eggs and muffins, just as, in an era of cholesterol consciousness, she boasts about the chocolate bars she eats, the ice cream she religiously purchases at least two times a week, or the aromatic coffee — high-test, not decaf — perfumed with hazelnuts, almonds, or Amaretto that she relishes daily. To her, eating is not just a matter of consuming enough calories to fuel bodily functions; it is an intense personal pleasure and an indispensable form of social glue. "Let's face it, if you want people to show up at a meeting," she says, "you have cookies there, you have food."

It is this insight, she tells the group, that also drives her care of patients like Hal and Lena. "We get so tied up in what path the food is taking, how big a bite do we give, do we need to suction, is it safe to feed the person, that we're missing the fact that food is central to life. Wedding banquets, feasts, birthday parties — that's what life is made up of. That's why withholding food from someone becomes so emotionally loaded. We study nutritional states and swallowing reflexes, but we miss the social experience, which can't be replaced with an infusion of calories," Jeannie says, concluding a profoundly emotional speech.

Her eyes have filled with tears and she pauses briefly. Like me, her colleagues are both moved and a bit surprised. Jeannie is so spare and steadfast in her self-presentation that such a show of emotion can take you off guard. But to her no aspect of patient care is more immediate, more meaningful than this. "Eating is one of my favorite things in the world," she acknowledges as she continues. "To have this happen to me would be one of my biggest nightmares. This is almost more painful than anything else that could happen to anyone."

If it's painful to her to think about such things, imagine, Jeannie says, how it must be for patients' families. Hal's daughter was his primary caregiver. But you couldn't simply reiterate the physician's orders — NPO, nothing by mouth. The woman refused to unflinchingly patrol his food intake because she felt that a regimen that caused him such unhappiness sometimes just wasn't worth it.

So yes, Hal would come in to the hospital terribly sick. You'd ask him what he ate and he would give you a sly smile.

Why? Jeannie asks rhetorically. Because he was happy as a clam after eating. And, she insists, everyone who really knew him understood why he would eat.

The problem, Jeannie says, was that doctors and nurses who did not know Hal well and who read only the medical record, not the record of the patient's life, would focus on the number of admissions and the reasons for them — aspiration pneumonia after cerebral vascular accident, or stroke (CVA) — and respond with frustration. As the nurses listen to Jeannie's story, Marion Phipps interrupts to ask how Jeannie helped to sensitize the house staff to the issues involved.

"I'd say, 'Well think about it for a while. Think about how you'd feel if someone said you can never eat another bite of food, never take another sip of water, or coffee, or wine, or Scotch. That you can never sit down and have another meal with your family or a friend,'" Jeannie replies with great intensity. "Think about how you'd feel and what you'd do."

With utter certainty she pronounces, "I would do what Hal did. They'd be digging ice cream out of my lungs. If it were me, I wouldn't just be sneaking a sip of coffee. I'd be eating something that grows bacteria especially well."

The members of the group smile knowingly at her comment. After several more questions about Hal, Marion asks Jeannie to comment on her choice of Lena. She chose Lena, Jeannie says, because the case illustrated a family problem. Lena's children just couldn't stand by and watch their mother not eat, even though they knew the food was not going to the right place.

"They were in such denial," Jeannie explains, "that they would say, 'Well, maybe this time it won't go down the wrong way.'"

Although they wanted their mother to eat, they refused what would have been the only solution — a tube into her stomach through which she would be fed. She had specifically instructed them never to put her on life-sustaining equipment, and they were determined to honor that wish. So they — and by extension Lena's caregivers — were caught between two untenable options.

"It was really hard for the nurses." Jeannie recalls the constant turmoil. "The children were very angry at them for starving their mother. You could give them all the data, but it didn't do a thing to change their minds. Feeding constituted a basic level of care for them and it was nonnegotiable. You had to feed her or she wouldn't live," Jeannie says, slapping the table to illustrate their adamant feelings.

As I listened to this discussion, I was suddenly transported twenty years into the past. It was the summer of 1970, and I was in my parents' apartment in New York City. My father had been diagnosed with pancreatic cancer and was undergoing chemotherapy. This treatment was a futile stab at survival, made even more torturous by the fact that there were then few antinausea drugs available to allay the side effects of the chemo. The idea of food was anathema to him. He could hardly bear to smell it, much less swallow it.

But to my mother food was more than the staff of life. She was convinced that if my father would finish just one meal, his tumor would magically shrink and the evil spell that engulfed our family would be broken. My father was, if not a great gourmet, at least a devoted gourmand. To appeal to the appetite that had added so many extra pounds to his large frame, she pleaded, cajoled, and tried to devise strategies that would lure him to the table. "Suzanne, call up and ask them if they'll make that special dish he loves so much for take-out," she would order me, naming one of my father's favorite neighborhood restaurants. I would obey, calling a restaurant that did not furnish take-out meals, imploring them to make an exception. If they agreed, I would hop into a cab and return home with a container full of bouillabaisse, or chicken Kiev.

My mother would set the table and reheat the meal. To please her, my father would force himself to sit down. But his revulsion was overpowering. He would look at the food, recoil, and push his plate away before leaving the table himself. Crestfallen but undaunted, my mother would implore, "Dan, just eat a few bites. You love this so much. Just try."

As she watched my father shed pound after pound, she grew as desperate as Lena's son and daughter. Right up until the end, she insisted that food was the cure. She was no longer the laughable Jewish mother begging a child to *"Ess mein kind, ess,"* but a frantic sorceress trying to conjure up one last miracle.

I watched these scenes in agony. I had sympathy for my mother's loss of a husband, but her persistent struggle to force my dying father to eat was a mystery to me. And now, twenty-five years later, sitting in this room, listening to these nurses and to the story of Lena and her children, I finally understood what food meant to my mother.

When I share these memories with Jeannie after the meeting, she nods in sympathy. Nurses and doctors and families, Jeannie says, all complain about "noncompliant patients." But they fail to ask why a patient is noncompliant. "Maybe," she ventures dryly, "it's because we told them to do something that is not acceptable to them. So they're not going to do it and what's more they don't have to."

When this happens, Jeannie believes it's her job — and should be every practitioner's job — to listen to that patient, rethink care and treatment plans, and come up with something that is acceptable. "Sometimes people do things that we think are not in their best interest, but they think *are* in their best interest."

Take smoking, Jeannie suggests. Nurses and doctors often get furious if somebody is smoking. But if people have smoked all their lives and are now sick — perhaps dying — maybe it doesn't matter that much if they continue to smoke. Maybe asking them to stop will be far more of a hardship than dying itself.

To illustrate, Jeannie tells another story about one of her patients. She was eighty-two years old and had been diagnosed with lung cancer two years before. She was waiting for a bronchoscopy — an examination of the respiratory tract by means of a lighted tube. Bored, restless, and miserable in the hospital, she confessed to Jeannie that she was going crazy because she hadn't had a cigarette in two days. All she wanted was one cigarette. But her doctor told her, "Don't smoke," her family said, "Don't smoke," and she was trying to comply. Which made it impossible for her to calm down, sleep, even lie still in her bed.

"I said, 'You know what? You've already got cancer. If a cigarette right now is going to help you get through this night, then let's go. I'll take you down to the smoking area and you can have your cigarette,'" Jeannie recounts. "I told her that she should still try and cut down and advised her not to exacerbate the disease. But at that point, one cigarette was not going to kill her, and it certainly wasn't going to prevent cancer not to smoke it."

The patient practically fell into Jeannie's arms with gratitude. The two women — one young and healthy, the other old and infirm — walked down to the smoking area. As the old woman relished each inhalation, Jeannie sat chatting with her. "We went back upstairs," Jeannie continues. "She felt much better. She slept through the night. She did better because she didn't have nicotine withdrawal to deal with on top of everything else."

Jeannie acknowledges that it is very difficult to step into the patient's shoes and feel how they pinch. But she believes the medical system renders this effort very difficult. Some feminists have argued that this would change if more women entered medicine and if the profession were to benefit from what some feminist scholars have called "women's way of knowing." The fact that 25 percent of all doctors and 50 percent of medical students are women has not altered medical reality much. I don't believe this transformation will occur when the balance between female and male physicians is equal or when more women attain power in the higher echelons of medicine. It is not so much the gender of physicians or nurses that makes them attend to the patient's experience of illness. What matters is how a particular discipline — medicine or nursing — defines its mission. If its mission is to defeat disease, then the patient may also be defeated in the process. If the mission is to acknowledge and deal with the reality of illness, then the patient's chances of emotional survival increase.

When Jeannie goes back down to Six Feldberg to care for patients, there is the usual mix of young and old, hopeful and hopeless, chronically and acutely ill. Late in the day, Jeannie goes into the room of an eighty-two-year-old patient named Salvatore Giancuomo.* He is a medium-sized man with a bald head, oval face, and the crooked nose of a prizefighter. For the past six years, Mr. Giancuomo has lived at a local nursing home. Confused, with a history of psychiatric problems, he is now in the hospital with a fever of unknown origin.

In his hospital johnny, Mr. Giancuomo lies in a bed in a semiprivate room. Next to him another male patient is studying the menus the nutrition department has left with him. Mr. Giancuomo's knees are bent and his sheet is crumpled beneath his feet. One hand is draped over the cold steel of the bed rail. Another rests at his side. His legs and arms are shaking. His eyes are riveted on the ceiling, as if by staring at the pattern of small dots on its soundproof panels, he can find an anchor that will attach him firmly to reality.

Jeannie begins to talk quietly with him. She asks him if he knows where he is and why. It is not a question merely intended to test and confirm his failing memory, but rather the first step in a process that will help him gain at least a temporary sense of security. She explains that he is at the Beth Israel, reviews the reasons for his admission, and tells him what the nurses and physicians are trying to do for him. While he was sleeping, she tells him, his son called to ask about his condition. When he seems agitated because he was unable to speak to his son, she promises that his son will call back. He seems to gain some comfort from her presence. The corners of his lips relax slightly.

Jeannie notices that he is sweating and reaches over to wipe his brow.

"Mr. Giancuomo," she says, "I am going out to get you a fresh johnny and sheets. Then I'll give you a bath to make you more comfortable." She walks down the long corridor to the supply room, pulls out towels, linen, a johnny, fills an aqua plastic basin with soap and water, and returns.

She begins with his head, wiping his bald pate, moving down across his forehead and stubbly cheeks. "Your face seems dry, Mr. Giancuomo. Do you use any skin cream at the nursing home?"

"Yes," he mumbles.

"Do you know what kind?" she queries. He tries to remember but cannot capture the brand name. "I'll call them and ask what kind," she says.

She has removed his johnny, using it to cover his body and protect him from the cold. Slipping it down to his navel, she begins to wash his chest in swift, low sweeps. To minimize the chill to his already vulnerable system, she rinses and dries an area as soon as she wets it and immediately covers him before washing the next spot.

"Mr. Giancuomo," she says, "I want you to turn over. Hold on to the bed rail while I do your back." She washes and dries his back, then his buttocks, thighs, and calves, and again covers him.

"You can turn over on your back now," she says. She lifts the sheet to reveal the front of his legs and his groin and moves the cloth up his leg, and under his scrotum. This could easily be perceived as an act of intrusion. Yet Jeannie deftly negotiates this intimate space so that her patient is neither mortified nor aroused.

Jeannie notices that he has wet the bed because he cannot manage to use the urine bottle that is attached to the bed rail at his side. To save him the considerable embarrassment of further bed-wetting, she asks him if he wants an external catheter put on so that he doesn't have to worry about going to the bathroom. Relieved, he agrees. After changing the sheets on his bed by rolling him gently from side to side, she goes out to get the catheter.

When she returns, she pulls up the sheet and begins to slip the condom-like rubber device over his penis. In the middle of the procedure, a dietitian walks into the room to ask Mr. Giancuomo's roommate for his menu choices. A minute later, a thin woman with short hair, a stethoscope draped around her neck, and a black canvas bag slung over her shoulder comes in. Abruptly she pulls aside the thin curtain that shields the patient from view and edges her way toward him. Barely acknowledging Jeannie's presence or the intimate activity she is engaged in, she briskly announces, "Hello, Mr. Giancuomo, I'm Dr. Jeffrey."*

Before he can respond, she begins a barrage of questions.

"Do you know where you are, Mr. Giancuomo?"

"In the hospital," he mutters.

"Do you know what day it is?"

He looks puzzled.

"Do you know the season? Is it winter, spring, summer, or fall?" He looks more baffled, as if he cannot comprehend why this woman would question him about the seasons while Jeannie Chaisson is manipulating his genitals. But the doctor — a resident assigned to the floor — seems oblivious to his discomfort. "Mr. Giancuomo," she prods impatiently. "Is it summer, fall, winter, spring?"

Desperate to satisfy her, he sputters, "I would like white rice and some tea."

With a look of disbelief, the resident turns to Jeannie for an explanation. Jeannie gestures toward the next bed, where the dietitian and Mr. Giancuomo's roommate are discussing the latter's meal requests. "He's listening to that." Jeannie interprets the appearance of white rice in a conversation about the seasons.

"Oh," the resident says without interest.

Jeannie has finished placing the catheter but remains at her patient's side.

"Can you put your right thumb up to your nose, Mr. Giancuomo?" the resident asks.

Trying hard to please, the old man pulls out his left hand and places his left thumb on his nose. The woman's eyes display her disappointment. As if to underscore his sense of humiliation, she asks the same question again. Again, he pulls out his left hand and puts it to his nose. "Yes," she observes in a judgmental monotone.

"Do you have any pain?" she asks.

"Yes," he stammers.

"Where?" she continues. He opens his mouth to explain but cannot.

"Fine. Well, thank you, Mr. Giancuomo," she says and turns to leave.

She sees me sitting in the corner taking notes and is caught up short. Thrusting out her hand, she asks me who I am. I shake it, introduce myself, and explain that I am writing a book on nursing.

"Oh," she says, and starts to walk out the door. Then she swivels. "What did you say you are writing?"

A book on nursing, I repeat.

She seems startled by the idea. "Oh, how nice," she asserts unconvincingly, and leaves.

Jeannie smiles ruefully. She bends over her patient and tells him she's going to see another patient. She reminds him that his son will call later and that the doctors will surely figure out why he's having the fever. Placing her hand over his, she squeezes it and tells him she'll be back again soon.

Grabbing an armful of dirty linens, she walks down the hall reflecting on the interaction that has just occurred. "She will never make a good doctor," Jeannie concludes. "She came in and saw me putting on the catheter and didn't figure out that this might not be a good time to ask him all these questions. He might, after all, be just a teeny bit distracted. When he said something inappropriate, she never tried to protect him from the realization that he'd just done the wrong thing. When she left, she did not try to comfort or reassure him. She just can't put herself in the patient's bed, in the patient's experience. She is too busy looking for clues to his disease or trying to assert her status. She will be a competent doctor and maybe people will think she's a good doctor. But that's only because most people don't know what a good doctor really is."

She shakes her head regretfully. Then she takes the bed linen, stows it in one of the containers along the corridor, and returns to the hubbub of the central desk area, with its crowd of physicians and nurses checking video screens, discussing cases on the telephone, and poring over patient charts.

Chapter 7

Collaborative Care

ELLEN KITCHEN

On Thursday mornings, the Beth Israel Home Care Department holds its weekly team meeting. There is no time for Ellen to fit in patient visits before this ten o'clock session begins. So she goes directly to the Home Care Department when she comes to work. A receptionist's desk sits immediately in front of the two glass doors. The large room is partitioned into smaller sections, each of which contains cubbyholes with a shelf, a drawer, and a small desk and phone for the nursing staff. The charts of the department's three hundred patients — most of them elderly, but some of them younger, shorter-term postsurgical or trauma patients or patients with AIDS — are kept in a large cabinet against the wall. At the back, to the left of the office, is a small conference room next to nurse manager Karen Dick's office, and there is another conference room next door.

None of the department's own conference rooms can, however, accommodate the congregation of physicians, nurses, social workers, occupational and physical therapists who attend team meeting each week to discuss their patients. The team reserves the pharmacy conference room in the bowels of the hospital. At ten of ten, Ellen and her colleagues head across a small parking lot behind the Beth Israel's main buildings. Entering through the heavy back doors, they walk through a maze of corridors to the Feldberg basement, where the meeting room is located.

Today, as usual, medical directors John Jainchill and Geraldine Zagarella are sitting at two long, rectangular Formica tables that have been pushed together. Both wear their standard uniform. For the fifty-four-year-old Jainchill, it's a rumpled suit and a white shirt with tie askew. His frizzy brown-and-gray-flecked hair is tousled. As he speaks, he occasionally runs his fingers through a graying beard. Gerry Zagarella, his wife and partner, is forty-nine. Her curly black hair masses wildly around her head and she wears a plain white cotton shirt, black slacks, and running shoes.

About five minutes later, psychiatrist Donna Mathias, a slender woman with short curly hair, comes in with Karen Dick. Social worker Mary Ann Wallace and physical therapists Helen Moulis and Sarah Harrington arrive a few minutes later. On occasion, a psychiatric resident accompanies Donna Mathias to team meeting. Similarly, when residents are working with Jainchill and Zagarella, they may attend. At times, the group may also have the help of a geriatric fellow.

For the next two hours, the team discusses a series of cases. The first half hour is devoted to patients' psychiatric problems. Today, for example, they discuss an elderly woman who is living alone and who has gradually stopped eating, bathing, and cleaning house. She has lost weight and refuses to take her medication for high blood pressure. The team speculates about the causes.

Did some event trigger the onset of this depression? Is it a bad time of year for her? Wasn't it at this time of year several years ago that her daughter died? Ellen asks. She could have an underlying medical condition — such as a thyroid problem — that hasn't been treated and that could account for such symptoms, someone else suggests. Or what about her medication regimen? With elderly patients who have multiple medical problems and take a lot of different medicines, medications could also be responsible. Questions fly: What's she taking? When did she start taking it? Has she had this kind of reaction in the past? Is this side effect common?

When Donna Mathias recommends an antidepressant, Ellen and other team members have additional concerns. How much does it cost? This woman is on a fixed income, and the cost of the drug must be considered. Because she may also be disoriented, it's important to know how many times a day she will need to take the medication. Many elderly patients lose track of pills they must take more than once a day.

When the discussion turns to medical problems, the nurses report on the patients they have seen during the week. They update other team members about the response of a variety of patients to treatment plans that were suggested at the previous meeting and advise them of new difficulties anyone may be experiencing. The team is always alert to any signs that a patient's condition is deteriorating so much that living at home is no longer safe. The goal of home care is to keep people at home, and the department's rate of nursing home placement is low. Nonetheless, the team members are constantly reassessing their patients' ability to function on their own. Their mission is to discover a patient's deteriorating condition before it results in an emergency — a fall that leaves the patient unable to call for help, a fire that starts because a patient forgets to turn off a stove, or a patient found wandering aimlessly around the neighborhood. If nursing home placement is necessary, the team wants that transition to be handled smoothly, on a nonemergency basis.

The nurses, physicians, and other staff members discuss their patients in a very collegial manner. The conversation is open and freewheeling. Sometimes doctors suggest a change in strategy on a particular case. Sometimes the nurses offer their ideas. During the course of this particular meeting, Ellen Kitchen talks about her patient Mac's failure to take his medication and her discovery that he had stopped taking his morning walk because of his problem with his diuretic. Then she describes Mrs. Beauchamp's dental problems.

Ellen's report on her handling of her patients highlights one of the big differences between nurse practitioners and bedside nurses. On the floor, nurses are much more bound by doctor's orders. Doctors are the ones who make the diagnosis and treatment plan, order the drugs and tests, write out the discharge orders, and dictate discharge summaries, although today, this process of giving "orders" provides nurses with greater latitude than it did in the past. For example, a doctor who is trying to manage a patient's postoperative pain may order pain medication within a certain dosage range. A surgical nurse will thus work within a set of parameters, adjusting the dosage of the medication to make sure the patient is comfortable. Similarly, a critical care nurse responsible for keeping a patient's blood pressure stable will be able to raise or lower the dosage of medication until the desired effect is achieved.

When nurses work closely with doctors, they often suggest the medications to be used or an alteration in the doctor's prescribed plan. But even if their input is accepted, it's often not publicly acknowledged. Only the doctor's orders — not the fact that the nurse may have recommended them — are recorded on the patient's chart. A nurse's participation in this aspect of patient care — and thus the collaborative nature of the health care enterprise — remains invisible. The written record, which reflects the formal chains of authority and command in the medical system, maintains the fiction that the doctor is solely in charge.

For nurse practitioners in Massachusetts, as in most other states, there is no such fiction. Nurse practitioners take patient histories, do complete physical exams, and use laboratory and related diagnostic tools to provide primary health care to their patients. Under physician supervision, nurse practitioners can also prescribe medications.

At Ellen's Thursday morning meeting with her colleagues, the entire team considers which drugs to prescribe, and which treatment plans to follow. The participating doctors recognize — and acknowledge — the fact that a nurse often knows the patients, their history, their financial status, and current physical and mental condition far better than they do. Can a patient tolerate a certain drug? Has he or she used it in the past? Will a patient find it too confusing to take medication that must be used several times a day? Will the pills be too expensive? All of these are questions the nurses may answer.

Home care nurses also have the knowledge — and freedom to use it — to help fulfill their patients' many other daily needs for shopping, feeding, cleaning, and social interaction. The team discussion, therefore, involves not only diagnoses and treatment recommendations, but patients' social and emotional functioning and the minutiae of their daily lives.

Successful home care work requires, wherever possible, both the construction of new social networks for the patient and the maintenance and preservation of their old ones. Maintaining healthy and helpful relationships between patients and their family and friends can be quite a challenge for team members. Sometimes it requires intervention on behalf of caregivers as well as patients. Consider, for example, a patient who is dependent on help from his sister. His sister does not live with him, but runs all his errands and does his shopping, laundry, and banking. Suddenly, the sister develops a mysterious resistance to leaving her own house. She thus curtails all of the life-sustaining excursions she once performed for her brother. In order to maintain their patient's independence, the team needs to know why this has happened.

The problem turns out to be incontinence. Like Ellen's patient Mac, the sister is afraid to leave the house because she keeps having embarrassing accidents. The team talks about this situation. The sister needs a medical workup to determine the cause of the incontinence so an appropriate treatment can be prescribed. If she gets help from an incontinence specialist and a clinical nurse specialist at the Beth Israel who assists patients with incontinence, she may be able to fully resume caring for her brother.

In many instances, the home care team must protect patients from family members. Another patient had a niece who was handling her finances and, in the process, stealing money from her. Sadly, the patient was completely torn about what to do. She was terrified that her niece would deplete her small savings account, but also afraid that — without some financial incentive — her niece would leave her and she would have no one to care for her. Ellen and John Jainchill talked about and with the woman for months. Finally the patient realized that the niece's thievery was too high a price to pay for her companionship and care. The team members arranged for someone else to handle the woman's finances.

In another case, a husband with mental problems was the primary caregiver for his wife — the victim of several serious strokes. Although she was unable to have sex, he kept pressing his attentions on her. The team had to work with both to calm the wife's resulting hysteria and defuse the husband's anger and misguided ardor.

Sometimes families endanger patients by deciding that their medications are not good for them and encouraging them not to take them. At other times, they think the medication is doing such a good job that more than the prescribed dose would be even better. "You name it and it's happened," Ellen says about the family situations the team has encountered over the past eight years.

Home care team members are also archivists of their patients' broader social community. "I get to know all of the people involved in helping my patients stay at home — from informal caregivers, like their family, friends, and neighbors, to their home health aides, who will be key in providing help with bathing, dressing, light meal preparation, and making beds, or their homemakers, who make meals and do shopping, laundry, and cleaning," Ellen explains. These people — not just family members — are critical to helping maintain a patient's independence.

This precarious independence is also contingent on the larger social web of private and public community, state, and national agencies that provide professional and financial assistance in the home and finance medical and other health needs. Nurses like Ellen become masters of the intricacies of state and federal regulations that can either help or hinder their patients.

"Nurse practitioners," says Karen Dick, "have to be familiar with the range of home health care agencies and services on the state and local level. For example, to get a homemaker, the nurse will have to make a referral to one of thirty-two different home care corporations that receive public funds for the provision and delivery of these services."

To get a home health aide, patients need to be in a home care program like the Beth Israel's. The program has two aides of its own, and it contracts with private agencies for others. There are also some community resources that will send volunteers into the home. "Nurses," says Dick, "are great at knowing which agency — the Little Brothers and Sisters, AIDS Action, hospice groups — can provide an added pair of hands or ears."

Home health care providers must also be experts in navigating the Byzantine, ever-changing regulations and requirements of private and public health insurance plans. Their patients depend on medical equipment, nutritional supplements, and of course medication, which are not always covered by these plans. When Mr. James came home from the hospital, for example, he could not keep any solid food down. He was becoming seriously dehydrated and malnourished. Ellen recommended that he take Megace, which is an appetite stimulant. The medication is quite expensive, and Medicare does not pay for drugs. Elderly patients who can afford it may have Medex coverage — private insurance that supplements Medicare. Mr. James didn't have the money to pay for such extra insurance. To make sure he had access to this medication, Ellen and John Jainchill worked with the Beth Israel pharmacy to obtain the medicine free.

Last year Mac needed a new bed. If he had been bed-bound already or if he had suffered a serious fracture that required a hospital bed, Medicare would have paid for it. Because what he needed was just a plain old bed — not a fancy hospital one — there was no help available from the government. So Ellen took Mac shopping to find the best possible deal on a mattress purchased with his own money. Then Bea McIntyre, the Beth Israel home health aide, and her husband picked it up for Mac, removed his old mattress, and installed the new one.

"You can't imagine how many hours you might have to spend on the phone trying to figure out the maze of private insurance benefits we have to deal with," Ellen says, raising her eyebrows. "A patient needs a hospital bed. So you have to find out if their private insurance will cover it. You call and ask. But insurers are not always forthcoming with the information. You are told that they can't have a hospital bed without having a certain diagnosis. Well, you ask, what is that diagnosis?"

The person on the other end of the phone hems and haws. "You have to ask for brochures that describe the insurance benefits. You have to press for an answer to find out what diagnosis a person needs to get what, what DRG they have to fall under."

The issue is not just ascertaining what benefits patients get, but the maximum benefits to which they are entitled. "You have to figure out what the bottom line is," Ellen adds. "And you can't do that without outright asking. It's very complicated. For example, if a patient is terminal and is not on Medicare, which would make them eligible for a hospice benefit, you have to know just what the benefits are. Sometimes for example, a person will be eligible for hospice care only if they are not admitted to the hospital. If they are admitted, they lose the benefit. That's an important thing to know."

Which means, Ellen says, that you have to keep up not only with current benefit determinations, but with changes in policy. What might have been true six months ago can change, Ellen says, and may no longer be applicable when the patient needs care again.

Although the media have tended to focus on the "newness" of the nurse practitioner role and the similarities between nurse practitioners and primary care physicians (a headline in the *New York Times* recently proclaimed, "The next doctor you see is a nurse"), when Ellen Kitchen rides her bike to visit the poor and elderly of Boston, she is a direct descendant of the public health nurses of more than a century ago. Those visiting nurses trudged through the tenements of America's big industrial cities, caring for poor and immigrant workers and their families. To reach their patients, they rode their horses through the mountains of Appalachia and other rural areas where they delivered some of the only care rural Americans received. Nurse practitioners are not some unexpected offshoot of medicine. The specialty grew out of the nursing innovations of the nineteenth and early twentieth centuries.

In the U.S., home care, or visiting nursing, has existed in some form for even longer. The first reported group of home care nurses was found in Charleston, South Carolina, in 1813 and was known as the Ladies Benevolent Society. Later, in the 1880s, the kind of home care nursing developed two decades earlier in England became the model for expanded home care for the sick poor in the U.S. The evolution of home care occurred in England after William Rathbone, a wealthy gentleman, hired a trained nurse to care for his wife at home. Rathbone was so impressed by the care his wife received that he felt trained nurses should also give such care to the sick poor. In 1859, he started an experiment in what we now call home care nursing for the sick poor. However, he was unable to recruit enough trained nurses to do the job. In desperation he approached Florence Nightingale with his plans in 1861. Nightingale was extremely supportive, and the two worked together to further develop the idea of the district nurse. These nurses operated in the community at large, serving impoverished patients in their own homes.

The district nurse concept spread slowly to America. Initially women in the urban, industrialized Northeast began to open small district nursing associations that tried to teach people how to get well and stay healthy. In America, visiting nursing exploded in the 1880s and 1890s when American pioneers transported Nightingale's concept of the district nurse to the United States. One of the major turning points for home care and community nursing was the Chicago World's Fair in 1893. There nurses from England and the U.S. met for the first time. They heard a presentation of a paper by Florence Nightingale entitled "Sick Nursing and Health Nursing," which articulated a vision of the role that nurses played in both the acute care setting and in the community and promoted the idea of health teaching.

One of the nurses at the Chicago World's Fair was Lillian Wald. Born in 1867, Wald grew up in a comfortable midwestern Jewish family who moved to Rochester, New York, when Wald was eleven. Like Nightingale, Wald began searching for a purpose for her life during adolescence. Through contact with a nurse who cared for her sister when the latter was ill during a pregnancy, Wald discovered her mission. Against her parents' wishes, Wald decided to become a nurse. She moved from Rochester to New York City to attend the School of Nursing of the New York Hospital and graduated in 1891. She then went to work for the New York Juvenile Asylum and after a year enrolled in the Woman's Medical College, not to become a doctor but to enhance her medical knowledge.

In 1893, Wald volunteered to teach a class in home care and hygiene for immigrant women at the Louis Technical School. One day, as Wald was showing her students how to make a clean bed, a young girl burst into the room in tears and explained that her mother could not attend class because she was too sick. Clearly, the child and her mother needed help. Wald excused herself. She followed the girl down filthy streets and up the stairs of a dark, bleak tenement. There she found the sick woman lying on a blood-stained mattress in a dark room. She had given birth two days earlier.

It was during this shocking encounter that poverty became a reality to Wald rather than an abstraction. She had stumbled on something she had never seen before — a family of seven living in two tiny rooms, leasing space to other immigrants, who slept on makeshift mattresses. The father, who was crippled, had to beg for a living. Wald later described her feelings. in these words: "All the maladjustments of our social and economic relations seemed epitomized in this brief journey and what was found at the end of it. The family to which the child led me was neither criminal nor vicious. . . . And although the sick woman lay on a wretched, unclean bed, soiled with a hemorrhage two days old, they were not degraded human beings, judged by any measure of moral values."

What they — and others like them — needed was help. And Wald resolved to give it to them.

She determined to move into the immigrant community and provide nursing care to those too poor to hire private duty nurses at home or obtain any other kind of medical care. She recruited Mary Brewster, a colleague from nursing school, to join with her in this project and approached the wealthy philanthropist Jacob Schiff, who agreed to finance their work for six months.

With Brewster, Wald moved to the Lower East Side and into a tenement home. Her work was so successful that Schiff continued to underwrite it. In 1895, she moved to larger quarters that would become the famous Henry Street Settlement. Like others associated with the urban settlement movement, she had begun to understand the connection between poverty and disease, between social conditions and personal conditions and illness. Joined later by nurses like Lavinia Dock, Wald and her colleagues coupled nursing, political activism, and the battle for the rights of women.

"What Wald did was critical," says University of Pennsylvania nursing historian Karen Buhler-Wilkerson. "She made a conceptual leap. She moved beyond a charitable to a social agenda by insisting that illness and poverty were inseparable. She had a bigger concept of why people were sick and a sense of the social agenda related to illness. She believed that poverty led to illness and that illness led to poverty. The two were inseparable in the households in which she was working, and she insisted that society had to address people's social needs and their physical needs or nothing would ever move forward. She called this new idea public health nursing."

Providing the kind of home care that nursing has pioneered is a multifaceted process. Solving the myriad problems of individual patients is like putting together a puzzle composed of many little pieces. Without a cohesive team, it would be impossible for Ellen or any of the physicians, nurses, social workers, therapists, and other personnel she works with to identify the different forms of support and care that each patient needs and assemble them into a coherent whole. Interdisciplinary collaboration is essential to her delivery of quality patient care.

Of course "teamwork" and "collaboration" are also the most popular new buzz words heard throughout health care today. Administrators, insurance executives, industry consultants, and public policymakers all extol the virtues of smooth-running interdisciplinary teams. Teamwork, they insist, is one of the keys to quality care and, more important, to the kind of efficiencies that produce cost savings. There is, however, a major roadblock that obstructs the fulfillment of this ideal: very few health care professionals have been taught how to work with one another or are encouraged to do so on the job. In most health care institutions, the infrastructure for teamwork is simply nonexistent. At the Beth Israel, more effort has been made than at many hospitals to promote cooperation between doctors and nurses. They are supposed to respect each other, get along with each other, share patients and information, and make important decisions about patient care jointly rather than separately. That's the ideal.

Because good professional relations do not automatically flow from good intentions, this ideal is not always translated into reality. When I observed Nancy on the Hematology / Oncology Clinic, for example, nurses met formally with their nursing colleagues to discuss the delivery of their care. They met with social workers. Similarly, social workers would routinely meet with each other. But nurses, social workers, and physicians never formally met as a group.

To move toward greater collaboration, in 1994 a group of nurses established practice groups. Three practice groups comprising one social worker, four, or sometimes fewer, nurses, and one fellow would share a particular group of patients. They gathered weekly to discuss these cases and patient care issues. The nurses hoped that such practice groups would allow new patients to meet a multidisciplinary group, rather than just an attending and fellow, as they came to the clinic. This would permit patients to ask questions of nurses and social workers and would give the latter the opportunity to discuss their perspectives and address patients' social and emotional needs.

In 1996, nurses proposed bringing attendings into these practice groups. But apart from this good beginning, the nurses, social workers, fellows, and attendings still do not meet together as a unit.

On the floor Jeannie Chaisson works on, collaboration may be inhibited by other structural constraints. As Beth Israel general surgeon Leon Goldman explains, "When you construct a floor of forty patients in a large rambling setting and make sure that attendings and house officers are always changing; when you never, ever keep them the same; when nobody has their name tag on, so nobody knows who's who; when it's always very busy and doctors and nurses don't meet together; then you're all set. Nobody will ever work together. No one will be able to because they never know each other."

While I was observing health care professionals at the Beth Israel, there was a serious effort on the inpatient units to break down the kind of barriers Goldman describes. At the instigation of clinical nurse specialist Adele Pike and her colleagues in nursing, a fourteen-bed unit was specifically designed to study and encourage nurse-physician collaboration. Pike recruited a number of experienced nurses and physicians to work to change the patterns of behavior that thwart collaboration between professionals. Among the original physician participants were Leon Goldman, Gerry Zagarella and John Jainchill, and a number of other physicians. In its four years of existence, the unit generated interesting models and research that demonstrated how physician / nurse collaboration could have a positive impact on patient care and staff morale. (Sadly, when the economic pressures of the early nineties hit the BI and other hospitals, this very successful unit was closed.)

Home Care is a living example of a genuine commitment to interdisciplinary collaboration. In Home Care, one element contributing to the cohesion of the group is the fact that all the nurses and doctors involved are very experienced clinicians and thus have the educational and professional qualifications that foster mutual trust. Home Care nurses are older and more experienced than the new grads on a floor like Jeannie Chaisson's. They are very aware of their strengths and their limits and are willing to acknowledge both. "Just as a doctor needs to recognize the limits of his or her practice and ask for help when he or she needs it, so, too, a nurse practitioner has to do the same," Ellen says. "If someone has a problem, they have to ask for help. We talk constantly with our physician colleagues."

The Home Care physicians also have a track record of working closely with nurses. Zagarella started doing home care when she was a resident at Boston City Hospital (BCH). When she had several patients who were unable to come to the hospital to see her, she went into their homes to care for them. In 1979, after the completion of her residency, she and a nurse practitioner, Cindy McCrystal, started the North End Community Health Center's home care program. Zagarella has been the medical director there ever since.

Her husband, John Jainchill, came to home care later in his career.

He did his training at BCH and Columbia Presbyterian Hospital in Manhattan. He then worked in neighborhood health centers in Boston and at the primary care training program at BCH. In 1977, he was one of the founding members of the Urban Medical Group. Urban Medical is an inner-city, private, nonprofit group practice dedicated to the care of the chronically ill — people with complicated medical conditions that our health care system tends to ignore. When Urban Medical was created, one of its first missions was to help revive the Beth Israel's then underutilized home care program. Eight years ago, Jainchill took over the medical direction of the Home Care Department. Seven years ago Zagarella joined him.

Respect flourishes easily in Home Care because the small cast of characters works together over time. Interdisciplinary communication is systematically organized in weekly meetings. Attendance is a priority of the program. "Everyone knows how important these team meetings are," Zagarella says. "It's not hard to get people to come. It's a given in our practice. We look forward to them and to seeing each other."

What this commitment to interprofessional communication breeds is a genuine desire to develop or enhance a colleague's skills. "The relationship that develops between physicians and nurse practitioners," says Zagarella, "is based on what we can teach them and they can teach us. In many cases, nurse practitioners are so knowledgeable that there's not a lot we can teach them. In some cases, there may be real gaps in knowledge of body systems and mode of action of medication. These bits of knowledge are easily imparted and go a long way toward enhancing satisfaction of patient and provider."

Because nurses are so expert in the care of their patients, Jainchill explains, home care physicians must adopt a very different patient management style. "Many doctors want to micromanage their patients. They want to control every detail of care. If you are in home care, that's the nurses' job, not yours. You macromanage. You back up the nurse if she needs it. You provide reassurance for her, maybe some knowledge base if you have it. But day-to-day care should be the nurse practitioner's job."

In my experience very few doctors publicly acknowledge the importance of nurses to their ability to provide quality care to their patients. But Jainchill and Zagarella explicitly state that for home care patients nurses are *more* important than doctors. "The medical model is a curative model." Jainchill explores the distinctions. "The nursing model is a care and comfort model. That doesn't mean that nurses don't want to cure or that doctors don't want to give care and comfort. But given where the two disciplines start from, if you have a patient who does not have curable illness, nurses are going to have a head start."

This kind of collaboration is a benefit not only to nurses and doctors but to patients, particularly when the patient is suffering from a terminal illness, or one that is difficult to manage.

As the 1995 SUPPORT study on the care of dying patients illustrated so strikingly, one of the times when lack of collaboration most inhibits nursing practice and quality of patient care is when a patient is dying. Ellen's work with terminally ill patients in the last stages of their life has been sustained by her physician colleagues in ways that are rarely reported by nurses involved in more traditional, professional relationships in the hospital setting. When Ellen and I talked about the problems of dealing with death and dying, she immediately recounted the story of a patient who had proved to be an unexpected challenge. In dealing with this patient, support from her physician colleagues, she said, proved to be invaluable.

Mrs. Marjorie Jeffries* — a patient Ellen shared with Gerry Zagarella — was a widow in her eighties. Her husband had been a corporate lawyer and she had been a librarian. Over the years, she had experienced problems with congestive heart failure and some kidney failure. But she had managed to remain active, live in her own house, and travel to visit out-of-town friends and relatives. Until the episode that brought her to Ellen.

Mrs. Jeffries had been planning an extensive journey to visit her children and grandchildren. She had planned to go to New York to visit a son. From there, she was supposed to fly to New Mexico to visit a daughter and grandchildren. Suddenly, she suffered a massive heart attack that irreversibly damaged her heart and kidneys, transforming her from a vital, independent woman to an invalid. Released from the hospital but bedridden at home, she could barely stand up without the help of family members and professional caregivers.

"The situation was terrible in many ways," Ellen recalls. "Unlike a lot of my patients, whose decline is long and slow, this heart attack happened so suddenly that she had no time to adapt."

In other ways, however, Mrs. Jeffries was more fortunate than most of Ellen's patients. Mac, Mrs. Beauchamp, and countless others live by themselves with little or no family support. They have no money to pay for surrogate family caregivers. Mrs. Jeffries had close relatives — both nearby and elsewhere in the country — involved in her care or decisions about her care. She already had a housekeeper, who had been working for her for years and was able to continue cleaning house and cooking. The housekeeper, Ellen found, knew some basic home health aide skills, such as turning, bathing, and massaging a patient.

Ellen quickly discovered that Mrs. Jeffries was also unlike many of her other patients in her clear understanding that the end was near and in her forthright expression of her wishes about how she wanted — and didn't want — to die.

"Mrs. J. was a very articulate woman," Ellen explains. "She could verbalize what she felt. With Zag and her cardiologist, she had been able to state her wishes quite clearly. She told them she wanted to die at home. She did not want to be on a respirator. And, at all costs, she wanted to avoid any trips to the ER. Many other people either haven't thought about these issues or don't understand what's involved with high-tech medical care. They think, 'Well, if I get pneumonia, I want to be treated for pneumonia. If I have a cardiac arrest, I want to be rescued.' They say this with no understanding of what it means to get CPR or be on a respirator. Mrs. Jeffries understood it all. She knew what the outcome of such decisions would be."

On a visit to Mrs. Jeffries's house, Ellen was sitting in the patient's comfortable bedroom. The woman's daughter was at her side. As Ellen was inquiring about the patient's health and state of mind, Mrs. J. interrupted. What would happen, she asked, if she stopped taking the cardiac medication prescribed to keep her from being in overt heart failure?

The question took Ellen by surprise. This was not an angry patient ranting about the necessity of taking medication or making idle threats about stopping it. Mrs. Jeffries stated her question in a sober manner. She was definitely engaged in a serious reflection about stopping life-sustaining treatment.

Ellen tried not to exhibit her surprise and responded, "What will happen is, you'll probably go into congestive heart failure and you'll have some trouble breathing. Then your lungs will fill up with water and eventually you'll die."

This prospect did not silence the patient.

"How long will that take?" she asked immediately.

"It might take weeks," Ellen responded.

The patient and her daughter said nothing. They were mulling over the information the nurse had provided so that they could make a momentous decision.

What Ellen found so unsettling was not the subject of death itself. As a nurse she had talked with many patients about death and dying. She is, in fact, grateful that a number of her patients have felt comfortable talking with her about the subject. In order to facilitate a discussion about the kind of treatment a patient desires at the end of life, Ellen says she usually asks, "What would your wishes be if you went out and were hit by a car and were unconscious? If you weren't going to regain consciousness, what would you want to happen?"

To better approach one of the last taboo subjects in American culture, Ellen often shares personal details. She explains that she and her husband have discussed their wishes about heroic treatment and have prepared health care proxies. These legal documents assign a relative or friend to act as a proxy who will make health care decisions when and if a person is unable to make them him or herself. Some patients recoil from any such discussion of death, Ellen says, because they fear that it means their condition and prospects are worse than the nurse or doctor has revealed. "My God," they tend to think, "this nurse is talking to me about death because she knows I'm going to die." She finds that confiding her own willingness to contemplate death and prepare for it helps to open the doors of communication with her patients.

"I advise patients to read all about health care proxies and living wills and have discussions about their wishes. I suggest that they find someone who could serve as a health care proxy. Most people appreciate this kind of conversation. Some people even anticipate this concern and raise it themselves."

But Ellen's bedside role with Mrs. Jeffries after the patient's heart attack was quite different from a chat about the hypotheticals involved in health care proxies. Over the next weeks, the subject was Mrs. Jeffries's major preoccupation. She repeatedly asked what would happen if she stopped her drugs. When would she die? What would it be like? How long would it take? Should she do it? If so, when should she do it?

Just before Thanksgiving, the patient made her decision. She stopped taking her medication for a week. Oxygen tanks had been brought into the home and morphine was prescribed, if she needed it, to ease Mrs. Jeffries's breathing. Nurses visited her daily to make sure she was comfortable and to support her family caregivers and cleaning woman. As the holiday approached, however, she relented. She was fearful that she would expire right before Thanksgiving, ruining that occasion for her family and also leaving them with a permanent association between the holiday and her death. But the patient's planning of that event soon resumed. Perhaps, she thought, she would wait until one of her daughters completed a move to the West Coast. That date would be her marker. But no, it would only make things more difficult for her daughter if, after just having gotten settled in, she was called back to Boston for her mother's funeral.

Finally, Mrs. J. just stopped taking her pills again. She waited, but nothing happened. She didn't die. But her breathing became more difficult and she was very tired. As she deteriorated, she developed bedsores on her legs that required frequent dressing changes. Ellen and her colleagues thus continued to see her daily. "During this time," Ellen recounts, "she slept more and withdrew from all the things that gave her pleasure."

She stopped listening to the classical music that had almost always played in the background. She stopped reading the *New York Times*, and the novels and biographies stacked at her bedside went unopened. "She stopped watching television and lost all interest in food. It was practically impossible to get her to eat or drink," Ellen says.

Mrs. Jeffries and her family also began to restrict the steady stream of visitors who had hitherto been welcomed into the house. "Whenever I went to see her," Ellen recalls, "she was always very cordial and sweet. But you could sense her gradual retreat from life."

As it became clear that her deterioration was accelerating, her children and grandchildren, who had visited frequently, came to stay.

About three and a half weeks after she stopped taking her pills, she died peacefully in her sleep.

Ellen says she will never forget Mrs. Jeffries. "What was different about her was her active involvement in deciding how she would die." For many patients it is the rhythm of disease and the traditional responses of the medical system that are the determining factors. Not so with Mrs. Jeffries. She was determined that she would not let a medical crisis — a cardiac arrest, congestive heart failure, pneumonia — put her in an intensive care unit. As Ellen emphasized repeatedly, she also had the financial and emotional resources to sustain that decision. And she had the respect and support of her physician and nurse, who made sure the necessary drugs, equipment, and nursing care were available.

Throughout this vigil, Mrs. Jeffries's nurse practitioner also had the support of her own medical colleagues. Ellen and Geraldine Zagarella were in constant contact. Ellen was able to talk freely with Zagarella about Mrs. Jeffries's medical management. And she was also able to express her own personal feelings of grief as she watched her patient decline. "I liked this lady and her family very much," Ellen explains wistfully. "It was just one of those relationships that clicked. So there was a personal link. Zag reaffirmed to me that I was really supporting her through this, because her quality of life had deteriorated and she was clearly miserable."

When both nurse and doctor share the same philosophy of care, Ellen and Zagarella both believe, it helps everyone involved — particularly the patient. In a truly collaborative practice, nurses and physicians can provide such support for each other in these situations because, as Zagarella puts it, "We have this understanding that at some point death is the goal. That's where our patients are going. That's where everybody's going. It's just a question of how we're getting there. Some doctors don't want to acknowledge that reality, and that makes it very difficult for the nurse practitioners and for patients. The nurses, of course, want their patients to live. But the difference between them and doctors is that doctors are trained to believe that if you're not fixing people, you're not doing your job. Nurses are educated to accept death."

The nursing model, John Jainchill once told me, is better suited to the kind of diffuse problems many of these elderly homebound patients have. A patient is depressed. Why? There are problems with family caregivers or children or other relatives. What are they? You try everything and nothing seems to work. What's really going on?

"With most of these patients, there are terrible difficulties getting them to do what you want them to do," Jainchill explains. "Nurse practitioners are a lot more competent than docs at dealing with this. The doctor model is, 'Patient, you do this,' and the patient is supposed to do it. But nurse practitioners assume that they must look at what's going on with the whole person in order to find out what's really going on. And they can often do this more easily because they go into the patients' home, onto their turf, where patients feel they have more control."

There is no better example of this than Mr. Elijah Fitch. When Ellen is making her rounds, she invariably tries to save a great deal of time for Mr. Elijah Fitch. "I can't run in and out on him," she explains. "He needs a good hour visit. He won't tolerate anything less."

Indeed, today, she will need more than an hour for Mr. Fitch. When she arrived at work this morning, she learned from reading the patient's chart that Mr. Fitch has missed two days of the steroids that control his emphysema, which he takes episodically for flare-ups, or in the summer and during pollen season. During these flare-ups, Ellen or another nurse visits him sometimes as much as three to four times a week. Although Ellen packages Mr. Fitch's medicine carefully in doses covering two weeks at a time, somehow Mr. Fitch managed to jump from one medication box to the other, skipping his prednisone in the process. Over the weekend, he phoned the home care nurse who was on call to say that he had no prednisone left.

"Who knows what really happened," Ellen says with resignation. "Whatever it was, it's just not a good situation, because when you're on steroids, you have to taper down very slowly because your body gets used to the increased amount of steroids. This is the first time this has happened with the steroids, but periodically he will call up and say, 'I've missed my dose of medicine, what should I do?'"

When she reaches Mr. Fitch's apartment at about four o'clock, he is stationed in a worn brown armchair next to a large picture window that looks out on the corner of a busy intersection near downtown Boston. It's a bright, sunny afternoon, but the sunlight does not penetrate his apartment. In spite of this, the lamp that sits on the small tabl next to his chair is unlit. Mr. Fitch, a wizened old man with close-cropped gray hair, greets Ellen with a barren smile and a look of disgruntlement.

There is little in his past or future to bring him cheer. His wife died years ago and they had no children. He was the youngest of four children, but has outlived them all by twenty or thirty years. To be nearer to one of his only remaining relatives — a niece — he moved from Chicago to Boston fifteen years ago. But soon after he arrived, his niece was diagnosed with cancer. After he was hospitalized for a heart attack, his niece called Mr. Fitch to tell him she had also been admitted to the hospital. Don't worry, it's nothing, she reassured him. But before he was well enough to visit her, the woman's doctor called to say she had died.

Now, in his late eighties, he is dependent on an elderly home-maker who is herself slightly demented and afflicted with agonizing arthritis in her knees. She lives in the same building as Mr. Fitch and manages to cook dinner for him each night. A home health aide also stops by four days a week — often to be told that there's nothing for her to do. "This really frustrates the heck out of her," Ellen notes.

For Mr. Fitch, old age has been a series of painful and humiliating blows. His body has, in fact, become his prison. As a younger man he smoked heavily and, like half of all smokers, will probably die of complications from smoking, such as emphysema and heart disease. He's had two recent heart attacks already. He spends his days tethered to a large oxygen machine that sits at the other end of the bare, buff-colored living room. Until last year, he was able to go outside and walk around the block. Now even walking out of his apartment and down the corridor is exhausting for him.

Not surprisingly, Mr. Fitch tends to welcome Ellen with a catalog of complaints. Why does he have to take one pill or another? Had he known smoking would do this to him, he never would have smoked all those years. Why didn't anybody tell him? Why is the food they bring him from Meals on Wheels so bad? Why isn't his breathing better? "How am I going to breathe if you don't give me nothing?" he demands grumpily.

Ellen has heard it all before. "One day," she recalls, "he got the idea that the inhaler manufacturers stopped putting as much medicine in the product he uses to help him breathe. He insisted that the inhaler just didn't have the kick it used to have. I said, 'Gee, Mr. F., I don't think that's what they're doing.' But he saw it as a conspiracy. Once in a while he relates it to race and insists they're not giving him the quality that they're giving other people. Sometimes he gets petrified that he's not going to be able to breathe, so he hoards inhalers, which is a problem because we can't monitor how much he is getting, how much he needs, and how effective the treatment is."

Today Mr. Fitch begins by complaining about the prednisone. Ellen takes it in her stride. "I know how hard it is to take the prednisone, Mr. F. But what it does is open everything up so you can breathe." She patiently describes the drug's purpose as she walks into the kitchen to crush some pills for him. Then, as the oxygen machine hums in the background, she listens to his chest.

"You're pretty tight, Mr. F.," she reports.

He gives her a look filled with anger and self-pity. "How do you like seeing a nice guy like me go down to nothing?" he says.

As she sits by his side holding his arm to draw blood, Ellen lists the positive developments that have occurred over the years. There was the victory of getting him off his arthritis medication, indications that the prednisone has helped him and is only taken for a short while, and the fact that his increased breathing difficulties are related to pollen season — which will be over shortly.

But Mr. Fitch is inconsolable. As Ellen leaves the apartment, he sits forlornly in the late-afternoon gloom, his head turned toward the window, where he can gaze out at life — tantalizing and untouchable — on one of the busy street corners in Boston.

As we walk down the hall away from the irascible old man, Ellen sadly sums up his plight. "He is always angry. He gets angry at me. Then he wants to see his doctor. When he sees her, he gets angry at her, too, even though I'm constantly reminding him that she also has asthma and her own breathing problems. It's inevitable," she sighs. "I'm the warm body he sees every week, and he blames me because he's not getting better. I feel bad for him."

I ask her if she gets frustrated when patients like Mr. Fitch use her as a verbal punching bag.

"No," she says sincerely. "I'm used to it. It's part of my job. He gets it off his chest. I try to bring him back to reality, but sometimes he just likes to vent. So I let him."

Ellen's empathic manner is, of course, the product of years of experience on the job, in both the hospital and the home care settings. But it also reflects her profound understanding of the impact of illness on a person's life — an understanding that is also derived from personal experience.

When she was in her mid-thirties, Ellen became pregnant with her first child. She and her husband, John Kitchen, who works in advertising, had, like many professional couples, put off having children until they were established in their careers. When they learned they were going to have a baby, they were thrilled. But Ellen lost the baby late in the pregnancy. As a result, she also developed some serious health problems.

Ellen recalls this period in her life as we sit in her new home in a suburb south of Boston talking about her many experiences dealing with the old and infirm. The entire ordeal, she says, with great emotion in her voice, gave her a new view of illness and death.

"Losing the baby was the greatest shock to us. It was the last thing in the world we expected, because until then we had led such an uncomplicated life. It made us realize how fragile human life is. I gained a lot of insight into what loss means to people."

Ellen does not advertise the basis for this insight. Although some of her patients know about her experience, she believes that "there's no point in telling people."

Similarly, being sick, she says, "helped me understand how people feel about illness. I learned first-hand how terrifying illness can be, how overwhelmed you can get." She says being a nurse did not make her experience any easier to bear. Because she knows more than the average person, it almost made it worse.

As I leave her house after this interview, she stops me. "I don't know if I articulated this well enough. But I think that everything that happened to me has helped me understand what it means to a family to have someone they love suddenly get a diagnosis of serious illness, to suddenly be sick. It doesn't matter if you're eighty-five or thirty-five, it's a terrible shock and a terrible strain on the family to have this happen."

When Ellen talks about her illness, you can feel the kind of anxiety she has lived with and to some degree will always live with. It is that shared feeling that also feeds her ability to relate so well to the Mr.

Fitches of the world. Mr. Fitch is eighty-eight and Ellen forty-four. He is poor, she is a well-to-do professional. He is black. She is white. On the face of it, there could not be two people more different than Ellen Kitchen and Elijah Fitch. Underneath, there are moments when they could not be more alike.

Chapter 8

A Good Enough Death

NANCY RUMPLIK

The United States is not winning the war against cancer. Despite advances in the treatment of some cancers, overall cure rates for most of the major cancers — lung, breast, colon, prostate — haven't changed much in thirty years. Patients whose cancers recur are likely to die of them. There have been, however, significant advances in keeping people comfortable, dealing with their pain and symptoms, and alleviating their suffering.

Each year, five hundred thousand Americans die of cancer. In addition, a relatively new group of patients suffer from AIDS-related malignancies. They die from AIDS and its complicating infections and cancers. Ralph Philmore* is one of those patients. Unlike Deborah Celli and Carol Benoit, he is not an easy patient to care for or about. His name first comes up during one of the nurses' Tuesday support group meetings. Eight nurses have crammed their chairs into the small family room. Nancy is among them, as is the clinic's manager, Ellen Powers, and the group's facilitator, psychiatric clinical nurse specialist Lesley Ail.

Today, Frances Kiel and Myrielle Whittle can barely wait to begin. The day before in the clinic, they were confronted with Ralph Philmore. He is an IV drug user with AIDS who is coming for treatment of Kaposi's sarcoma. The nurses in the clinic are no strangers to AIDS. But their typical KS patient has been a gay male in his late thirties to mid-forties, middle class to upper middle class, well-educated, both in general and about his disease. These patients tend to become partners in their care and assert their right to make decisions in a firm but nonetheless polite manner. But as the AIDS epidemic changes, so do the patients who come to the Beth Israel. Suddenly these nurses are seeing some of the kinds of patients that fill public hospitals. Often homeless, poor, and in trouble with the police, they are IV drug users who were unable to cope with life before they got the disease. Afterward — particularly as the disease progresses — they are even less able to do so. They present an entirely different challenge to the nurses, physicians, and social workers who care for them than the gay HIV / AIDS patient.

Ralph Philmore fits this description completely. Although Nancy had signed up as his primary nurse, she was out of the clinic when he came in to receive chemotherapy for KS the day before this meeting. Myrielle and Frances were in the clinic while Ralph was sitting receiving the IV medication. Other patients were seated in the clinic's blue high-back chairs. Philmore was seated right in the middle of this group of patients. He was anxious, uncomfortable, and fidgeting in his seat. But he seemed tractable enough. At the support group meeting they describe what happened next. Suddenly, Myrielle and Frances turned around and saw that Philmore was standing up, trying to leave. Myrielle asked him to wait and then noticed, to her horror, that his IV was no longer in his arm. The needle, covered with lethal blood, was dangling off the tubing, and his arm was dripping blood on the floor.

"I didn't have gloves on," Myrielle explains — the anger still fresh in her voice. "But I had to stop the bleeding, so I grabbed some gauze and tried to put on a bandage. He took the gauze, pushed it off, and just stalked out."

Nurses are used to danger, but Myrielle and Frances are furious about being put in a situation that compromised their safety and that of the other patients in the unit. Nancy enters the discussion, commenting that she felt from the first that there was something "off" about this patient. After a short discussion, they decide that they need to have a meeting with the patient's oncologist to find out more about the patient and figure out — as a team — how best to deal with him.

That session, involving the doctor, the clinic's nurse manager, Ellen Powers, and Nancy, proves to be very enlightening. It turns out that Ralph has had three hospital admissions for psychiatric problems. On one occasion he had expressed homicidal feelings. "So what's he going to do next?" Nancy raises her eyebrows and posits a worst-case scenario. "Pull out his needle again and spurt blood or use the needle as a weapon?"

This was not such a far-fetched scenario. One AIDS patient in the hospital had apparently done just that. While he was on one of the floors, he "flipped out," stood up, removed his IV needle, and deliberately spurted blood while threatening to poke someone with the needle. She shudders at the thought of it. The doctor suggests that he and other staff members should perhaps refuse to treat Ralph Philmore anymore. But Nancy demurs. She wants to talk with Ralph further before taking such a final step.

"What I learned is that people who try to control you do that because they feel so out of control themselves." Nancy explains her reasoning after the meeting. "It's important to give him a chance, to let him get to know me and see if that can decrease his anger. I think we have to anticipate and have a plan in his case so that he doesn't get out of hand and lose control. He represents a danger because of the HIV and the fact that he pulled the needle out. He had infectious blood dripping out of him, and a patient walking by or a nurse could have been hurt. This increases the risk of caring for him a hundred percent above normal."

Several days later, Ralph shows up in the clinic again. Hearing the staff talk about him in his absence, I'd imagined an imposing, frightening hulk of a man. Instead, he is small, frail, clearly on his last legs. His face is blotched and pale, his gait faltering. "Can I sit down and rest?" is the first thing he says when he sees Nancy.

Nancy pulls the curtain around a chair so that he can have some privacy. She rolls in a stool and sits next to him. Lowering her voice, she immediately addresses her concern and that of other staff. "I wasn't there when you pulled the needle out," she says, referring to this recent incident. "But it wasn't properly done. Some blood was spilled and the needle wasn't capped. That's a major concern to anyone in health care," she explains patiently.

Barely able to muster the energy to listen, he shrugs. "I've pulled needles out before, it's not a big deal."

"Well, we have to address this," she counters firmly. Then, in a more empathic voice, "I just want you to know, I'm glad you're back, and I want to reassure you that your care here won't be affected by this incident. We just have to worry about the safety of the other patients and staff. We care about you. We know you need your chemo, and you'll get it."

When he hears those words, Ralph seems to dissolve. "I don't know if I can handle the chemo again," he says softly, beginning to weep. "I know I'm going to die soon. All I wanted was a week or two with my wife to feel better and I never do feel better." Nancy places her hand on his and just sits with him.

About an hour and a half later, he quietly leaves the clinic. Three days later, Nancy visited Ralph again when he was admitted to the ICU, where he died.

Although Nancy Rumplik is an intensely private person, she willingly talks about her work with patients, about what it means to her to be a nurse. She is deeply committed not only to her patients, but to passing on nursing expertise to a new generation. That is why, after taking years to get both two-year and four-year nursing degrees, she was once again in graduate school in nursing administration and family nursing in the early nineties. Over the years, she had observed nursing management and had had nurse managers whose inspiration informed her own practice. As she became more confident of her own nursing expertise, she also wanted to pass that on to new nurses. It had taken her over twenty years, but in late 1994, she earned a master's degree in nursing administration with a specialty in family issues from the College of Nursing at the University of Massachusetts, Boston.

What her years on the job and her education have taught her are both the skill of involvement and the kind of coping skills necessary to maintain that involvement with sick, dying patients over the long term. She often refers to the coping mechanisms she employs to avoid burnout from her emotionally draining work. Even though graduate school was difficult, it was for Nancy a diversion from the often enervating emotional work she does on the job. Other coping strategies she employs, she says, are taking long walks, going to the movies, gardening, and visiting with friends and relatives — particularly those with children. And she relishes her vacations. When she returns from a two-week vacation, she says, "I feel great. I couldn't do this job if I didn't take a vacation. One week away from here doesn't do it. You just stop thinking about work and then you have to come right back to it. Two weeks really helps you separate from here. Which is mandatory."

On the cancer clinic of the Beth Israel Hospital, she is never far from the daily reminders of human vulnerability and mortality. "It certainly makes you set priorities about who you want to be with, how you want to spend your time," she muses.

Even patience-trying patients like Ralph Philmore elicit her sympathy and understanding. "I always say, you gotta love 'em," she says. "You have to find out if there's a reason they are acting out. There's so many things that happen to these people. You have to be open."

Several years ago, for example, she had a breast cancer patient who was on adjuvant therapy. "Her husband would come with her every time she got chemo," Nancy recalls. "She wasn't that sick, but I sensed that there was something wrong. I felt there was some tension between them.

"It turned out that her husband wouldn't have sex with her because he was afraid he would catch the cancer," Nancy continues. "He was not an ignorant man. He was a professional, but nonetheless he was afraid. So I asked Frank [the social worker] to talk to him. Frank couldn't get him to go to a support group for the husbands of cancer patients that he was conducting, but he was able to help him in other ways."

Nancy, meanwhile, spent time talking with the wife to enable her to deal with the problems in her marriage stemming from her disease.

The ability to use what nursing scholar Patricia Benner has called skilled intuition is no more critical than when helping terminally ill patients navigate the last days of life. In late summer, Nancy is caring for Herb Clark.* He is an internist who admits to another teaching hospital. However, when he was diagnosed with cancer in his mid-fifties, he did not seek treatment there. His hospital, he confides to me, was a factory. Rather than endure the kind of impersonal care he would get there, he chose an oncologist at the Beth Israel and became a patient of Nancy's.

As we talk, Herb leans against the high countertop around the island of desks, computers, and phones in the middle of the treatment area. Although a patient himself now, with an Irish wool cap covering hair thinned by chemotherapy, he still looks the part of the impeccably dressed medical academic, with his natty tweed jacket, sky blue Oxford button-down shirt, and teal blue tie. In deference to the patients and staff around us, Herb speaks quietly — but with intensity — about his experience at the BI. Dealing with his own illness has clearly given him new insight into the healer's art and the importance of having good hospital care, rather than the assembly-line variety.

In some institutions, he says ruefully, the whole system is so mechanized that patients feel as though they have been put on a conveyor belt. If the chief of service just wants to move people along, they don't get much caring, he explained. Doctors and doctors-in-training get points for writing papers, not for talking with patients. Here at the BI, he notes, staff members spend more time and energy building the more human relationships with patients that the latter need and want.

Which is why, as Herb's cancer spreads and there is less medically to *do* for him, Nancy's efforts to *be there* for him do not diminish but intensify.

The role that Nancy plays in the period prior to his death reflects the orientation of nursing. While many physicians do assist people when they are forced to come to grips with their own mortality, the medical model of diagnosis, treatment, and cure makes it difficult for doctors to cope with the dying and death of their own patients. The physician often experiences the loss of a patient as a personal failure, a defeat in the daily battle against disease. This may be as painful as the loss of any further human connection with the deceased. Avoiding dying patients, after efforts at active medical intervention have ceased, becomes a way of avoiding a continual affront to doctors' professional self-esteem.

Doctors are sadly given little guidance about dealing with the complex feelings that suffering and dying provoke. Expressing and dealing with feelings is typical of a culture of nursing that stands in direct contrast to a culture of medicine, in which feelings tend to be avoided, unexplored, and suppressed. Their practice has developed from a "male" model that values doing, not being, acting, not talking about feelings. Forty-four-year-old oncologist Glenn Bubley remembers his training and the socialization process that flows from this model. "When I was in medical school, exploring feelings was actually looked down on," Bubley says. "People used to make jokes like, 'Have you touched base with your feelings today?' There was a value judgment placed on how you responded to your work. If something went wrong, most people felt you were stronger if you sublimated your feelings and worked harder, and that you were weaker if you explored those feelings."

Nothing in the formal medical school curriculum or in his residency or fellowship programs taught him how to deal with his feelings about his difficult work.

A generation later, younger physicians and fellows are not given much more help in dealing with the dying. According to a 1992–93 survey conducted by the AMA, of the nation's 126 medical schools, only five have a required course on the care of the dying. One hundred and seventeen of the schools said that the care of the dying is included in other required courses or in elective courses. The *Cecil Textbook of Medicine*, a volume used by most medical students, devotes only three of its 2,300 pages to the care of the terminally ill. Or as another classic, *Harrison's Principles of Internal Medicine*, put it, "The discovery and cure of potentially serious disease represents a far greater service to one's patients than ministrations in the course of an incurable condition."

Harvard Medical School offers an elective course for medical students called Living with Life-Threatening Illness. It is run by physicians J. Andrew Billings, Susan Block, and Lynn Peterson and is much appreciated by those students who take it. But only a handful of the three hundred or so students do so each year. For those students who have benefited from such tutorials, there is little systematic follow-up effort to help them develop emotional skills during their professional apprenticeship. But novice physicians need to do more than remember what they learned years ago in a medical school class. They need to work out their feelings when they are dealing with the individual patients who are suffering and dying.

At the Beth Israel, in the physicians' conference room just outside the doors of the Hematology / Oncology Clinic, attendings hold discussions with fellows, residents, interns, and medical students. With only few exceptions, Bubley explains, the conversations focus on topics like "What was the patient's hematocrit? What was the platelet count? Should we give her this drug or that drug? Sometimes, some attendings will talk about whether we should pull the plug. How aggressive should we be? But only rarely does anyone ask, 'How are you feeling about this?' There are certainly no formalized discussions about what it's like to take care of people who are so sick and who so often end up dying."

This reflects the priorities of the cancer research and treatment community. In 1995, the National Cancer Institute devoted only $26 million of its total $2.1 billion budget to research on issues of concern to the dying, such as controlling pain and palliative and hospice care.

A medical culture based on a relentless war against disease tends to influence everyone within it — biomedical researchers and physicians — regardless of gender. Thus, some of the female attendings in oncology are no less averse to talking about feelings, holding meetings with patients' families, and dealing with the dying than their male colleagues are. This means that the fellows they train may also get little or no education in "the skill of involvement."

Paola Rode, a second-year fellow who works with Nancy in the clinic, talked to me one afternoon about her frustration with the medical world's lack of emotional guidance. "Going through the course of the patient's disease is more intense than I or, I think, any of the fellows would have ever predicted. It's really tough at times. You have a lot of patients who are very ill. About halfway through the year, you start to see people who are really sick and some start dying or failing their therapies. It's a really tough time.

"You start wondering, 'What am I doing?'" said Rode.

With the exception of individual conversations with colleagues or particularly sensitive attending physicians, younger doctors-in-training have nowhere to turn for emotional support. "I've noticed that the nurses are very smart. They have groups where they meet and discuss their feelings about these issues," Rode said. "We don't have anything like that. There is nothing formal. You're left to talk to your colleagues or track down social workers and talk to them. I've tried to coordinate people to meet and talk about these things. We are able to coordinate people to go to conferences on medical matters."

But somehow, she says, meetings about emotional issues never get scheduled. "I think that's because of this attitude that it's no big deal. But it *is* a big deal. There's a lot of burnout in oncology, a lot of alcoholism and suicide, because there's no one to vent and discuss things with."

It is thus not surprising, Rode adds, that teaching future specialists how to talk to and be with dying patients and their families is not part of their training — even for a field like oncology, where the need for these skills is, unfortunately, very great. As a result, when a fellow must deal with the dying and their close relatives, he or she is thrust into situations almost entirely unprepared. "To a certain extent," Rode said, "you're winging it in each conversation."

Rode also attributes this gap in training to a "macho" attitude. The idea is that we don't need to waste time on this. There are more important matters at hand. Also there is a suspicion of anything that appears to be "touchy-feely."

It is no wonder then that so many physicians flee the dying and that nurses must often pick up the pieces. One day in the clinic, Paddy Connelly, one of Nancy's closest colleagues, is reeling from a recent experience. She had arrived at work on a Monday morning to find one of her patients in the clinic. She knew the patient, who had terminal cancer, had been in the hospital the previous week and had been discharged over the weekend. She did not know she was supposed to appear that Monday in the clinic.

But right before her discharge, the first-year fellow "in charge of her case" had told the patient and her husband that the doctors had done all they could. He informed the couple that "there was no more hope, nothing further to be done."

Awkwardly, like a gawky teenager, the fellow stammered out the lack of options. He said that there was no need for further clinic visits and vaguely proposed hospice services at home as a makeshift alternative to what the patient and her husband clearly perceived to be a total medical abandonment. The wife and husband, like so many Americans, had little understanding of hospice care. (Hospice nurses, physicians, social workers, and other personnel manage the pain and symptoms of dying patients and help patients and families deal with overwhelming emotional suffering and feelings of guilt and loss.) Instead of concrete help, the couple interpreted this as an offer of spiritual guidance. They already went to church, they said, and could talk to their minister anytime. Spiritual help was hardly what they needed at this point. To this definition of hospice-care services, they said a frustrated thank you, but no thank you.

The fellow, Paddy continues, seemed to have as little understanding of hospice as the patient and her husband and no medical encouragement to find out more. The very fact that he raised the issue of hospice so late in the patient's illness process demonstrated this ignorance. Hospice is not designed for patients who will literally be dying in two or three days and for families who are inevitably in desperate straits. Hospice has been far too narrowly defined in the U.S. Here it tends to be viewed as comfort care in the very last days of life — as in just two or three days before a patient dies.

But this radically restricted definition of hospice care, Connelly exclaims, is ludicrous. Family members often can't cope with the idea of introducing a whole new set of players — hospice nurses, social workers, and volunteers — when they are trying to deal with the fact that their loved one is actually dying and will be dead in only a few days or weeks.

Although the patient and her husband did not agree to a consultation with a local hospice, they were terrified of going home alone. They begged to come back to the clinic the following week for further blood products.

"They obviously looked at blood products as . . . hope . . . of what?" Connelly gropes for words.

Although the fellow knew that further treatment would be useless, he nonetheless relented and told the patient to come in the following Monday for the blood products. That's when Connelly saw her. The patient was sitting in her wheelchair in the waiting room. "She looked deathly ill, like she was dying in front of my eyes. Which in fact she was. We got her into the treatment room and gave her platelets. And I talked again with her about hospice and explained more fully about being cared for and made comfortable at home by hospice. Although she was understandably confused, she agreed. So I immediately called the hospice and set that up. I also talked to the fellow and told him in no uncertain terms how upset I was by all this."

The fellow shrugged it off.

Unfortunately, Connelly said, the attending physician who supervised this fellow provided little guidance. This attending had little skill in mentoring a fellow at this stage of a patient's illness. The system hasn't taught them to deal with death, and they can't teach others to deal with it, Connelly explains.

The patient died two days later. Connelly tried to talk with the fellow again about the patient's treatment. But he said huffily, "I don't have the time for this," slamming the door with irritation on his way out.

Connelly sighs with regret. "We've given the patient aggressive treatment. But just when she needs palliative care and a team that won't abandon her; just when she and her family need help understanding the dying process and getting through it, they feel like we're washing our hands of them. And to make matters worse, the fellow — who only knew the patient for a few months — decided to make decisions on his own without consulting the other caregivers on the team, some of whom had known the patient far longer."

Her observations are sadly confirmed by numerous medical studies. In 1989, for example, in an article that appeared in the *New England Journal of Medicine* entitled "The Physician's Responsibility Toward Hopelessly Ill Patients," Dr. Sidney H. Wanzer and eleven other physicians argued that doctors "have a specific responsibility toward patients who are hopelessly ill, dying, or in the end stages of an incurable disease." According to the authors, "the care of the dying is an art that should have its fullest expression in helping patients cope with the technologically complicated medical environment that often surrounds them at the end of life."

But, in many hospitals, "implementation of accepted policies has been deficient in certain areas, including the initiation of timely discussions with patients about dying, the solicitation and execution in advance of their directives for terminal care, and the education of medical students and residents and the formulation of institutional guidelines." The article observes that "only a minority of physicians" consistently engage in such "timely discussions about life-sustaining treatments and terminal care." As a result, patients' pain and suffering is often ignored and measures to minimize suffering are not intensified, and as the authors state, "patients are too rarely cared for directly by the physician at or near the time of death."

Wanzer and his colleagues concluded that "dying patients may require palliative care of an intensity that rivals even that of curative efforts." Such care includes keeping the patient free of bedsores, treating depression, dealing with the swelling of limbs that results from fluid absorption, reducing nausea and vomiting, administering intravenous medications, and helping to keep families together.

"Even though aggressive curative techniques are no longer indicated," the authors conclude, "professionals and families are still called on to use intensive measures — extreme responsibility, extraordinary sensitivity, and heroic compassion."

More recently, in late 1995, the *Journal of the American Medical Association* reported on a major study that was supposed to improve the care of the dying. As mentioned earlier, it was called "The Study to Understand Prognoses and Preferences for Outcomes and Risks of Treatments" — or SUPPORT. The multimillion-dollar four-year study included five major medical centers nationwide — one of which was the Beth Israel — and 9,105 patients. The study documented the inadequacy of physician-patient communication when dealing with the dying and tried to remedy this by providing physicians with information about their patients' prognoses. It also recruited expert nurses to communicate with patients and families, help educate them about possible outcomes of their disease, and relay information about pain management and patient preferences back to physicians. The study's principal investigators had thought this would help patients receive less-aggressive treatment before death, spend less time on intensive care units, and suffer less pain. The study, however, failed miserably. Principal investigators reported that patients' pain was not adequately relieved; patients often expressed wishes — like the fact that they wanted to have a Do Not Resuscitate order (DNR) — that were not heeded; and too many patients spent their last days of life aggressively treated on intensive care units.

When the SUPPORT study appeared in *JAMA*, it received enormous media attention. Researchers, other practitioners, and health care observers evinced a great deal of shock and surprise that such good intentions should yield such poor results. But how could it have been otherwise? Nurses played a central role in this study. Specially trained nurses spent hours with patients and relayed information about the patients' conditions and wishes to their doctors. As the principal investigators themselves acknowledged, in many instances, doctors simply did not listen to or act on the information nurses brought them. And in our medical system, nurses cannot openly overrule physicians decisions or preferences and protect patients from well-intentioned efforts to defeat their diseases. One of the nurses involved in the SUPPORT study was so troubled by her experiences that she called me after I had written an article analyzing some of the study's conclusions. She described the time and effort she had put in trying to talk with and honor the wishes and needs of her patients. The pain in her voice was palpable, when she also related how often she — and by extension her patients — were rebuffed by her physician colleagues.

Although few of the medical researchers involved in the study seemed to have publicly acknowledged the deeper meaning of its conclusions, the study was, in fact, a $28 million experiment that shows how patients suffer when doctors do not listen to nurses or treat them as colleagues rather than subordinates.

What is rarely studied is what nurses can do for dying patients when they are given the time to get to know them and the freedom to act on that knowledge. Nancy Rumplik's care of Herb Clark is a case in point. Herb's physician certainly continues to play an active part in supporting him throughout the final stages of his illness. But it is the patient's nurse who works with the physician to organize and maintain the support network that helps him to die in comfort.

Organizing community support is, for instance, crucial to helping Herb live out his last days more comfortably. In the families of many of Nancy's patients, the woman of the house provides and / or orchestrates the demanding professional and family caregiving that an ill family member requires. Herb, however, was divorced and a married daughter, Joanna,* tried to help care for him while also caring for her own young children.

Fortunately, Herb has a wide circle of friends. The catch? Neither the patient nor his friends are used to dealing with this kind of situation. "It's like a stereotype of intellectuals." Nancy laughs when she presents the cast of characters. "He's an intellectual, and, as he says, he can't remember to take a pill. So I make it very concrete for him. He also can't deal with day-to-day things like making a meal or going to the grocery store. He's exhausted. So his friends call and ask, 'What can I do?' but they don't know what to do either, so they're not helpful. And he can't tell them, 'Why don't you go grocery shopping?' So he ends up not getting help."

Nancy encourages Herb to call a meeting of his friends to decide what, specifically, each should do. To facilitate this gathering, she helps him divide the week into a series of chores — each of which will have a name and day attached to it. If it's Tuesday, Richard goes to the cleaner. On Wednesday, Mark does the shopping. Thursday, Florence cooks a meal. "It seems amazing," Nancy comments, "but you have to get down to that level of concreteness and write it all down on a piece of paper so he doesn't forget."

Later Nancy reflects that Herb is typical of many of her patients. "A lot of what I do is to help people identify what their needs are, what they are having trouble doing," she says. "One of the biggest things they have trouble asking for is help. I'm the same way. I'm single, I'm independent," she adds parenthetically. "People need to learn that it's all right to call someone up and say, 'I need this. Can you help me?'"

People in crisis need help learning how to husband their energy and make choices. "Family caregivers are sometimes so overwhelmed they can't prioritize. You have to say, 'Don't worry about this, you're spending too much energy on this, don't worry about that now.'"

Another crucial component of Herb's care will be hospice, which is particularly important for cancer patients, whose deaths can be long and drawn out and who suffer from considerable pain, weakness, and depression.

Nancy is very familiar with the concept of hospice, or palliative care. In 1967, Dame Cicely Saunders, a nurse turned social worker and then physician, launched the modern palliative care movement when she founded St. Christopher's hospice in London. Saunders, who personally embodies the multidisciplinary approach of the hospice movement, consistently argues that hospice is not, as many people believe, a special place where terminally ill patients go to die. "The care of the dying demands all that we can do to enable patients to *live* until they die," she writes. "It includes the care of the family, the mind, and the spirit as well as the care of the body. All these are so interwoven that it is hard to consider them separately."

The hospice philosophy acts as a much-needed counterweight to the modern trend toward the overmedicalized death. In confronting rather than denying the reality of death, hospice and palliative care programs believe patients should be helped to die in comfort and dignity. Palliative care services may be provided either at home, in a residential center, or in an inpatient hospital unit like the kind commonly found in Canada, the United Kingdom, and Australia.

The United States, however, is years behind these countries in its care and treatment of patients with incurable and terminal conditions. Only 17 percent of the nation's 1,168 accredited medical residency programs offer their residents training in hospice. And fewer than 9 percent of these rotations are required. Studies show that residents aren't rewarded for showing concern about the physical and emotional suffering of patients with incurable illnesses and are not taught the basics of palliative care. It's hardly surprising that those doctors who finally refer a few of their patients to hospice programs do so far too late in the dying process. At the Hospice of Galveston County, in Texas, for example, 40 percent of patients die within five days of their admission.

There is only one World Health Organization–designated demonstration project in palliative care in a United States hospital. That is the integrated palliative care service directed by a physician, Declan Walsh, at the Cleveland Clinic Foundation. It provides consultation services to patients on other units of the hospital as well as outpatient consultation and follow-up. It has a twenty-three-bed unit to which patients can be admitted if their pain and symptoms are difficult to manage or if they are dying and cannot be cared for at home. The program also trains fellows and offers courses for doctors, nurses, and other health care professionals. Finally, it has a hospice service that cares for patients in the home.

In the past few years, a number of other programs have opened around the country. They include programs run by physicians: Carlos Gomez at the University of Virginia Health Sciences Center in Charlottesville, Charles Von Gunten at Northwestern University Medical School in Chicago, Susan McGarrity at Milton S. Hershey Medical Center at Pennsylvania State University, and Marcia Levetown, who began a pediatric palliative care program at the Hospice of Galveston County and the University of Texas in Galveston.

Although Boston teaching hospitals are some of the richest in the country, until 1996 not a single one had devoted any of its immense resources to creating such a program. In the spring of 1996, the New England Deaconess Hospital teamed up with an agency, HealthCare Dimensions, that delivers hospice services in the home and has run a residential hospice for AIDS patients, to open a fifteen-bed palliative care unit at the Deaconess. And in August, a physician, J. Andrew Billings, started a palliative care consultation service at the Massachusetts General. (At this writing there is no palliative care service at the BI.)

Unfortunately, many hospital administrators erroneously believe that their hospitals will not be adequately reimbursed for providing palliative care and many physicians are either ignorant of or scorn palliative care. In cancer treatment, as in many other areas of high-tech medicine, some practitioners actually view attentiveness to the patients' "illness narrative" — their story of their pain and suffering — as mere "hand holding" that distracts them from their main task. There are oncologists who consider too much TLC to be a kind of capitulation to cancer, a symbol of defeat, a response that doesn't produce triumphs of the human spirit. "We don't do a lot of pain management here," said one doctor to a nurse who was watching her friend die in agony at a major cancer center. "That's just palliative care!"

It is often the nurse who raises the issue of hospice care and certainly the nurse who, with the social worker, arranges for hospice services. In midsummer, Nancy is scheduled to go on a two-week vacation. Anticipating that Herb will need hospice care either during the time she is gone or shortly before she leaves, she brings up the issue of hospice with Herb and his daughter. It is not a hard sell. Herb understands what is suggested and asks Nancy to make the initial call.

She calls the hospice, and contacts the nurse who will be taking care of Herb. By the time she returns from vacation, Herb is using the service intensively. He is also markedly weaker and sicker, his daughter far more worried and less able to cope.

On a Friday afternoon, Herb comes into the clinic for a blood transfusion. Paddy Connelly, who'd been taking care of him while Nancy was away, quickly informs Nancy of what has happened during that time. Standing at the back of the clinic, outside the door of Herb's treatment room, Paddy tells Nancy about a meeting Herb has just had with his oncologist. The physician told Herb that he was nearing the end and suggested he start to make some time for himself to think about death.

"Herb asked me whether a lot of my patients had been able to find comfort in religion," Paddy whispers. "I told him frankly that a few found a great deal of comfort in religion, but only those who had been religious before."

"He isn't religious," Nancy affirms. "In fact, he comes from a long line of staunch atheists."

"When I came into his room an hour ago to hang the blood," Paddy continues, "he told me, 'I feel confused. I don't know how I'm supposed to feel. Am I supposed to feel reconciled? Angry? How am I supposed to feel?'"

After hearing this, Nancy walks into the treatment room, where Herb is groggy from the morphine he has been taking for pain and is resting while getting a blood transfusion. Herb lies on the narrow bed, his bald head thrown back on the pillow, his eyes closed and mouth open as he dozes. The nattily dressed academic is no more. He wears a pair of faded wine red pants, a blue short-sleeved shirt open at the neck, and a pair of frayed black-and-white plaid socks. One pant leg is pushed up, revealing the white, almost hairless skin on his leg. He seems very vulnerable and alone.

Nancy moves the IV pole aside and gently pats his arm. "Herb, are you asleep?"

He opens his eyes. "Just dozing," he replies.

Sitting down next to him, she begins what she suspects might be their last conversation. At first she tries to catch up on the details of his daily life — where he is staying in his house (upstairs); how he likes the hospice nurse (a lot); whether an electric chair has been successfully installed in his stairwell (it has); if he is having trouble bathing or getting on and off the toilet (yes, he is).

"It's difficult," he says, referring to the latter two activities. "I just don't seem to have the strength to get in and out of the tub, although I do it."

Nancy suggests getting a shower chair for the tub, which he can slide onto from the rim, and a toilet seat extender that will make it easier to get on and off the toilet.

He seems enlivened by the suggestions. "Those are really good ideas," he says enthusiastically. "Both of them."

Then he pauses and observes sadly, "That's what life has become — worrying about getting up and down the stairs, eating, bathing, making it to the bathroom in time. All those things you used to take for granted."

Nancy nods and Herb returns to the subject of how impressed he is with the hospice's ability to get him the things he needs — a commode for his bedroom, a reclining chair, a hospital bed — without delay.

Nancy asks how he has gotten to the clinic — via an ambulance or chair car? He explains that he came in a chair car and that two men helped him into and out of the house. "Having those two husky guys help you up and down the stairs is a real convenience," Herb observes matter-of-factly. "It's something I wouldn't have even thought about a while ago."

Finally their conversation turns to the fact that he is dying. "You know, when you have a disease as complicated as this, and you're so busy fighting it, all you think about is this stuff," he says, glancing at the IV tubing, the chest of needles and bandages, the large tank of oxygen stored at the end of the bed.

"Do you have trouble talking?" Nancy asks. "Is it tiring you?"

"No, it's not hard to talk, in fact it's energizing. In fact," Herb says, "I really want to tell you about something that hurt at the time. A very close friend, I've known him for years, called the other day. He just can't talk about what's happening and how I feel about it. He's getting older. He's in a panic about that. It's crazy, he calls up all the time to ask how I am, and he really doesn't want to know. My sister is like that, too. They can't handle it."

"It's difficult," Nancy acknowledges. "Sometimes people just don't know what to say or how to deal with it when someone is seriously ill."

Herb and Nancy continue to talk about his friends and family for a few more moments until she deftly steers the conversation away from his illness and back to the stories of his own career in medicine that she has heard many times before. Herb begins telling her once again about one of his most interesting cases. More and more animated, as if the sedating effects of morphine have been temporarily overcome by the sheer power of conversation, he recounts his triumphs and failures as a doctor and muses about the limitations of his profession. Listening attentively and asking polite questions at all the right moments, Nancy lets Herb's mind wander back and forth from his sad and disorienting current situation to the anchoring points of his past.

After fifteen minutes, the blood finishes dripping into his vein.

Herb's daughter, Joanna, comes into the room to tell him the chair car is waiting.

As he walks out of the clinic, Nancy turns to me. "When I take fifteen minutes to talk about his work, it affirms the validity of his life. He is not just a person with cancer, he is a person who has an identity that extends beyond his illness, even beyond his death. I hate this stage, because this really could be the last time I see him. You can't really say that to them. But you watch when you say good-bye. It's in their eyes. They know it."

Nancy is right. This was her last visit with Herb. Over the weekend, he gets much sicker. At one point, his daughter says later, he cried out in his sleep, exclaiming emphatically, "I can't do this."

During his months in the clinic, Herb and his daughter have come to trust their nurse. As the end nears, Joanna relies heavily on her to act as interpreter. Each day, as Herb's condition worsens, Joanna calls to question Nancy about the signs of his decline.

On Monday morning, for example, as soon as she comes to work, Nancy receives a call from Joanna reporting that Herb is bedridden, his hands are cold, and he refuses to take any fluids. Joanna is worried that Herb will be subjected to heroic measures to keep him alive and reiterates that this is not what she, Herb, or the rest of the family want. Nancy reassures her that the hospice will only make sure that Herb is comfortable.

The next day — Herb's last — Nancy is in constant touch with both the hospice nurse and Herb's physician. As the physician and Nancy talk in the corridor outside the exam rooms, he debates whether to ask the hospice nurse to give Herb IV fluids.

Nancy gently reminds him that ordering fluids this late in the dying process will simply delay the inevitable. Will it really make Herb more comfortable, she wonders out loud, or will it prolong his death? The physician considers her comments and decides against hydration.

After this exchange, Nancy turns to me. "Sometimes there are considerations like this. On the one hand, the physician says, we shouldn't intervene, we should let him go. On the other, he considers giving the patient fluids. If he wasn't conflicted about it, he'd say, 'Absolutely nothing, don't do anything.'"

Herb dies later that afternoon. Early the next morning, in the clinic, Nancy stops to engage in what has become, for her, an important ritual — remembering. Some nurses do their memorializing at the funerals they attend. Only in rare instances does Nancy attend a patient's funeral or memorial service. Instead, she constructs her own memorials to the dead. Talking quietly, almost reverently, with her friend and colleague Mary Whitley, she recalls her experiences with Herb. She tells Mary about his sense of humor. She describes that one case he kept telling her about over and over again in their talks and admires the graceful way he faced his own impending death. "It's hard," she admits. "In the last two days there was such a flurry of activity. I was on the phone six times a day." And now, there was nothing about Herb — just silence.

Later, she delves further into her feelings about this part of her work. You learn a lot about dying in this job, she explains. You learn that there's a window of opportunity when it comes to talking with the dying. And you have to take advantage of it. If you talk to them too soon about their death, they feel you know something that they don't know. But if you wait until the last minute to say good-bye, they may slip into a coma and you will never be able to talk with them again.

"I was so happy to talk to him in the clinic on his last visit," she says. Even though she and Herb had talked about this all summer, she says that talking once again restored Herb's sense of self, of who he'd been before he became a patient with a terminal disease.

"I knew that visit might be the last opportunity. I didn't really get a chance to say good-bye to him the way I wanted to," she continues, her eyes filling with tears. "I didn't get to give him a really good hug and look him right in the eye. Many times, people will look at you and have tears in their eyes and you know they're saying good-bye in their own way. But with him I feel okay that it happened so quick. I really believe that, spiritually, he was ready to go."

Later that week, Joanna comes into the clinic. Finding Nancy in the hallway between the waiting room and treatment area, Herb's daughter draws the nurse into a quiet corner. "Nancy," she says, embracing the nurse, "You were it. Whenever we needed anything, you were there." Gripping Nancy's hand, her whole body shaking, she talks about Herb's last moments. "He died holding my hand, Nancy. And you know, it seemed as though he was smiling."

*   *   *

Herb's death was what I have come to think of as a "good enough death." Nancy has helped patients and their families navigate this crucial transition. To illustrate the various roles she plays when a patient dies, Nancy tells me about Roxanne,* an African American woman in her early thirties. Roxanne was married and had one young child when she was diagnosed with an aggressive form of breast cancer. For over seven years, Nancy cared for her through cycle after cycle of chemotherapy, through another pregnancy, and finally through the dying process. At the end, Nancy says, her primary role was that of family mediator.

As Roxanne's disease became more invasive, she realized it was incurable. She reconciled herself to the fact that she was going to die. This was, however, a conclusion her husband, Al,* was unable to accept. She watched with growing distress as he kept approaching Steve Come and begging him for another drug or experimental treatment. Meanwhile, Al was unable to talk with Roxanne about arrangements for the future, including their children and how her death might affect them. This plagued her and left her no peace.

Finally, she asked Nancy for help. Please, she implored the nurse, do something to help my husband.

Nancy, of course, agreed. Because she knew that Steve had a much closer relationship to Al than she did, she suggested that the best way to deal with the situation was to arrange a meeting among the three of them — Al, herself, and Steve.

On one of the afternoons when Al accompanied Roxanne to the clinic, the patient quietly excused herself so that her nurse, physician, and husband could meet.

When the three were together in a small exam room, Steve asked Al how he was coping.

Instead of evading the topic or brushing it off, Al seemed to crumble. "He started crying," Nancy recalls. "In fact, he knew she was dying. But it took a softer approach to help him finally admit it."

Their conversation made it possible for Al to talk, for the first time, about his feelings about Roxanne's impending death. This, in turn, made it possible for the couple to speak together about their children and the family's future without a wife and mother. Finally, Roxanne had some solace. "She died very peacefully," Nancy remembers. "She was able to work things out she would not have been able to work out with him. And because of that conversation, I was able to keep talking to him."

Thinking back on her years in oncology, Nancy notes that there are many permutations on the experience of dying. There are people, she says, who are ready to deal with the reality of their imminent death but are constrained because friends and relatives around them can't give up. Or sometimes, it's the other way around. A spouse or relative wonders why doctors and nurses are giving chemo at all. After all, the patient is dying. They want to know what point there is to giving it another try.

"If I've learned anything, it's that every patient is an individual," Nancy concludes. "You can't generalize about any part of their living or dying. And I don't care how many people you see dying. The more you see and deal with this, the more you realize you don't know."

In dealing with terminally ill patients and their families, Nancy draws on her own personal experience. When she was twenty-eight, her father died. She'd been a nurse for eight years at the time and was working in the Surgical Intensive Care Unit. Suddenly, the parent who had been so important to her — who constantly encouraged her and wouldn't let her quit when her applications to nursing school were initially rejected — suffered a massive heart attack. He was taken to the Medical Intensive Care Unit (MICU) in a hospital near her family's home in western Massachusetts. For two weeks, Nancy drove back and forth from Boston to see him.

He was on the MICU for a week. After that, he was transferred to a regular floor. And after another week, he went home — presumably on the mend. He arrived home on Friday. On Sunday, he had another heart attack and died.

"I wanted to think he'd be better," Nancy said. "But I knew and I wasn't surprised. He was so weak. He'd had such a bad heart attack.

"Going through this myself gave me insight that I didn't have before. I learned about the whole process of dying — getting sick, being in the hospital, how to be available to someone who's sick, thinking about who is the primary caregiver, about what happens afterward. It's like you think you know something and then you really know it. You have the experience behind you. Your whole life experience is part of nursing. Now, as a nurse, it's second nature to me how a son or daughter feels when a parent dies. I have more empathy."

To illustrate how her own experience feeds her ability to care for her patients, Nancy refers again to one of her current cases. "I talked with a patient's husband today. I've been taking care of his wife for three years. She had metastatic breast cancer. Before I went on vacation, I visited her up on the floor. I was worried that she wouldn't be alive when I came back, and she wasn't. When I got back, I found out she died and I called him up."

It was really a bereavement call, she says. She wanted to make sure the husband understood that she and the physician and social worker were still available to him. Above all, she did not want him to feel that as soon as his wife died, he had been forgotten.

Nancy also called because she knew he was probably having trouble dealing with feelings of guilt arising from his response to his wife's cancer. "She had a terrible tumor growing on her chest wall, and he found it repulsive," Nancy explains. "Finally, he would not sleep with her, and they had to have separate bedrooms."

Over the course of the last few months, the man's wife seemed to improve. Then, suddenly, she took a very dramatic turn for the worse. One complication followed another until the cancer was everywhere in her body. Now, in her husband's mind, there was only one explanation — his own revulsion and withdrawal had actually hastened his wife's death. On the phone, he asked Nancy if stress had made her die so quickly. Did stress have anything to do with it? he asked again and again.

"I told him no. It wasn't stress — it was the disease," Nancy says. "I knew what he was feeling. He was feeling, 'Oh God, it's my fault.' I told him to talk to his wife's physician because I knew that would help, too."

Although she says she has never had to deal with this kind of guilt herself, Nancy is no stranger to lingering memories and emotions that the death of a loved one engenders. "I know from having experienced the death of someone close to me that it's not over in a day. It keeps coming back. Because of my father, the feeling of what it's like to have someone close to you die has never left me. Never."

Chapter 9

Final Checkups

ELLEN KITCHEN

In February of 1994, Ellen Kitchen discovered that she was pregnant. It was obviously a much welcomed event. But it also led to a difficult decision. What should she do in the months before she delivered, and how long would she take off work afterward? While she wanted to continue caring for her patients, she knew she also needed to care for herself. She could, she recognized, continue to see her patients until only weeks before her due date. But she worried about the effect of stress on her pregnancy. Summer months are some of the most highly charged and burdensome for home care nurses. Many of her colleagues would be on vacation, and she would be asked not only to handle her own caseload, but to cover for them.

Ellen finally decided to leave work in July, well before her baby was due. Her decision to leave early was due not only to the increasing stress of the summer vacation load, but to the new pressures in health care. During the period in which I observed Ellen and other nurses' work, enormous cost-cutting constraints were surfacing in health care. Moreover, many more patients were being seen in the home, as hospital stays had been dramatically shortened. Home care nurses like Ellen were seeing not only patients with chronic illnesses, but acutely ill patients who'd been ejected from the hospital while still unstable.

"It's so crazy in the office now," Ellen comments. It's become such a busy place. When I started, we used to see four patients a day. Now it's up to six or eight. We used to be able to spend a good hour with people. Now it's about forty-five minutes. There's been a dramatic increase in volume. We're taking so many different kinds of patients. On top of this, we have a professional responsibility to educate other nurses. Each year I have a student to teach, which adds to the work-load."

As we talk about her decision to take early maternity leave, an uncharacteristic note of pessimism informs her comments. She says she doesn't know if nurses who follow her will have the benefit of the kind of mentoring relationships she enjoyed or if they will be able to take the time to educate themselves as she did. "At the time I was in the hospital, staffing was up, and you could take educational days and personal days," Ellen recalls. "You could go to the library and read and do research. Now, I don't know . . ." She frowns as her voice trails off.

Several weeks before she is to go on maternity leave, I follow Ellen as she makes penultimate visits to some of her patients. I had asked if I could come with her on her last visits to her patients. But she demurred. Saying good-bye to people whose lives she had shared so intimately for so long would be a wrenching and thus a very private affair.

Although Ellen knows that her patients will be shifted to other colleagues who are as expert as she is, nonetheless she knows how much she will miss them and they her. She is well aware that health care is not just a service to be delivered by interchangeable pairs of hands. It's a relationship that is difficult to uproot and reestablish. "I have had a relationship with some of these people for years," she explains her concern. "I have known them so well, for such a long time, and have had a positive impact on their lives." Similarly, she says, it is hard to contemplate leaving the physicians and nurses with whom she has worked for so long.

As before, the schedule includes Mr. Cousins, Mac, and Mr. Fitch. In the winter, Mrs. Beauchamp was admitted to the hospital following another stroke. Over the past year, Mrs. B. had greatly deteriorated. She had to work much harder just to get around the house. She was often confused, and it was hard for her to figure out how to get through the day. It was even difficult for her to dress and bathe.

Ellen had visited her at home a few days before her final admission. Mrs. B. had told Ellen and Zag that she did not want to be put on life support, but her stroke occurred at night, and in the tumult and confusion of the emergency admission, she was put on a mechanical ventilator and admitted to MICU before anyone could ascertain her wishes.

Ellen visited her in the hospital. To see the woman she had known for so long lying in bed, the long gray hair a disheveled mass around her head, her breasts hanging down near her belly, her face pallid, and a breathing tube protruding from her mouth, was a shock. Even the voice, whose strangled, labored utterances had become such a fixture, was silenced.

Over the course of the days following her stroke, Ellen visited with Mrs. B. as much as she could. Although Mrs. B. was taken off the ventilator twenty-four hours after her admission, and sent to a general medical floor, she was frightened and felt alone. "She had gone through the time with me when I was sick," Ellen remembers fondly, "and most of my patients didn't know that. And I knew how isolated she felt. She had never expressed such feelings of isolation before. But during this period, she felt alone." About a week later, Mrs. B. died.

Today, Ellen goes to Mr. C. first. Mac is next, and she again saves the inconsolable Mr. Fitch — who has been recuperating from yet another heart attack and is extremely frustrated with the slow pace of his recovery — for last.

As we approach Mr. C.'s building, Ellen spots the old man out for a walk in a small nearby square. We arrive in his lobby at about the same time and go up in the elevator together to his apartment. Mr. Cousins is dressed in brown slacks and a multicolored shirt in blue, fuchsia, black, and gold. More pictures of his children and grandchildren have been added to the display on his walls and windowsills. Proudly exhibited among them is a card addressed to "Dear Grandfather."

Then there is Ellen's handiwork. Attached to the refrigerator door is her poster-like reminder to Drink Water — 6 to 8 Glasses a Day. On a small table in the living room is another sign near Mr. C.'s plastic pillbox. Take Your Heart Pills! *Two* Times a Day from the Box. *Do Not* Take the Heart Pills from the Bottle. On the front door there's a final warning: Don't Forget to Take Your Pills!

Conversations with Mr. C. always include warm but sorrowful reminiscences about his deceased wife. Ellen is important to him because she is essential to his independent living, but also because she is a repository of his last conjugal memories. He shares these memories easily with her because he knows that Ellen knew and cared for his wife as well.

Today, as soon as Ellen enters, Mr. C. begins worriedly rifling through a pile containing all the documents relating to Mrs. Cousins's last illness and death. There are hospital bills, funeral papers, and cemetery papers, for Mrs. Cousins's grave. For some mysterious reason, Mr. C. says, he just received a bill pertaining to his wife's burial, and he can't figure out why. "I haven't looked at this for years," he says, his eyes misting. "I didn't want to touch it."

"I had the money at that time, and I put it in the bank. I took care of all that. I paid for her funeral so no one would have any trouble. It was five thousand dollars. I don't understand what all this is about."

Ellen volunteers to sort through the papers to try to find the receipt. After a few moments, she pulls out a piece of paper. "Here it is, Mr. C.," she announces, "forty-three hundred dollars for the funeral parlor."

His face smooths with relief. "Thank you, thank you so much," he says.

As they discuss the matter further, she tries to reassure him about the fact that she will no longer be available to help him sort through such matters in the future. "The social worker and new nurse can help you with anything like this. I don't want you to get into a tizzy about this," she says.

These tizzies have increased over the last months, and Mr. C. seems to be getting somewhat confused, Ellen says. He has angrily related stories about helpers and relatives trying to steal money from him. Sorting out which accusations are true and which are false is often no easy task. In one case, someone who was helping with meals did seem to be taking advantage of him. When it comes to accusations against grandchildren and daughters-in-law, that is harder to fathom. "It's difficult to sort all this out," Ellen comments. "You never know because you have never met the cast of characters. Sometimes families do take advantage of a relative. Sometimes it's just paranoia related to dementia. Sometimes it's depression and isolation."

To help disentangle this skein of cause and effect, Ellen has enlisted a Home Care Department social worker, who has come for home visits and has brought students with her. They spend time talking with Mr. C. about his life. "He loves it. He never remembers the students' names, but it's a way of bringing people into his life."

Ellen is also concerned about his physical condition. She takes his blood pressure, which seems fine. Ellen asks about his eating. A woman in the building cooks him meals and brings them up every night. He had a fall several months earlier. Ellen wants him to maintain his strength, and she wonders whether he's getting out enough. He laments the fact that he can't get to his church as easily anymore. For twenty years, he was on its board and now he can rarely get there, even for services.

Can't someone pick him up? Ellen asks. He seems to feel this will be too difficult and changes the subject to speak about the people he once knew in his fraternal order, the Masons. Then he and Ellen talk about his son who lives in Michigan. "Both my sons were very close to their mother," he reports with a canny laugh. "I couldn't get a word in edgewise."

Ellen does not interrupt his reminiscences. Just listening, she knows, represents some of the most important work she accomplishes with Mr. C. Deftly, however, she introduces her medical and nursing concerns.

"Mr. C.," she asks, "how is your knee feeling?" Ellen bends near him and lifts his pants leg so that she can check for any swelling or pain. She has been worried about Mr. C.'s arthritic knee and wants to make sure he will have a new brace by the time her leave begins. They have experimented with a variety of elastic knee braces; she and the physician feel he should have a sturdier variety, but Mr. C. has resisted. He has also resisted using a walker. "I don't know if it's pride or just the unfamiliarity of new equipment, but the only thing he will tolerate is his cane, which he uses about fifty percent of the time," Ellen has told me.

She asks him if he has been using his cane when he walks. She keeps reminding him that a weak and painful knee can lead to the kind of fall he's recently had. What she wants to prevent is a more serious incident. "You could fall and be lying on the floor for twenty-four hours — in this building, thank God, it wouldn't be for more than that because they come to check on you. You could have a hemorrhage or skin breakdown and an ulcer over a bony protrusion. Or you could have a hip fracture." As she gently explains all this, Mr. C. nods less than enthusiastically.

Before Ellen goes, she asks Mr. C. for a urine specimen. He's had problems with urinary tract infections in the past, and she doesn't want another one to crop up during the transition between caregivers. Dutifully, he goes into the bathroom and returns with a filled specimen cup.

When he comes back, he sits down and stares at a picture of his late wife. "I've never missed a person so much in my life," he says. "She was so good to me. There was nothing I wouldn't have done for her."

"And you did do everything for her, Mr. C.," Ellen affirms. "You took such wonderful care of her. Now we have to take care of you."

Across the street, Mac has grown progressively weaker. He had a setback several months earlier. Because of problems with congestive heart failure and an elevated blood pressure, he was admitted to the hospital. Like many elderly patients, he became disoriented, confused, and dependent there. Ellen continued to visit Mac in the hospital. One of her jobs was to relate her long history with him to his hospital caregivers. She wanted his nurses and physicians to understand that his severe disorientation and confusion were not permanent, but temporary results of his hospital stay.

Some nurses listened to her. Ellen recounts that one particular nurse — a nurse who had a great deal of experience with the problems of the hospitalized elderly — diligently read her notes and respected her recommendation that Mac once again be discharged home. Other, newer nurses, unfortunately, were not so attentive. "One nurse ended up telling me that Mac needed to go to a nursing home," she said.

Ellen could sympathize with the nurse's concern. What this nurse was observing on her daily hospital rounds was a dysfunctional ninety-year-old who simply could not make it on his own. Ellen did not disagree with that judgment. What she tried to explain was that the other nurse's view of Mac was only partial. Over the years, Ellen has amassed a broader picture of this particular patient. She knows that he's gotten confused every time he's been in a hospital. And she also knows that he gets better as soon as he gets home.

Ellen tried valiantly to explain this to the nurse in question. "I asked her if she had been reading my notes," Ellen recalls. "She obviously hadn't. That struck me as one of the problems. They're so busy in the hospital today. She didn't have time to look at the home care notes, so she really didn't understand what we do in home care and how we evaluate patients. She didn't know I'd been seeing Mac for seven years and that I really knew the situation at home."

Ellen and Mac's physician, John Jainchill, prevailed. Mac came home.

Ellen and John Jainchill know that this is only a temporary reprieve, and their goal is to keep Mac at home for as long as possible. "Even though it goes against everything we try to do in home care, we know there comes a time when a person will be safer in a nursing home than at their own home," Ellen comments. "But there's no cookbook recipe that tells you when that time has come."

Ellen instead will carefully observe what may be a gradually evolving progression of small signs that must be deciphered by someone who has known the patient over time and has the knowledge to interpret their significance. Because Mac is even more forgetful, Ellen has to assiduously survey his medications. She talks to him about his physical therapist and makes sure he does the exercises she prescribes. He needs physical therapy because he has lost a lot of muscle tone, is now unsteady on his feet, and has increased difficulty getting in and out of the shower. She is also on the lookout for red flags — weight loss and the fridge full of rotting food that indicates Mac isn't eating; bruises on legs, arms, or hips that signal a fall he's forgotten about; odor from his body or clothes that suggests he's no longer able to bathe or has forgotten to change his clothes; or the repeatedly wet sheets that are evidence of urinary incontinence.

In someone who is increasingly demented and who cannot answer direct questions — did you fall yesterday, are you eating enough, when did you last do your laundry — such signs must be read from the patient's body and environment. Ellen also counts on Mac's homemaker and home health aide and his friend Harry for vital communication about his deteriorating condition.

When we arrive at Mac's apartment, he is again seated on his bed. He wears green boxer shorts and a loose undershirt stained with sweat. Harry, a spry character in his late sixties, is also visiting. He wears a baseball cap, a neatly pressed shortsleeved shirt, and light summer slacks. As Ellen talks to Mac, Harry putters around the apartment, washing dishes, opening and closing cupboards, gathering laundry like a frantic Jewish mother. In a raspy voice, he barrages Ellen with questions. When is Mac's homemaker coming? How many times a week does Mac have to have physical therapy? When is the therapist going to be here? She better come a lot, he cautions as he throws more laundry into a pile near the front door.

Ellen answers Harry's questions in a level tone. Then she turns to Mac. He's taken a few walks since he got home from the hospital, and she wants to know how they've worked out. He complains about feeling weak, and she explains that it's because he hasn't been out much. "You'll get your strength back," she assures him.

Mac's main preoccupation seems to be how he is going to get his laundry done and obtain his latest supply of pills.

"That's all right, Mac. I'll get your pills and Bea will do the laundry. Don't worry."

"Yeah," he interrupts, "but what about quarters for the laundry?"

"We'll get you those, too," she says.

The laundry is a particularly tricky issue. Bea has been doing the laundry and Ellen wants to make sure that she reports any important information about Mac's condition that she gleans from it. But Mac has been reluctant to allow Bea to venture into the basement, where the washer and dryer are located. Prostitutes have been found selling their wares in the basement, and Mac worries for Bea's safety. Mac would insist on doing the laundry himself, but would then forget to do it.

"Someone's been ringing the doorbell at nine in the morning," he complains, adding to a list of problems that are beyond his capacity to solve.

"Well, don't answer it, Mac," Ellen suggests.

"Does Bea call before she comes?" Harry shouts through the archway to the kitchen.

Ellen explains that she does. Mac sits passively on the bed while Harry continues to question Ellen and then disappears into the kitchen to wash some more dishes. Mac's hands shake ever so slightly. In the corner, his cat sits silently licking his paws.

Ellen reaches into her backpack and pulls out her blood pressure cuff. "Did you get your groceries this week, Mac?" Ellen inquires as she takes his blood pressure.

"No," he replies.

Overhearing this conversation, Harry emerges from the kitchen and irately demands, "Well, who brought the hamburger, half gallon of milk, and the quart of orange juice?" Mac sits idly by utterly bewildered by his questions.

Noting the blank look on Mac's face, Harry turns to Ellen like a prosecutor who has just proved his case. "You see," he exclaims and points accusingly at Mac, "you ask him these questions and he don't remember."

Deftly ignoring Harry, Ellen congratulates Mac because his blood pressure is 134 over 70. Then she listens to his heart and pays him another compliment. "Good, nice and clear."

"Can you stand up for me, Mac?" she requests. Instead of getting off the bed, Mac points to his cat, who is now scarfing down her food in the kitchen beyond, and smiles contentedly. Ellen smiles back.

Ellen asks Mac to stand on the scale. He has lost more than twenty pounds in the last year and she wants to make sure that he is not losing more. After weighing him and congratulating him on maintaining his weight, she carefully looks over his arms and torso and legs and thighs to make sure there are no signs of bruises.

After she finishes the exam, Ellen goes to the phone, explaining to Mac that she is trying to call Bea to make sure she comes later that day. She speaks to an office staffer and stresses the importance of a timely visit. "If she gets here in the afternoon, she'll have enough time to shower him."

Meanwhile, Harry has become obsessed by the problem of laundry bleach. There is no bleach in the house, he announces. How can anyone do laundry without bleach? he asks sharply. Rather than responding impatiently to his carping, Ellen humors him.

Harry has been an indispensable link in the social safety net that has allowed Mac to remain at home. As Mac has gotten weaker, Harry has increased his visits and sees Mac daily. He is an objective observer who offers her a great deal of information about how Mac is doing, and she values his input. Harry also brings Mac a home-cooked meal every day. Mac is supposed to get one meal a day from Meals on Wheels, but for reasons they have not been able to ascertain, there are gaps in the service, which Harry fills in.

When Harry initiates a search for the bleach, Ellen walks into the kitchen and with a pleasant "Well, let's see where that bleach could be," checks the broom closet and the cupboards under the sink for bleach and calmly promises to leave a note for the homemaker reminding her to get some bleach for Mac when she goes grocery shopping. Harry looks content.

Throughout this exchange, Mac looks baffled. He repeats Bea's name several times. "Do I know her?" he asks Ellen.

"Yes, Mac, she's the lady who helps you bathe and who used to walk your dog."

He smiles vaguely.

While they are talking, Harry puts on his jacket, picks up a shopping bag, and announces that he is leaving. Ellen and Mac politely say good-bye. After he goes, Ellen helps Mac go over some of the exercises the physical therapist left for him.

"I want you to start going out again soon," she tells him, and he nods obediently.

Then she goes into the kitchen. While she makes him a cup of coffee and cuts him a slice of the banana cream pie that Harry brought for him, Ellen uses the opportunity to look inside the refrigerator and cupboards. She doesn't only want to make sure Mac has enough food and note if any staples are missing, she also wants to make sure the food he has is actually used. When Mac came home from his last hospitalization, he insisted that he was eating. Yet he was losing weight. The solution to this riddle lay in his fridge: he had the food, he simply didn't prepare it.

When she brings Mac the pie, she sits next to him companionably while he eats. Mac chews hungrily and smiles up at Ellen. Licking the last tastes off the spoon, like a kid savoring the last taste of a candy bar, he stares at the door. Turning to Ellen, his closest confidant, he lowers his voice as if Harry might hear. "Ellen, I'm glad to have Harry around, but" he adds, shaking his head with dismay, "I just can't understand him."

Right before lunch, Ellen reaches Mr. Fitch's apartment. Earlier that morning, he called to make sure she was coming. She assured him that she would be with him soon and also took some time to make an eye appointment for him. Mr. Fitch's calls and concerns have escalated because he knows that Ellen will soon be leaving him. Of all her patients, she knows that Mr. Fitch will have the greatest difficulty with these last meetings. So she has tried to allot extra time to spend with him even if it means cutting into her own lunch hour.

The door to Mr. Fitch's apartment is open, but his apartment is stifling. Ellen grimaces at the stagnant air. Over and over again, she has urged Mr. Fitch to use his air-conditioning. Instead, she often finds him sweating through the heat of a humid Boston midsummer afternoon. Mr. Fitch is not at his usual post in his chair by the window. Ellen hears sounds in the bathroom and calls out, "Mr. Fitch, are you in there? Are you okay?"

The old man grunts in the affirmative.

"Well, let me know when I can come in. I want to weigh you."

She hears yet another grunt and soon the door opens a crack. Ellen goes in to weigh Mr. Fitch, and after a few minutes, he shuffles out in front of her. Hearing the rasping in his chest, she asks him how his breathing has been over the week and reminds him to turn on the air conditioner. She starts it up while she is talking to him. On his way to his chair, Mr. Fitch seems to stumble. "I feel dizzy," he complains.

Ellen moves toward him to help him along and hands him his cane. "You should be walking with this, Mr. F., especially if you feel dizzy," she suggests.

He accepts the cane, and as he gropes toward the chair, Ellen remarks that she hasn't seen him so unsteady in a long time. "How are you, how have you been?" she asks with growing concern.

Mr. Fitch moans in reply. "You're asking how I am? I don't even know myself, doll, it's up and down with me."

He slouches into his chair and moans again. Ellen squats at his feet, slips off his worn slippers, and begins to feel his legs and ankles. "Do your legs hurt? Do you feel pain in the hip when you walk?

He mutters vaguely with frustration.

"Remember, you stopped taking your arthritis medicine because you said it gave you heartburn, and now you're using Tylenol. Have you had to take many Tylenol this week?"

"I don't know," he replies gruffly. "When I walk around, it gets better."

Ellen nods. "That's what happens with arthritis," she explains.

Mr. Fitch refuses to be consoled. "I never had none of this until I went to the hospital," he blurts out angrily.

Again, Ellen tries to help him understand his condition. "You felt pretty lousy for the past couple of months, since you had your heart attack. You haven't gotten your strength back yet. Sometimes that happens with a heart attack, Mr. Fitch. Sometimes you get your strength back quickly. Sometimes you don't."

To check on his condition, Ellen stands up and reaches into her bag for her stethoscope. Mr. F. lifts up his V-neck undershirt and stares out of the window, dutifully breathing in and out as she listens to his weary heart and lungs.

"You sound a teeny bit better than you did the other day. Do you feel better?"

"No improvement, no way!" he practically shouts. "It makes me feel so bad. I never felt like this till I went to the hospital."

"It's hard to believe that was only seven years ago. You were a mere eighty-one and three-quarters," she says, trying to cheer him up.

But he remains in a bitter, cantankerous mood. "You people keep talking about heart attacks. What is a heart attack, anyway?" he asks as if he cannot, will not, believe this medical jargon.

"What happens is that blood and oxygen don't get to the heart," Ellen explains. "There's hardening of the arteries. Sometimes an artery gets blocked. Sometimes a little piece of fat breaks off." She continues to explain the physiology of the three heart attacks he's had since 1987.

"I never had heart trouble. It never bothered me. Now you're telling me I have a heart attack. All through my life I never even knew I had a heart," he says, with no pun intended.

He leans his hand on his chin and stares morosely at the flowered plastic tablecloth on the small lamp table near his chair. "How in the world can I do something to get better?" he inquires of no one in particular. He pauses and seems to ready himself for another outburst. "It's hard for me to say, but I'm going to say it. Every time you come, I don't get better. I just go back to where I am. Who's the fool? Me or you?"

Ellen does not skip a beat. "It's hard for you. You started out with emphysema. Then there were the heart attacks. You've had to become more dependent on other people. You feel like a fifty-year-old trapped in an almost ninety-year-old body."

Ignoring her words and the concern behind them, Mr. Fitch begins to rock back and forth in his chair, getting more and more agitated. Then he announces an epiphany. His problem, he insists, is being treated by a nurse instead of a doctor directly. "It's just not like hearing things from doctors, hearing things from the horse's mouth. You're not the horse. You're just relaying messages from the doctor. She's the big gun," he concludes. And then again, as if for emphasis, he repeats, "She's the big gun."

Mr. Fitch's angry rebuke of his caregiver is stunning in its cold-hearted embrace of the myth that only a doctor can provide real patient care. But he doesn't stop there. "The patient always feels better going to the doctor. The doctor's name alone lifts the person up. Not the nurse."

Ellen does not interrupt, object, or even betray any reaction by her facial expression. She doesn't get defensive. She just listens and finally asks gently, "Would you like to see the doctor?" There is no hint of rejection or abandonment in her tone. "What do you want me to do, Mr. F.? Do you want to go and see Dr. Zagarella or would you like her to come here?"

The very fact that she shows such readiness to heed his wishes seems to strike a deep chord in the old man. His angry face crumbles and reflects only regret. "I don't want to keep going to the hospital all the rest of my life," he says dejectedly. "The sickness is making a fool of me. I smoked cigarettes, but I never dreamed it would make me not able to breathe."

Ellen continues to listen. As he talks, she goes into the kitchen, checks the refrigerator, and asks Mr. F. if he would like a couple of eggs. Yes, he tells her. Ellen cooks the eggs and serves them with toast. He smiles wanly at her and remains in a mournful, depressive state. Ellen sits at his side while he eats. When he is finished, she washes up, collects her bag, and then sits again in front of him. With a hand on his arm, she asks, "So how about it, Mr. Fitch? Would you like Dr. Zagarella to come here or do you want me to make an appointment to see her in her office?"

Like a bewildered child, he looks at her for guidance about what to do, then ventures a reply. "I kind of think it would be better for me to call on her."

"Okay, Mr. Fitch. Then that's what we'll do. You keep that air conditioner on, all right. I'll be back soon." She again pats his arm before leaving.

In the hall, she turns to me and says with sympathy, "It's so hard for him. He's so sick. There's nothing that will really make him better. And now I'm leaving and he's really angry at me."

She turns and walks down the long, barren hallway, takes the elevator to the lobby, unhooks her bike, and rides back to the Beth Israel on a journey she will make for one of the last times.

In August 1994, after Ellen had been on maternity leave for two months, Mac was finally put in a nursing home. Ellen and John Jainchill had been trying to prevent this for as long as possible. But living at home just wasn't working out. Mac needed a regular homemaker, but the agency couldn't get him one expeditiously. Bea couldn't fill in. He was getting too confused, and he was unable to continue on his own. John Jainchill visits Mac in the nursing home and has told Ellen that he has adjusted fairly well.

Mr. Cousins is still doing fine on his own. On the day of his ninetieth birthday, Ellen called to wish him well. Sad and bitter, Mr. Fitch still watches life pass by underneath his window. For him, little has changed.

On the eighth of November, Ellen went into labor. After eight hours, she gave birth to a girl — Samantha — who weighed eight pounds and one ounce. There were no complications.

When Ellen left on maternity leave, she planned to return to work after a year. But, like many professional women, she was torn between family and career. When it came time for her to go back to work, her daughter and son were ages one and four. In order to maintain her medical coverage and other benefits, she would have had to work a minimum of four days per week. The thought of ten-hour days — dropping her children off at day care in the morning and picking them up at six or seven at night — was unbearable. In the fall of 1995, she asked Karen Dick if her leave could be extended. Unfortunately, hospital policy precluded such an extension.

Ellen decided that she would just have to risk severing her ties with the BI. In a year or two, she may reapply for a position. But she worries that there may not be a job for her in the Home Care Department when she is ready to get back to work. And she also worries that, given the current changes in health care, whatever job she returns to — whether it be at the BI or elsewhere — may not be a job she will like.

Ellen says she relishes doing the kind of case management that she did at the BI — case management that embraced the heart of primary care and primary nursing. To her, case management is doing everything that needs to be done for the patient. But, she wonders, is that what the words "case management" mean to many health plans and insurers today? "For a lot of them, case management means you call them on the phone and give them the information and they tell you what they deem to be appropriate," Ellen comments sadly. "To me that's not case management, that's just dispensing the goods as they deem necessary.

"I'm used to fighting for what patients need," Ellen says. "But I wouldn't want to have to go into a home with blinders on, and just do a dressing change or tracheotomy care and ignore the other things a patient needs." Morally, she says, that would be unacceptable. To her, that is neither primary care nor primary nursing.

Chapter 10

A Good Enough Death II

JEANNIE CHAISSON

There are days, Jeannie Chaisson says, when Six Feldberg slips into battlefield mode. This week is a perfect example. First a ninety-seven-year-old woman was admitted after having had a massive heart attack. The woman, who was unconscious when she was discovered on the floor of her apartment, never woke up during her admission. She could not make her wishes known. There was no advance directive registered in her chart — no Do Not Resuscitate order to indicate she did not want to be resuscitated should she have a cardiac arrest. She was thus being fed through a feeding tube; her blood chemistries were being monitored and her vital signs recorded every four hours.

It was later ascertained that the woman hated doctors and had rare visits with a doctor. Her only recent contact with the health care system had consisted in episodic encounters with a visiting nurse who checked up on her from time to time. The nurse explained to Beth Israel staff that the old woman had clearly told her that she never wanted to end up in a hospital. So adamant was she about avoiding the medical system that she refused to countenance any of its legal and ethical paraphernalia, like living wills and health care proxies. In spite of the Visiting Nurse Association (VNA) nurses' assurances that the patient had made her wishes known, the situation was still ambiguous, and physicians chose to continue fairly aggressive care.

The old woman did have two elderly nieces who lived in the Midwest, and Jeannie talked with them. Did they know their aunt's wishes regarding care at the end of life? she asked. Had she ever voiced what she wanted to happen should she be incapable of deciding her medical fate herself?

The nieces were unable to answer. They were elderly themselves and hadn't seen their aunt in years. Their sporadic social contact had not produced the kind of information the medical system now demands. Lengthy discussions about life-supporting technology during a terminal illness is hardly the stuff of idle dinner table conversation, Jeannie notes. "Most of us don't sit down with our relatives, ask them to pass the mashed potatoes, and then turn to them and say, 'By the way, don't ever put me on life supports. I would never want a PEG [percutaneous endoscopic gastrostomy] tube inserted in my stomach to feed me artificially. And absolutely no antibiotics if I get pneumonia. Got that? Now I think I'll have some gravy and catsup, please,'" she says archly.

This was why the woman's nieces could not guide medical professionals. What they themselves wanted was guidance from those professionals. This produced an impasse. You tell us. No, you tell *us!* And the woman languished in the hospital.

Then two days later, there was another elderly patient who had a similar medical emergency. This woman actually did have a DNR order in her chart. She did not, however, pin it to her chest when she went out to do errands. When, on one of them, she had a cardiac arrest, she was raced to a different ER near her home and given cardiopulmonary resuscitation (CPR), even though she had explicitly forbidden it.

And finally, to top off the week, there is the third elderly woman, who is already on Six Feldberg for complications due to cardiopulmonary disease and cancer. The sick old woman goes into respiratory failure. Although she isn't Jeannie's patient, Jeannie joins staff as they crowd around the bed to intubate her. Her johnny has slipped down to reveal her chest. Several EKG leads to provide a continuous read-out of her heart rhythm are pasted on various parts of her sternum, her legs, and arms. While the commotion escalates around her, she is fully conscious, staring in mute terror. The story of this heroic intervention comes out in spurts as people cluster in the doorway and move in and out searching for equipment and debating what should or should not be done. The woman was being seen by a respiratory therapist when suddenly she couldn't breathe. So it was rescue time.

Or was it?

As one intern standing at the foot of the bed angrily tells a resident, he had a long talk with the patient on Saturday. She told him quite clearly that she had been intubated before and never, ever wanted to go through that again. She wanted to be DNR. He then conveyed that message to the woman's attending physician, who came to visit her sometime that weekend. The intern assumed that the patient and physician formalized this decision, that she would be DNR and would not be intubated or given CPR or other aggressive measures.

But just a few minutes before, when he was leafing through the chart to make sure the DNR order was in fact written there, he found that the attending had written the complete opposite. "The patient is *not* DNR." The "not" was underlined. Totally baffled, he could not imagine what had happened, why she had changed her mind. More to the point, the intern wants to know why the attending failed to come to him and explain the patient's change of heart. What if he had not had time to see the note in the chart? What if they had not intubated her?

The resident, too, is stymied. As Jeannie hears the story, she is astonished. "An attending can't write a note like that in the chart and not verbally convey the message to the house staff. Not on a busy weekend when there are so few people around," Jeannie hastily explains as she moves in and out of the room to help with the intubation.

In spite of all the confusion, it is clear that the intubation will proceed. The woman's primary nurse holds her hand while a tube is inserted down her throat. The respiratory therapist is standing next to the head of the bed, manually manipulating what is called an "ambu bag," which delivers air into the woman's lungs until she can be shuttled up to the Intensive Care Unit, where she will be put on a mechanical ventilator.

No one in the room seems at all happy about this medical rescue. Jeannie stands at the head of the bed holding the woman's hand. The emergency medical consult (EMC) — the physician in the hospital who is sent to any code or arrest — appears and begins to ask questions. More nurses and doctors congregate in the door and mill around the bed. Crammed into this tiny space, it seems as if someone is shooting a Cecil B. DeMille movie and has ordered a cast of thousands.

In the hubbub, someone notices that the patient is not sedated. A brief discussion ensues. Sedation might depress her respiration further, someone offers. Rationalizations fly about the room. She doesn't really know what's going on. She can't really feel the horrible pressure as they are inserting a tube down her throat and into her lungs. Someone shouts out for morphine and Jeannie rushes off to get it.

While the procedure is being done, the attending arrives. He looks briefly and nervously at the patient. Then he turns to the young intern standing at his side. The intern looks hesitant, then suddenly seems to make up his mind and begins to question the attending about his change of order.

It is one of those quintessential David and Goliath scenes. Even the costumes and size of the characters seem to highlight their different roles. The intern, dressed in wrinkled hospital scrubs, is slight, diffident, clearly anxious about leaping over the barrier of status that separates him from the attending physician. The senior doctor is dressed imposingly in a dark suit and tie. To make matters worse, the intern has to state his case in front of residents, nurses, respiratory technicians, and, incidentally, it seems, the patient — who appears more and more to be the object — rather than subject — of all these ministrations. The conversation is radically abbreviated — a slightly extended version of a sound byte, taking place in a crisis situation, conducted in staccato bursts of frustration and defensiveness.

Having gathered the courage to air his concerns, the intern blurts out, "The patient told me that she didn't want to be intubated. We thought your conversation with her would result in a DNR order, not in *not* Do Not Resuscitate."

The attending's gaze seems to career off the intern's face and flit around the small room. Uncomfortably, he explains that he and the patient had talked. She simply changed her mind about code status. She decided she wanted "everything," after all — intubation in case of arrest, CPR — in other words, a full code. The intern nods skeptically and, clearly disgruntled, leaves the room.

He stops outside the door, still fuming. Another doctor-in-training approaches, pats him on the shoulder, and applauds his action. "I heard that. I admire you for that," he says, referring to the challenge to an attending physician.

"I had to tell him," the intern repeats, as if trying to diminish his awareness of the chance he took questioning this medical authority by reasserting his moral obligation to the patient. "He should have told us when she changed her mind."

They share the commiseration of the powerless. The question hangs in the air — who changed whose mind? Who was really resistant to the DNR order? Was it the patient who decided she couldn't give up another crack at life, or the attending who couldn't give up on another crack at saving her? What did the attending say to this woman after the intern's conversation with her? Whose death is it, anyway?

After listening to this exchange, Jeannie steps back into the room. After the briefest of visits, the attending has gone. So have most of the residents and interns and nurses. The respiratory therapist remains at the head of the bed pumping the ambu bag.

Jeannie begins to take off the woman's telemetry leads, one by one. Then she notices that the woman has no catheter through which her urine could flow. Going outside to get the equipment, she double-gloves and then lifts the sheet and carefully separates the woman's legs. She washes her off, and looking up at the patient, advises her that she will feel a little pressure. When the catheter is inserted, the urine starts to flow down into the bag. Jeannie and the EMC then go to fetch the gurney that will carry the woman upstairs to the ICU and the long plastic plank that is used to slide patients off of their beds and onto it. The nurses carefully accomplish the transfer and hook the woman up to a portable heart monitor, defibrillator, and an oxygen tank.

About forty-five minutes have elapsed. Only the two nurses — Jeannie and the patient's primary nurse — and the respiratory therapist remain. Jeannie holds the woman's hand. On the other side of the bed, the patient's primary nurse grasps the patient's other hand and runs her fingers through the woman's hair. "I'm so sorry this had to happen to you," she whispers, leaning close to the patient and trying to calm her. As if divining the old woman's concerns, she assures her she will call the niece who is her nearest relative. The old woman clutches both nurses' hands. Alert, but unable to talk because of the tube down her airway, she mouths, "Do you have her number?"

Adept at lip reading, the primary nurse nods. "Don't you worry about that. I don't want you to worry about anything except your breathing. We'll take you up to the ICU and get you settled in just a few minutes. I'm going with you to get you settled," she reassures the woman once again.

The nurse and Jeannie linger at the patient's side. A few moments later, when Jeannie is certain that she is no longer needed, she leaves the woman with her nurse.

At lunch, about an hour later, this incident dominates the nurses' conversation. One of the nurses asks Jeannie what happened. Acting in her role as nurse educator, she uses this informal exchange to explore the ramifications of the incident. "It's a question of how much do you want to put yourself through as a patient. It may be that she'll pull through and have another couple of months. Maybe. That's a big maybe," she suggests. "It may be very difficult to get her off the vent."

One of the other nurses looks up. "And you just have to wonder how it is that a woman who said she never wanted to be intubated again on Saturday suddenly wants to be a full code on Monday."

As we finish our sandwiches, I say to Jeannie, not totally in jest, "It makes you want to have 'DNR' tattooed on your forehead, doesn't it?"

"Yeah," she says, and, pointing to a spot just above her heart, "and 'Don't even think about it!' plastered right here." Then, more seriously, she adds, "You know, half the time people say 'I want everything,' but they have no idea what 'everything' means. Most people don't know what CPR really involves."

In the hospital, when a patient gets cardiopulmonary resuscitation, the first thing that happens, Jeannie explains, is that somebody compresses the chest to force the heart, which is not beating, to circulate blood. In elderly patients whose bones are very brittle, this usually causes multiple rib fractures. Then may come defibrillation, in which two paddles are placed on the chest. These are attached to a machine that delivers a large jolt of electricity to the heart to shock it into beating. Meanwhile, a tube is placed down the patient's throat so that oxygen can be directed into the lungs. "Most people don't know that when you press so hard on the chest of an elderly person or a person with bone metastases from cancer, the result is that their ribs crack. It's such a great feeling," Jeannie says sarcastically, "to bear down on their chest and hear that lovely sound of ribs cracking. God, if that happens to me, just give me morphine and leave me alone. When I go, I'm not going to argue with Saint P. I'm outta here."

The last patient in this particular run of heroic efforts was exceptional because of the fact that a physician discussed her wishes at all. According to a study conducted at the Beth Israel itself, physicians may be quick to start CPR on patients, but few actually take the time to talk to them about their wishes before such an event takes place. In his book *Examining Your Doctor: A Patient's Guide to Avoiding Harmful Medical Care*, Timothy B. McCall describes the study. "Doctors at the Beth Israel Hospital in Boston looked at how often physicians talked with their patients about cardiopulmonary resuscitation (CPR). . . . The doctors discovered that less than 20 percent of patients who had been resuscitated with CPR had discussed it with their doctors beforehand.

"Of twenty-four patients who survived CPR, fifteen had wanted it, one was ambivalent, and eight had not wanted it done. The patients who didn't want CPR were worried about further suffering or a life hampered by chronic disease. Significantly, only one of the doctors who cared for the patients who hadn't wanted CPR correctly anticipated the patient's desire. Some doctors apparently can't imagine that a rational person could refuse throttle-to-the-floor medical technology. One of the doctors even said, 'Who wouldn't want to be resuscitated?'"

It is to this kind of throttle-to-the-floor, no-questions-asked-either-before-or-after treatment that Jeannie takes such strong exception. She is deeply concerned about a system that will do everything to keep patients alive but will deny them the benefit of sustained guidance and / or the advances in pain management that can make their days less anguished.

One morning at the Knotty Pine, as I read over a breakfast menu listing, as Jeannie puts it — "eggs, eggs, and if you like them, more eggs," she tells me about one of the most distressing cases she has witnessed. The patient was a man in his sixties. Because of bad heart disease and little angina attacks, the man was a frequent visitor to Jeannie's floor. The nurses on the unit had known him for years. He had always been a perfectly gracious, meticulously groomed gentleman who took great pride in his appearance. Which is why the disease that finally killed him was such an affront. It was a totally disfiguring tumor. "Think of it," Jeannie describes it, "as the worst red-oozing, protruding grotesque thing you can imagine. Well," she pauses for effect, "it was worse. It was the size of a baseball on his upper chest. It was like something out of *Aliens*, or one of those science fiction movies where things are pushing through a person's body and gushing outside. And it was causing him incredible pain."

Everyone knew how much pain he was in. No one denied the fact. Not even the physicians who staunchly refused to treat it.

"The resident was the biggest problem," Jeannie explains as she picks at her scrambled eggs and home fries. "He was obsessed with being sued, and he passed that obsession on to the intern who was writing the orders. He, in turn, had just gotten out of medical school and was interested in going into dermatology. He had no experience with the management of the pain and symptoms of cancer patients. What he did have was an interest in preserving life, which is why he went to medical school in the first place and what was reinforced there.

"Preserving life is a wonderful thing when life can be preserved. But there are instances when it can't. And there are instances when the pain involved in extending life is more than most people are willing to accept. It's important to learn the strategies that help people live. But it's also important to learn the strategies that are available to help people die comfortably. The problem is that these latter strategies aren't highlighted in medical school, or nursing school, for that matter."

This isn't hard just on patients, Jeannie says, it's hard on the young doctors who are ill prepared to confront the realities of the human condition and who feel a patient's death is a professional failure. "It's amazing," Jeannie reflects, "to think that you can get through four years of medical school without understanding that people actually die." She shakes her head and comments, "I've seen medical students who have come to the hospital to practice doing history and physicals on patients with cancer and who burst into tears when they discover that there is no curative treatment for this patient's cancer. They thought they were going to be 'saving lives.' They've been taught what medicine can do, but not what we can't do."

In the case of the man with the tumor, the resident reinforced the intern's dream about saving lives and fed him his own legal nightmare. His message was, if a cancer patient's pain is treated with too much morphine, breathing will be depressed. If the patient dies in comfort, the result may be a lawsuit. "Anybody can sue you. It doesn't have to be the patient or family, it can be the dietitian. He even told the intern that one of us — one of the nurses — might sue him," Jeannie recounts with one of her can-you-top-that looks.

So, Jeannie sums up, we have a man in agony whom we can help. His care is entrusted to an inexperienced young intern. At his elbow is a slightly more experienced resident warning him that if the patient dies in peace, the family won't send him a thank you note, but rather a subpoena. The intern doesn't know how to go check this out with more-experienced physicians and nurses. After legal tutorials from someone with no legal knowledge, the intern is terrified to do anything to treat the patient's pain because it might decrease breathing rate and blood pressure.

As I listen to the story, I ask the obvious questions. Where was the attending? What about other physicians on staff?

Drumming her fingers impatiently on the feathered red Formica tabletop, she responds. Yes, of course, other physicians who were competent and familiar with palliative care tried to intervene. They spoke to the physicians involved in the patient's care. They referred them to articles that documented the need for pain management and urged them to treat the man's pain. It didn't do any good. Jeannie assumes the patient's physicians felt defensive and were reluctant to forcefully advocate for better pain control.

To justify their course of action, they insisted that the patient wasn't clearly terminal and therefore couldn't have the type of aggressive pain management that might suppress respiration. To this Jeannie retorts, "You could have taken any five people off the street and asked them to look at the patient and describe what they saw, and they would say, 'Yup, this man is dying, he's in agony, do something!'"

But the intern, resident, and attending were observing the patient through a different lens. "When we reminded them that he was in agony every time we turned him to put a bedpan under him, they just said, 'Well, don't turn him, then.'"

As we are speaking, a waitress appears to ask if we want more coffee, but Jeannie is so involved in this memory — the kind that does not dull and then recede — that she does not notice. Instead she continues. When the physicians in charge of a case like this refuse to alter their course, it's very hard to influence their decisions. The family would have had to intervene. But in this case, the family didn't live nearby. Relatives visited only sporadically and didn't understand what was going on. Moreover, they held doctors in such high esteem that they were afraid to challenge their orders.

The result? The patient died two weeks later — with no effective pain management.

"Doctors in America have a terrible record when it comes to managing pain," she says. "When they don't treat pain well, it is — in my opinion — the moral equivalent of battery. What is incredible is that many don't look at it that way. They manage to convince themselves that their refusal to treat a patient's pain during a terminal illness is not, in fact, causing the patient's pain. That pain, they argue, is caused by the disease, not by their inaction."

Jeannie again shoots me a look filled with incredulity at the human capacity for denial. Obviously the technical distinction they make could be construed as accurate. But hospitals are supposed to succor and comfort as well as heal and cure. In this case, the sin of omission is, Jeannie feels, a sin of commission. Deciding to do nothing when you could do something is, itself, a form of taking action.

Soberly, Jeannie explains how terrible it feels to know you can help a patient and yet you aren't allowed to do so, to be tethered to a hierarchical structure that deprives patients of caregivers with wisdom and experience and places their fates in the hands of people who may have little of either.

To improve the quality of care of dying patients, Jeannie recently gathered with a small group of nurses and physicians — including oncology nurse Paddy Connelly, oncologist Glenn Bubley, and fellow Paola Rode, general surgeon Michael Cahalane, internists Geraldine Zagarella and Elizabeth Kass, Karen Dick, nurse manager of the Home Care Department, and medical nurse Deborah Jameson. The group was interested in starting a palliative care consultation team at the BI.

The group formed in late January 1995, after Paddy Connelly

came across an article in the *Boston Globe*. One of the foundations created by international financier and philanthropist George Soros, the article reported, had just announced a new initiative to "understand and transform the experience of dying in the United States." The Open Society Institute had set aside $14 million for "The Project on Death in America." Connelly was particularly intrigued by the Project's interest in palliative care initiatives in hospitals.

While meeting to plan a proposal, Jeannie suggested that it would be important to gather data that would benchmark where practice at the hospital was now so they could tell whether a palliative care service would be effective in helping patients. To do this, she designed a study that would collect information about the types of care received by patients with late-stage chronic illness who were hospitalized at Beth Israel. This is a group for whom palliative care options would often be appropriate. "We wondered," Jeannie explains, "whether the option — focus on comfort rather than cure — was routinely offered to patients and whether their care looked different than the care of patients with less-serious illness."

To find out, Jeannie proposed a study that would review the charts of a sample of patients with significant chronic illness who had died at the BI within the last year. "We would know they were end-stage because they died," Jeannie says with a smile. "And we could go through their charts and find out what type of care they received. Everything from numbers of blood draws to types of medications to how many tests the patients got to how care providers characterized the significant issues — were they calling the problem breast cancer or were they calling it pain control — all of these things would help us to learn more about what is offered and given to this population, and equally important, what is not offered."

The group met for almost half a year but did not ultimately get an Open Society Institute grant. In the summer of 1996, Glenn Bubley, however, headed a committee of nurses, doctors, and social workers whose goal is to provide better palliative care options, in a more timely fashion, to cancer patients at the Beth Israel. The team's mandate was to prepare guidelines for physicians that would help them better navigate the transitions in cancer care. Jeannie also proceeded with the study she suggested and got a small grant to help cover part of the time it takes to prepare the data as she and her coinvestigators — Karen Dick, Geraldine Zagarella, and Elizabeth

Kass — move forward with the study. "I hope the results of the study will show us how to design teaching strategies so that all physicians and nurses in the hospital will know when to seek palliative care options for appropriate patients. Right now it's hit or miss."

One of the patients who was almost missed is an eighty-five-year-old woman, Mrs. De Marco.* The elderly woman is demented and has been living at home with twenty-four-hour care for a number of years. Like so many of Jeannie's patients, she has been in and out of the hospital. Several months ago, she was admitted to Six Feldberg following a major stroke that had paralyzed one side of her body. Now she has been readmitted with infected decubitous ulcers, otherwise known as bedsores, on her heels and backside.

We tend to apply the word "sore" to minor abrasions or other less-significant aches and pains. These "sores" are, however, awful red craters that penetrate her limbs. Both heels have been abraded to the bone and are a raw mass of oozing pus. The bedsores on her backside are inflamed holes almost half an inch deep and two inches by two inches square. They are not her only afflictions. Because of her dementia and the stroke, it has been almost impossible for her care providers at home to feed her. These awful sores are a result of malnutrition, not neglect. In the hospital, Mrs. De Marco had a nasogastric tube inserted into her nose and down her throat into her stomach to provide nutrition.

When Jeannie first walks into her room, she finds a woman lying in bed with a desperate look in her eyes. When she reads the chart, she discovers that the two craters on the woman's backside have been surgically debrided (the dead skin removed) and require dressing changes every four hours. Mrs. De Marco's only mobile hand is tied to the side of the bed to prevent her from ripping the tube out of her nose. She also has a high fever; she is in pain and thus on morphine.

Looking through the patient's medical record, Jeannie discovers that three days hence the patient is scheduled for the insertion of a PEG tube, or permanent feeding tube. A gastroenterologist will push a fiberoptic endoscope through the patient's throat and into the stomach. Once the instrument is in the stomach, the physician will be able to push the stomach up against the abdominal wall. Then a simple stab wound will be made in the abdominal wall and the feeding tube will be directly inserted into the stomach. The use of the endoscope will make this procedure less invasive than a surgical one, but it will nonetheless be invasive and uncomfortable.

When Jeannie leafs through the patient's chart, she comes upon something that makes this planned gastrostomy difficult to countenance. Years ago, Mrs. De Marco had gone to the trouble of making a living will, which had been affixed to her chart. It says, as Jeannie analyzes the document's intent, "Don't prolong my life. I don't want to be dependent. I don't want to be in pain."

The woman Jeannie sees in the bed is not getting what she has asked for. Not by any stretch of the imagination.

Jeannie immediately determines her plan of care, which she puts into action the following day. As soon as she gets to work, she finds the resident and asks her to join her for a few moments in the solarium. As they sit and converse in the long, narrow room she points to the DNR order in the chart with a finger. "Hello, is anybody home here?" she asks. "What are we doing here? She's dependent. She's in pain. We're prolonging her life. What's this for? This makes absolutely no sense. Why are we scheduling for a PEG tube insertion this week? Why are we debriding these ulcers? Why are we aggressively treating this woman who is at the end of her life?

"This is absolutely against everything that is behind the patient's living will." Jeannie states what should be the obvious. "It may be a very general one-paragraph document," she concedes. "It doesn't contain a list of everything you can and cannot do. But it's very clear that this is not what this woman wanted when she was lucid. It's very clear that our treatment isn't working. What we really need to be discussing with her family is withdrawing the feedings, not putting in a permanent feeding tube."

The resident does not disagree. In fact, over the course of the day, it becomes clear to Jeannie that everybody involved in caring for the patient thinks the insertion of a feeding tube is a terrible idea. But institutional inertia has prevailed and nobody has mustered the energy to oppose it. Similarly, no one has investigated the patient's wishes or those of the elderly sister who is responsible for the patient.

Jeannie can imagine how confused and intimidated the patient's sister probably feels. "If you have an eighty-year-old woman, she'll tend to do whatever the doctor says needs to be done," she tells the resident. "She'll probably go along with it, even if she thinks it's a shame. She doesn't know that she has options, that she can choose to follow the recommendations or not follow them."

Jeannie continues to appeal to the resident's common sense. "Listen, we need to talk to this lady," Jeannie advises. "We need to tell her what it's like for her sister. Her sister is in pain. She's miserable. She's probably aspirating. She's febrile. This is ridiculous. She's got a living will in there that says 'Don't torture me' and we're torturing her."

The young woman agrees that a family meeting is definitely in order and says she will talk to the attending to arrange it quickly. When Jeannie learns, later in the day, that the family meeting will take place the following afternoon — a day before the PEG tube is slated for insertion — she seeks out Mrs. De Marco's primary nurse. It will be this young and less-experienced nurse, not Jeannie, who will sit with the family, the resident, attending, and social worker in the meeting in which Mrs. De Marco's fate will be decided. Jeannie recognizes that the nurse will need some coaching from someone with more experience if she is to be a forceful advocate for the patient.

To underscore the problems the family might have withdrawing feeding and propose how to deal with them, Jeannie suggests that she and the nurse talk in the conference room during a lull on the day shift. "It will be very hard for the family to say, we're not going to feed her anymore." She explores the process with the nurse. "The reason that people kind of bumble along saying, 'Well, okay,' we'll put an NG [nasogastric] tube in and feed her, or place a PEG tube in, is that this is a huge, socially loaded issue. This woman needs to hear what we're going to do, not what we're not going to do."

In a fluid arpeggio, Jeannie runs through each of the positives. "We are going to keep her comfortable. We are going to maintain her dignity. Feeding won't help any of this. The sister needs to hear that many families make this decision because of their concern for the patient's comfort. She needs to hear that withdrawing feeding is not uncomfortable for the patient. She needs to learn that all the medical and nursing research that has been done on this issue shows that withdrawing nutrition does not cause discomfort for a patient in her state."

The patient's sister, Jeannie adds, also needs to understand another benefit of removing the feeding tube: "The restraint can be removed. The patient will be able to move her hand. Plus instead of looking for a nursing home, we'll be able to keep her here and care for her really well until she dies."

A day after she meets with the nurse, and two days after she talks to the resident, the family meeting takes place. Confident and thus emboldened after their conversation, the patient's primary nurse reports back to Jeannie. She says she spoke forcefully in the meeting, which went extremely well.

Jeannie later relates the details. "The NG tube is out. The feedings have stopped. We can make a new care plan, a new Kardex, and focus on comfort. Thank God! It just shows what can happen with the appropriate coaching and communication between the attending, nurses, GI service, and medical team. We were able to head off the catastrophe that was supposed to take place this morning."

About a week later, Jeannie cares for Mrs. De Marco. It's eight in the evening, and the unit is particularly quiet. Jeannie has a moment to go into Mrs. De Marco's room and sit with her as she breathes laboriously. While Jeannie is holding her hand, the old woman dies. She bends over the bed and silently brushes her hand over Mrs. De Marco's forehead and bids good-bye to her patient. Then she goes to notify the attending physician, who will, in turn, call the patient's sister to tell her of the death.

Soon, Jeannie knows, Mrs. De Marco's sister will arrive at the hospital. "The main thing now," Jeannie explains, "is to make things look as good as possible. I always want families to be able to come in and see someone recognizable."

In this case, Jeannie goes back to clean the body. First she pulls out Mrs. De Marco's IV and her catheter. Had she been receiving oxygen or been attached to a heart monitoring unit, she would have taken out those tubes and lines. Jeannie removes the old woman's hospital johnny and bathes her from head to foot, removing the dressings covering her ulcers. She opens her mouth and brushes her teeth. "Sometimes, if someone has been very ill, it's been hard to clean their mouth because it's too uncomfortable, so I like to give their teeth a good scrub," Jeannie explains. She also puts a new johnny on Mrs. De Marco. She lowers the bed rails so that friends or relatives can easily reach her.

Jeannie does this for all her patients who die. The only exception are orthodox Jews. "In the Jewish culture," she explains," you have to check with the burial society. Usually, they don't want us to clean the body in any way. They don't even want us to pull the tubes. The members of the burial society come to the hospital and prepare the body themselves."

Jeannie then waits for Mrs. De Marco's sister to arrive. When she does, Jeannie escorts her into the room and allows her to sit with her sister. "I always let families stay as long as they want, no matter how loudly the admitting office is screaming that they need the bed," Jeannie says.

When the sister leaves, Jeannie goes to find one of the white plastic shrouds used to cover the dead. Before placing it around the body, she affixes a name tag to Mrs. De Marco's toe. In arranging the body in the shroud, Jeannie is again aware of cultural differences. Because the old woman was a Christian, she crosses her hands in front and ties her wrists and feet with the gauze cord used to wrap corpses. (Had she been Jewish, she would have placed her arms at her side.)

"We once had a Gypsy die in the Emergency Unit," Jeannie comments. "In their culture, they open windows so that the soul of the dead person can escape and is not bound to their body. It's difficult to do this in a place where windows don't open." She smiles. "They opened all the doors leading to the front door at the ambulance bay, which was also left open. That way the family felt the woman's soul could be freed."

Jeannie then folds the plastic over Mrs. De Marco's head. "This is the hard part for some people," she explains. "You have to remind yourself that the person is dead and no longer breathing." After making sure there is also a tag identifying Mrs. De Marco on the outside of the shroud, she calls transport to take the body down to the morgue.

A few minutes later, two men arrive. In some hospitals, transporters take the body down to the basement morgue unaccompanied by a nurse. At the Beth Israel, nurses accompany their patients on this last hospital journey. When the attendants have shifted Mrs. De Marco's body onto the morgue stretcher and covered it with a large plastic sheath that conceals its contents, Jeannie and the two men roll the gurney to the elevators and down to the bowels of the hospital. Wheeling their load through a maze of corridors, they stop at a small square room across from the autopsy suite. A bank of refrigerated lockers — most for adults but two set aside for babies — awaits. With Jeannie watching, the men pull out one of the stainless steel drawers and carefully place the body within.

Jeannie explains that many people who are not medical professionals are understandably nervous about being around dead bodies. They may deal with their discomfort with inappropriate joking and / or rough treatment. She has seen gurneys rolled too quickly and banged into walls, bodies unceremoniously dumped into morgue drawers, heads banged against the drawer's edges.

Jeannie does not believe that her dead patients can feel pain or suffer from any of this unseemly behavior. And she is certainly not a religious or even a "New Agey" person. But she does believe that there is something awesome, beyond one's understanding, in the moment of death and its aftermath. One moment a person is there. Their spirit is occupying their body. Their body is still vital, even in the worst agonies of illness. And then, suddenly, they are gone.

"Sometimes, you can actually feel that something is different about the room when a patient dies — especially if you're alone with the patient and there is no one else there muddying up the energy," Jeannie says. "I'll be standing, looking at a chart, or out the window — not looking at the patient — and I can feel the change in energy in the room. You turn around and the patient is dead."

To Jeannie there is a dignity and solemnity to death. In extending her care beyond the moment of death, she ensures that this is respected.

When Mrs. De Marco's body has been safely sheltered, Jeannie leaves the room to return to the care of the living.

Chapter 11

Unraveling the Tapestry of Care

When I began researching this book in the late 1980s, it seemed that nursing was finally on the cusp of true societal recognition and far greater financial rewards. In the mid-eighties, hospitals reported high rates of unfilled positions for registered nurses. Press and scholarly accounts documented the negative impact this nursing shortage was having on patient care. Public attention was drawn to the important role nurses play in health care. As a result, hospitals raised nurses' wages and offered better benefits and working conditions. As the new decade began, the nursing shortage ebbed. By the late eighties, most hospitals had low RN vacancy rates. In a number of areas, salaries for nurses had increased, and working conditions and benefits were much improved.

Hospitals also developed a variety of ways to keep educated, experienced nurses at the bedside. More and more hospitals were shifting to the primary nursing model pioneered at the Beth Israel. Many hospital nursing departments had allocated the resources to run education and empowerment programs. It seemed that hospitals were ready to recognize that nurses as well as physicians are learners in hospitals. The nursing profession was refining and designing new roles for hospital nurses, such as the clinical nurse specialist. Nurse practitioners were gaining more prominence. Some hospitals were even developing promising experiments in nurse-physician collaboration. As mentioned previously, for four years the Beth Israel devoted a fourteen-bed unit known as the Collaborative Care Unit to the study and promotion of nurse-physician collaboration. Nurses were also gaining a greater voice in the public debate about reform of our health care system. As if to underline nursing's steady progress, nursing school enrollments were up.

Just as I was finishing my research, Jeannie Chaisson, Nancy Rumplik, and Ellen Kitchen were suddenly affected by trends that have been unfolding continually for over a decade. Hospitals were struggling to adapt to the rapid ascension of a corporate version of managed care that focuses increasingly on profit maximization. To do this, many have chosen to sacrifice care at the bedside. Although the Beth Israel has tried to maintain its culture, fierce marketplace competition makes it difficult for any hospital to remain an island of caring in a sea of cost cutting.

In the Hematology / Oncology Clinic at the Beth Israel, the volume of patients is higher and the patients are sicker. Because most insurers are trying to decrease hospital stays, they want more chemotherapy given on an outpatient basis. "Some of my patients may be in the clinic all day long," Nancy explained regretfully in the winter of 1995. "In our unit, we run out of chairs. We're getting backed up because people are staying four to five hours getting their Taxol. With cisplatin, that's another two hours. That makes eight hours."

Home care departments like Ellen's are also feeling the pinch as nurses are asked to see more patients and do less for them. But nowhere are the changes in health care more visible than on the inpatient units where nurses like Jeannie Chaisson work. Over the past several years, the Beth Israel has reduced through attrition the number of its clinical nurse specialists and closed the Collaborative Care Unit. Jeannie Chaisson saw patients one or two days a week and acted as an educational resource three or four days a week. She now cares for patients four days a week and acts as an educational resource only one day a week. Most distressingly, she feels profit-driven health care is now transforming the definition of hospital. "There is more and more pressure to push people out of the hospital. Insurers are telling you to discharge a patient at eight-thirty at night because they don't want to pay for another day in the hospital. And nurses, like everyone else, are asked to get involved in that. Hospitals now feel their survival depends on getting patients in and out."

On October 1, 1996, the Beth Israel Hospital — as an individual entity — became an artifact of the past. In the merger mania of the period, it had joined forces with the Deaconess Hospital to become the Beth-Israel Deaconess Medical Center. In the summer of 1994, the Deaconess had formed the Pathway Health Network, including the New England Baptist Hospital, the former Glover Memorial Hospital in Needham, Nashoba Hospital in Ayer, and Waltham-Weston Hospital. Then the Beth Israel and the Deaconess merged into a single hospital and Mount Auburn Hospital in Cambridge also joined the fold. Their parent organization is called the CareGroup. Mitchell T. Rabkin is now the CEO of the CareGroup.

Many nurses are worried about the fate of the BI's culture of caring in this new, larger corporate structure. Some of the articles in the *Boston Globe* have discussed the change in terms of the system's competitive advantage in the new health care marketplace. They also mentioned plans to cut beds in the two new hospitals from eight hundred to four hundred or five hundred — the kind of downsizing that has brought increasing job loss for nurses and other hospital employees. "We're all very anxious," one nurse told me. "We're taking it one day at a time."

When President Clinton fashioned his health care reform proposal of 1993–1994, his main concern was to avoid expanding government while, however, expanding health care coverage. To do this he relied on a theory that Theda Skocpol, a Harvard professor of government and sociology, has called "inclusive managed competition." This approach combined private, employment-based health insurance with "universal coverage and publicly enforced cost controls." The President proposed a system of mandatory employer contributions to health care and large regional health alliances in which privately run health care plans would compete with one another. The plans offered by these regional health care alliances were mainly health maintenance organizations (HMOs) of the type that have functioned by significantly limiting patients' choice of physicians, restricting their ability to see medical specialists, radically shortening hospital stays, strictly micromanaging physician behavior, increasingly offering physicians a financial incentive to underserve patients. The proposal also included some modest regulation of the health care industry.

The Clinton proposal sent a message to the health care industry. To gain a more advantageous position in the competitive new health care marketplace, hospitals accelerated a trend toward merging or closing that had begun earlier. And insurers and health maintenance organizations also continued similar mergers and consolidations. Although Congress refused to act on the Clinton proposal, the stage was set. When the proposal failed, there was no return to a larger public debate about government-funded universal health care. Instead, the corporate version of managed care — minus government regulation and any increase in the uninsured's access to health care — has become the cosmetic solution to our nation's long-standing health care crisis. In our uniquely American health care system — one that depends on private insurance provided as a benefit of employment — employers large and small are trying to save premium dollars by pushing employees into health maintenance organizations or other forms of managed care.

By the end of 1995, health maintenance organizations had 56 million subscribers. Another 70 million Americans have more traditional insurance retrofitted with managed care features such as preferred providers and utilization review. Over 70 percent of HMOs are for-profit and many not-for-profit HMOs are converting to for-profit status. This means that more and more Americans now depend on profit-making corporations for their health care.

Investor-owned managed care companies are legally mandated to increase profits for shareholders. The terminology of HMOs reflects the orientation toward profit maximization. The percentage of premiums spent on medical care in HMOs is known as "the medical loss ratio." According to the *New York Times*, the large not-for-profit HMO Kaiser Permanente of California spent all but 4 percent of its 1994 revenue on patient care. U.S. Healthcare, the largest for-profit HMO in the Northeast, spent less than 74 cents per dollar on care. The rest went for administration, advertising, executive salaries, and shareholder dividends. The lower the "medical loss ratio" — that is, the less spent on patients and caregivers — the more a plan is attractive to potential investors.

As reports in the *New York Times*, the *Wall Street Journal*, and the trade publication *Modern Healthcare* have documented, managed care companies have become some of the most profitable in America. Revenues in the largest HMOs have been astronomical. A recent story in the *Wall Street Journal* discussed the multibillion-dollar surplus that for-profit managed care plans have amassed that they simply don't know how to invest. The salaries of CEOs and stock options for the top seven for-profit HMOs averaged $7 million in 1994. Leonard Abramson, the CEO of U.S. Healthcare, owns over half a billion dollars in company stock. When Abramson negotiated the merger of U.S. Healthcare and Aetna in 1996, his personal fortune increased by just under $1 billion (that's enough to pay for the extra care for all the uninsured children in the state of Massachusetts for twelve years or for all the uninsured in the Commonwealth for three years or the salaries of about twenty-five thousand nurses for one year).

We have heard about some of the excesses of managed care — no choice of physician, difficulty in seeing specialists, barriers to emergency room care, gag clauses that prevent physicians from speaking honestly about a patient's diagnoses, prognoses, and treatment options. But two other phenomena accelerated by managed care, radically shortened length of hospital stay and hospital restructuring that targets nursing, are having a devastating impact on the quality of care nurses like Jeannie, Ellen, and Nancy are able to provide.

One of the chief strategies that insurers have deployed to save money is either to keep people out of the hospital entirely or to shorten their hospital length of stay. Part of this trend is due to new technologies and chemotherapies that are far less invasive and toxic and allow people to have outpatient surgery, recover more quickly from inpatient surgery, or be cared for at home. But much of this is due to what the noted Princeton University health care economist Uwe Reinhardt has called "our obsessive quest to gut the hospital" and has led to radical and inappropriate reductions in admissions and lengths of hospital stay. Health care insurers recognize that their plans can potentially save billions of dollars if patients are not cared for in the hospital, but are transferred to rehabilitation facilities that hire fewer nurses and more LPNs. Even greater cost savings can be generated if the cost of patient care is borne by unpaid caregivers in the home.

"Between 1980 and 1995 total inpatient admissions per thousand population and average length-of-stay declined by about 20 percent each; consequently, inpatient days per thousand declined by about 40 percent," Reinhardt wrote recently in an article in *Health Affairs*. As Boston University health care ethicist George Annas has pointed out in an article in the *New England Journal of Medicine*, childbirth is the most common reason for hospitalization. Yet over the past twenty-six years, average length of maternity stay in the U.S. for all vaginal deliveries has gone from four days in 1970 to two days in 1992. For many it's now twenty-four hours. In California, some mothers and newborns are being discharged as quickly as eight hours after delivery.

This decades-long trend of shortening length of hospital stay has not curtailed soaring health care costs. In fact, as Reinhardt points out, from 1980 to 1993, real per capita spending on hospital inpatient care rose by nearly 53 percent even though inpatient days plummeted by 36 percent. This apparently paradoxical rise in costs accompanied by declining hospital stays occurs because the hospital days that have been cut really cost very little. Yet the way hospitals price their services disguises this fact.

Hospitals have traditionally negotiated their services at a flat average per diem rate — thus trying to capture in that rate some or all of the hospital's fixed and variable costs. This means that a hospital day that actually costs $300 because the patient needs fewer medical interventions and less monitoring is still billed at, say, a $1,000 rate. HMOs also often demand that hospitals accept a flat daily payment. This gives HMO's — through their physicians — the power to pay for fewer days and thus avoid paying for some of the hospital's legitimate costs.

Reinhardt calls this system "perverse pricing." It encourages insurers to try to kick patients out of the hospital — or not admit them at all — as quickly as possible. Often these unstable patients are sent to facilities like nursing homes and subacute facilities that actually charge more per day (on average about $400) than the hospital would charge for a less intensive day of recovery and monitoring if it priced its services more accurately. The HMO may save money, but we, as a society, actually end up paying more for the care of acutely ill patients than we would if they stayed and recovered in the hospital.

Because of this "perverse-pricing" system, cutting inpatient days and length of stays has become almost a religious principle in the United States. We now have the shortest length of hospital stay of any industrialized country in the world. In a country that spends 14 percent of its Gross Domestic Product (GDP) on health care, patients spend 20 to 40 percent less time in hospitals than they do in countries with single-payer universal health care systems that devote only 9 or 10 percent of GDP to health care.

In managed care plans, patients are discharged from the hospital twice as quickly as people covered by traditional indemnity plans. Indeed, today, some HMOs are linking physicians' pay to their ability to keep patients out of the hospital, or to discharge them quickly. Kaiser's own southern California business plan details how the HMO wants to cut its costs by $800 million over the next five years. The Kaiser plan proposes to do this, in part, by cutting its hospitalization rates by about 30 percent and by early discharges of patients.

In the summer of 1996, the California Nurses Association and the Los Angeles–based Consumers for Quality Care exposed a particularly egregious practice by Sharp HealthCare — a California hospital chain that employs ten thousand people at seven hospitals and twenty-six clinics in San Diego and Riverside Counties. The company's hospital handbook contained a section on conflicts of interest and stated that "all employees have the responsibility to place the interests of Sharp HealthCare above their own and those of others." Such conflicts, the handbook said, could occur when the best interests of Sharp differed from those of a "vendor, supplier, patient, friend, relative, visitor, applicant or competitor."

As Rose Ann De Moro, executive director of the California Nurses Association commented, "Provisions like this are chilling. The message they send is that patient care is for sale, and doctors and nurses should check their responsibility to patients at the door and not protest when patient care is jeopardized by HMO policies like, for example, shortened length of hospital stay."

The shorter lengths of stay that result give Jeannie and her colleagues all across the nation a mission impossible as they try to provide quality care for patients in only the briefest periods of time. "You don't have that period with patients when you can work with them on teaching, on how they're going to take care of themselves when they get home. You don't have time to walk with an elderly person who has pneumonia, to make sure they're steady and you know they're going to be okay. You send them home before you know they're going to be okay," Jeannie explains.

The healing encounters Jeannie and her patients value so much, she says, are becoming rarer and rarer. Sometimes a patient is lucky enough to spend sufficient time in a hospital. But when that happens, Jeannie says dryly, insurance companies brand them an "outlier" — someone who lies outside the statistical norms insurers deem appropriate for hospital care. So, Jeannie concludes, you're either abandoned or you're an "outlier."

What makes the work of nurses like Jeannie Chaisson much more difficult is that shortened length of stay has led to what is called higher patient acuity — or higher intensity of patient needs — in hospitals. Today, no one who is not very sick is admitted to a hospital. Patients no longer go into hospitals for observation. Nor are they admitted a day or two before surgery or invasive diagnostic procedures. Similarly, after such operations or tests, they do not remain in the hospital to be fully stabilized. Nurses are no longer caring for one patient who is waiting for surgery, another who has been out of surgery for four or five days and is relatively stable, and another highly unstable patient just returned from the operating room. Everyone in the hospital is acutely ill and unstable.

In November of 1996, Boston College nursing researcher Judith Shindul-Rothschild released the final results of a study based on a survey of over 7,500 nurses conducted in collaboration with the *American Journal of Nursing*. Responses to a questionnaire printed in the *American Journal of Nursing* were analyzed for this report. Nurses all over the country had been asked about their experiences on the job. Sixty-six percent said that patient length of stay had decreased. Seventy-three percent said they had less time to teach patients and families and to comfort and talk to patients, and 69 percent said they had less time for basic nursing care.

Jeannie and other nurses are not only worried about the impact of heightened acuity while patients are in the hospital. They are worried about the well-being of patients who are being sent home or to a burgeoning new industry of "subacute facilities." Nursing homes are designed to handle elderly and chronically ill patients or patients well on the road to recovery after surgical or other medical procedures — not acutely ill patients. Now that hospitals are discharging this class of patients so quickly, a new kind of facility — the subacute facility — is emerging. Many of these new facilities are just old-style nursing homes refurbished with the high-tech equipment necessary to deal with patients who are immediately postoperative or still acutely ill and who have more complex medical needs. Others are newly built centers or new businesses that have taken over hospitals that have been shut down in the merger mania of the last several years. Largely run by for-profit companies, this industry is now worth $1 billion and it is projected that it will be worth $10 billion by the year 2000.

The problem with this exploding new field is that many of these facilities lack the kind of expert nursing staff needed to take care of the acutely ill patients they are actively seeking. A major study conducted by the consulting firm Lewin-VHI revealed that many of these facilities fail to hire adequately trained nursing staff. Lewin-VHI said that claims that subacute facilities were more cost effective than acute care hospitals were unsubstantiated. Similarly, it said there was no basis for the claim that patients fare better in these facilities than in hospitals. Indeed, the report noted that there were no major studies evaluating the outcomes of subacute patients who had complex medical conditions.

Those patients who are not sent to subacute facilities are sent home. "You would not believe what people are going home with today," says Ruth McCorkle, professor of nursing at the University of Pennsylvania School of Nursing and a prominent researcher on the home care needs of cancer patients. "We're doing mastectomies on an outpatient basis. Mastectomies!" She pauses almost with disbelief. "Women are going home with complex dressing changes, with drains from their wounds, with injections they have to give themselves. Men are going home after prostate surgery with inadequate education about the consequences of their surgery. And I haven't even gotten to the emotional needs of these patients, who are faced with life-threatening illnesses and whose bodies may have been dramatically altered."

McCorkle and her colleagues studied the nursing activities involved in the care of elderly postsurgical cancer patients. In an early stage of their study in 1993, they discovered that a fifth of their one-hundred-person sample had deep vein thrombosis, or blood clots in the leg. Out of that group of twenty patients, four were readmitted with pulmonary emboli — a catastrophic complication that occurs when blood clots that break off from the leg travel to the pulmonary arteries that feed the lung, where they can cause instant death. "This means," says McCorkle, "that we're getting patients out of the hospital so fast that we're forgetting the fundamentals about the dangers of blood clots after surgery and the need for nurses to initiate walking with supervision after surgery."

As she is presently completing the study with 301 additional patients, she has documented a 15 percent mortality due to a number of complications, including pulmonary emboli. "We find these figures alarming," McCorkle says and speculates that "early discharge without adequate follow-up nursing care in the home puts these patients at increased risk for premature death."

Advocates of competition and a private, corporate-driven health care system argue that many patients will be fine after their discharge from the hospital because of the care that will be available from nurses in the home. In reality, home care for the acutely ill is also being turned into a no-care zone. Because the kind of nursing care that will ensure patient safety in the home is not cheap, the goal of managed care companies is not to cut hospital labor costs and redistribute savings to home care. Their goal is to squeeze the system in every setting — whether it be hospital or home — and redistribute any savings to shareholder dividends and executive salaries.

The catch-22s in which patients and their caregivers are entrapped, says Jeannie, are nothing short of incredible. Insurers regularly ask Jeannie to send home patients who are unstable and still need nursing care. Will the insurers pay for quality care in the home? No way.

Take the first day of discharge. This period is crucial to the patient's recovery. Nurses often need to visit the patient's home immediately after discharge to make sure the patient is safe. Can the patient make it to the bathroom or up and down the stairs? Will he or she receive meals? Are complex drug regimens laid out in a way that makes it possible for patients to take medications correctly? Do patients understand how to use any high-tech medical equipment — a ventilator, an infusion pump for IV medication, suctioning devices? Neither a hospital nor a visiting nurse can make these determinations without visiting the patient's home.

Instead of welcoming the nurse's role in ensuring quality of care in the home — the new "locus of care" — insurers seem to consider home care just another arena of denial. "If I send someone home on a Tuesday and want a nurse to check up on that patient on Tuesday,

most insurers won't pay for it," Jeannie says with mounting frustration. "They say the patient can do without a nursing visit until the
day following discharge because they have just seen a nurse in the
hospital."

Home care nurses, Jeannie says, must also argue for every visit,
every minute of care. "I was working with a nurse yesterday who does
home care and works with us a couple of days a week," Jeannie recounts. "She told me that she actually had a patient with three draining abdominal wounds after complicated surgery. This patient
required very skilled dressing changes and evaluation and she was ar-
guing on the phone for an extended period of time with the HMO to
get this care."

Instead of agreeing to provide the nursing care in the home that
was no longer available in the hospital, the insurer blamed the nurses
in the hospital for the patient's problems. An angry utilization re-
viewer wanted to know why the hospital nurses were unable to teach
a man who had just had major abdominal surgery and was thus exhausted and groggy from pain medication to do his own dressing
changes at home.

"My question," Jeannie asks, equally angrily, "is, 'Is this patient
stable enough to be in the community, and if so, why do you think a
patient should be able to know how to evaluate a wound?' Don't
these people get it?" she demands. "It's not just a matter of taking a
dressing off and putting another on. It's a matter of knowing how to
tell if they're developing an infection or what to be concerned about.

"The people who run health care these days seem to think that because a person has a Ph.D. from Harvard, they can be sent home
from the hospital acutely ill and do okay," Jeannie comments on the
brave new world of health care. "They think people can administer
their own drugs, that they can give themselves antibiotics with a
high-tech device like an IV infusion pump and that they'll be just
fine."

But just because a person is intelligent does not mean that he or
she has the knowledge or confidence to master high-tech medical
equipment and procedures. Because they did not go to nursing
school and have no job-related experience, her patients often fail as
"nurses" because they don't have the knowledge or confidence to do
at home what professionals do for them in the hospital.

"This isn't something you learn in twenty minutes while you're walking out the door of your hospital room," she says. "It's not just a matter of intelligence. It's a matter of practice and having a repertoire of different experiences that show you what happens when something isn't going right."

All of this is complicated by a fact that seems to elude the new health care managers: patients leaving the hospital for home are not operating from a position of strength. They are vulnerable and anxious and so are their family members — if, that is, they're lucky enough to have anyone to take care of them at home.

Jeannie tells me about a visit she recently made to a woman in her own church who was recovering from an illness. The woman had had surgery to correct a restricted esophagus. Her physicians had put a tube down her throat to try to expand the stricture. Unfortunately, one of the rare and unpleasant side effects of this procedure is an esophageal tear. This is a serious condition that requires surgical repair.

The woman had the second procedure, could not eat, and was sent home with a feeding tube through which nutritional formula was pumped. After the woman recovered, she and her husband gratefully accepted a meal Jeannie brought to their door and invited her in for a cup of tea. After the three chatted amicably, Jeannie asked how the woman was faring.

"Very tentatively and apologetically, as if it were her fault, as if she wasn't being a good patient, this poor woman told her story," Jeannie explains.

Before she left the hospital, both the physician and social worker assured the woman that the home health care equipment company furnishing the pump would come and show her how to use it. She assumed this meant that someone with experience would stay with her to make sure she understood how to master the technology.

She was to be sorely disappointed. A young man arrived at her door, placed this mysterious piece of equipment into her hands, hastily explained how to use it, and turned to leave. When the woman panicked and asked if he would come back to check on her, he told her that the company offered no follow-up lessons. If she had problems, here was the number to call, he said, thrusting a piece of paper into her hands. Then he rushed off to go to his next appointment.

"She and her husband had about twenty years of graduate studies between them," Jeannie comments dryly, "but they had no idea what to do with this equipment. The woman felt awful. She was running fevers. She was worried. She had no idea if it was okay to be feeling the way she felt. She didn't know if this was the normal course of recovery or if something was really wrong."

Finally, the woman called her physician, who concluded that she was too sick to stay home. After a five-day readmission, she returned home. But even two weeks later, when Jeannie visited with her, she was fragile and anxious.

"It was so tragic to see her blame herself," Jeannie recounts. "I felt it was important to tell her that no, it was not her fault that she had not done well at home and had to be readmitted. She wasn't crazy to think they were asking too much of her by sending her home like that. The fevers and trouble with the feeding could have happened in the hospital. But if she had been in the hospital, a nurse would have seen what was going on and intervened far earlier in the process.

"I have to assume that what insurers are doing is saying, 'Well, if there's a hundred people and we send them home early, then maybe five people will have the kind of experience this woman had. So we're still saving a lot of money," Jeannie says with a harsh laugh. "The problem is, we're saving it at the expense of patients' agony. It might be okay to send someone home who's stable. But in my book, she wasn't a stable patient."

Many of the studies on home care that do exist have been conducted by nurse researchers. These nurses have found that patients followed in the home by advanced practice nurses, such as nurse practitioners, often fare better than hospitalized patients. Unfortunately, many patients today aren't even being seen by a registered nurse, much less one with an advanced degree.

If a patient does not die following discharge or suffer a serious complication that requires either significant medical attention or hospital readmission, that patient's home health experience is largely uncharted. Because hospitals and HMOs and others that initiate and fund research have not adequately funded or studied this phenomenon, we can only rely on anecdotal reports from patients and providers. These indicate that there is a significant amount of invisible pain and suffering — unmanaged postoperative pain, poorly managed side effects of medication and other treatments, anxiety because family members cannot adequately assess and monitor their loved ones' complex medical conditions or utilize high-tech medical equipment — that goes unrecorded.

Another phenomenon affecting nursing is cuts in hospital nursing staff. Today, insurers control huge blocks of patients. In order to attract these patients, insurers must, in turn, be attractive to the employers who purchase health care and whose major concern is cutting premium costs. To compete for employer dollars, HMOs must cut their own costs by extracting massive discounts from the hospitals with which they contract. As Alan Sager, a professor at the Boston University School of Public Health, explains it, "Managed care organizations work to dodge any costs they can. They shun paying their fair share of the costs of the hospital. This includes paying their fair share of a hospital's fixed costs and their fair share of the training of new physicians and nurses, the cost of medical and nursing research, and the care of the uninsured."

Managed care companies do this, says John O'Brien, CEO of the Cambridge Hospital Community Health Network and chairperson of the Massachusetts Hospital Association, by seeking discounts of up to 30 and 40 percent on hospital services. Hospitals are agreeing to these discounts because they feel that they will make up in volume what they lose by procedure or by raising their prices later — after their competitors close (or merge with them). But, O'Brien says, this means hospitals feel they must "squeeze down on our costs at every possible level. Nursing has been hit hard. Nursing is the backbone of the hospital. But the pressures we're putting on our nurses are inordinate. I have done it like everyone else. It certainly can't continue."

Hospitals are also anticipating cuts in the Medicare and Medicaid programs. One of the ways hospitals are making up for their losses — both losses of patients in hospitals and losses of revenues for services — is to "redesign," "restructure," or "reengineer" their organizations by downsizing.

According to a study conducted by the American Hospital Association, three-quarters of all American hospitals are restructuring, which means they are laying off nurses. In February 1996, a report in *Modern Healthcare* noted that "from 1993 through January of 1996, 140 hospitals or systems laid off a total of 23,910 workers, or an average layoff of 171 workers per hospital." Another issue of *Modern Healthcare* published an article entitled "Jobs Go First." A survey of hospital administrators revealed that more hospital executives said they would save money by cutting staff than by limiting capital improvements or research and development. (This mind-set is certainly reflected in a city like Boston, where expensive new hospital buildings spring up while nurses and other hospital employees are laid off.)

Only a few years ago, many hospitals staffed units with 90 percent registered nurses and only 10 percent ancillary personnel. Today, hospitals are spending millions of dollars hiring consultants like American Practice Management to help them cut RN staff. And the AHA recently reported that 97 percent of hospitals were using some kind of nurse extender.

In 1994, when the American Nurses Association (ANA) surveyed its members, 70 percent of all respondents said their employers were cutting back on staffing by leaving vacant positions unfilled, and 66 percent said hospitals had already laid off nurses or were planning to do so. In Judith Shindul-Rothschild's 1996 study, 60 percent said the number of RNs providing direct patient care had decreased, and 66 percent of RNs said the number of patients assigned to them had increased and that the patients were sicker.

This downsizing is coming at a time when many teaching hospitals are also reducing their residency programs. These reductions are a result of a number of factors. There are fewer patients in hospitals today. Hospitals are also anticipating reductions in the funds used to support the teaching of novice doctors — Medicare's indirect teaching adjustment. Hospitals are also trying to give physicians more experience in doing primary care by moving them out of the hospital and into doctors' offices and community clinics. Thus, the number of residents actually listed on the books may not actually be available for patient care duties in hospitals. And residency programs for certain subspecialties — like anesthesiology — are drying up as the country tries to move toward a more rational balance between generalist and specialist physicians. Whatever the reason, the result is that intensely ill patients simultaneously have fewer physicians and fewer experienced nurses to care for them.

By no coincidence, the two states with the highest penetration of managed care in the nation — Massachusetts and California — also lead the country in cuts in nursing care. Over the past few years, Boston's prestigious Brigham and Women's Hospital has announced nursing layoffs. Although patients today need more help making the transition to life at home, the hospital wiped out its entire Continuing Care Department, laying off five clinical nurse specialists, one nurse practitioner, and one staff educator. They were replaced by less-expensive social workers. (The hospital insists its nurse-to-patient ratio is still very high.)

The Brigham and Women's announced its historic merger with the Massachusetts General Hospital in December 1993. In 1994, the general director of the General Hospital Corporation and the president of the Brigham and Women's earned $1,326,390 and $639,755 respectively. The hospitals proudly trumpeted that they were going to cut 20 percent of their budgets, which would entail the loss of at least four thousand hospital jobs. In September 1995, the Brigham and Women's initiated another round of nursing layoffs. Brigham and Women nurses say they have been required to work mandatory overtime and have had to give up the kinds of flexible scheduling arrangements that have made marked improvements in nurses' working conditions and job satisfaction. The Massachusetts General has already begun laying off its most senior and therefore most expensive nurses as well as nurse managers, and bedside nurses report short-staffing of units and difficulty caring for patients.

In 1994, Howard Berliner and Christine T. Kovner, a professor at the New School for Social Research and an associate professor at New York University's Division of Nursing, with their colleagues, projected that the demand for registered nurses would decline by about three thousand in New York City's hospitals. They estimated that this decline would be offset by a growth in demand for two thousand nursing home and home care nurses. This would nonetheless mean a net decrease in a thousand RN positions in the city. Although Kovner says there is unfortunately no current research to document that the kinds of changes occuring are associated with decrease in the quality of patient care, anecdotal reports from nurse colleagues seriously concern her.

Since that time, New York City's Health and Hospitals Corporation has eliminated twelve hundred RN jobs from the city's public hospitals. In only two years, the agency has cut its RN workforce down from eight thousand to sixty-five hundred.

In California, nurses say the ratio of RNs to patients has declined so precipitously that the California Nurses Association and other nursing organizations have been asking both state legislators and congressional representatives to mandate safe minimum staffing ratios for all units in hospitals. Even on critical care units — developed specifically to provide intensive *nursing* care — nurses insist staffing has suffered. Because patients on critical care units are so ill, they require one-to-one nursing care. Sometimes one nurse will take care of two patients. Now some hospitals have gone so far as to rename units to disguise the intensity of patient needs so that they can give nurses responsibility for more patients. Or patients may be transferred out of critical care units prematurely in order to justify a reduction in the number of RNs employed on those units.

The hospitals that are laying off nurses may be some of the richest in the nation. On the cover of its October 1995 issue, *Modern Healthcare*, one of the leading health care industry business publications, ran the following headline. "We're in the Money — Hospitals Sit on Big Cash Reserves." While nonprofit hospitals were claiming they did not have enough money to pay for RN staff, the cover story stated that "like never before, not-for-profit hospitals are in the money" and were sitting on the biggest cash reserves of their history. The Brigham and Women's Hospital was listed as one of "the top ten cash rich acute-care hospitals in 1994." Its cash reserves totaled $308.7 million.

In an increasing number of hospitals, many floors are so short-staffed that nurses are no longer able to take time off — even to learn about new techniques, equipment, or drugs. Yet, the very same hospitals are cutting or eliminating the positions of nurse educators, researchers, and clinical nurse specialists — like Jeannie Chaisson — who provide bedside nurses with easy access to clinical updates and in-service training. "There's no one to cover for a bedside nurse if she wants to go to a lecture or in-service that keeps them up to date. So when you rely on lectures and in-services to educate people, it just places more stress on them, not less." Hospitals argue that the support personnel who help nurses acquire greater clinical knowledge — and thus improve patient care — are expendable because they don't provide direct hands-on care. Within the Beth Israel, for example, when units have been closed, clinical specialists have left the hospital for jobs elsewhere and other vacancies created by attrition have not been filled. "In the face of cuts in health care payments, it is difficult for a hospital like BI to support a role like mine," Jeannie says.

Instead of providing care by expert registered nurses, hospitals are, however, changing the kinds of people giving direct care to patients and are replacing nurses with lower-wage and less-skilled employees, like nursing assistants and technicians — called unlicensed assistive personnel (UAPs). In 1991, for example, the American Hospital Association reported that 97 percent of hospitals were using some form of unlicensed aide. (Echoing the terminology of the functional and team nursing of an earlier period, these aides are once again termed "nurse extenders.")

These little-trained and less-educated aides generally earn 20 to 40 percent less than RNs. Because about two-thirds of any hospital's employees are nurses, this can clearly represent huge savings for hospitals searching for either profits, surpluses, or survival. According to the Institute of Medicine (IOM) report on nursing staffing, "the RN skill mix [that is, the proportion of RNs to other nursing staff] appears to be dropping in many settings, from a range of 76–100 percent to a range of 52–79 percent." Some of the "nursing assistants" who are now delivering care are hospital employees who have been cross-trained to perform nursing duties. In other words, the "nurse" at one's bedside may actually be a housekeeper or a transport or kitchen worker who also changes a patient's sterile dressing.

Forty-two percent of Shindul-Rothschild's respondents said that their health care organization is hiring unlicensed assistive personnel to provide direct patient care previously provided by RNs. Or according to the Institute of Medicine, "RNs have moved from direct patient care to coordinating and supervising patient care in hospitals. In some institutions, nurse assistants are assuming greater responsibility for direct patient care under RN supervision."

Training these RN replacements is not regulated by state licensing boards. There are no minimum requirements governing the amount of training aides or "cross-trained" workers must have before they can be redeployed, at least part of the time, to do nursing work. Training periods can range from a few hours to perhaps six weeks. One 1994 study cited in the IOM report "found that 99 percent of the hospitals in California reported less than 120 hours of on-the-job training for newly hired ancillary nursing personnel. Only 20 percent of the hospitals required a high school diploma. The majority of hospitals (59 percent) provided less than 20 hours of classroom instruction and 88 percent provided 40 hours or less of instruction time."

Aides can have an important role to play when they do not perform skilled nursing duties, but in many hospitals, these workers now insert catheters, read EKGs, suction tracheotomy tubes, change sterile dressings, and perform other traditional nursing functions. The remaining bedside nurses have less time to care for more — and sicker — patients and must supervise untrained techs as well. A day-shift nurse may care for seven or eight patients and, at the same time, be responsible for supervising an aide assigned to care for four or five others. This means that the nurse will be effectively in charge of twelve patients, because RNs are legally responsible for techs as well as for any of the mistakes they make.

What is worse — and completely unjustifiable — is that patients are often deliberately kept in the dark about the qualifications of those who are caring for them. In some hospitals, nurses are no longer allowed to identify themselves as RNs. The RN initials are taken off their identification badges, and all nonphysician personnel are referred to as "patient care associates," "patient care technicians," "multi-skilled caregivers," or some other variation on this theme. MDs still retain their identification. In other hospitals, nurses protested so loudly about this policy that hospital administrators have retreated. The nurses must wear the patient care associate badge but can now add their RN qualifications to it. Patients, however, may still confuse registered nurses and aides.

Hospitals are also increasingly using temporary, agency nurses or hospital "float nurses" to deal with unpredictable fluctuations in patient demand. On one day a unit may have relatively few patients and need fewer nurses. The next day, a flood of patients may be admitted and the demand peaks. (These problems are, of course, exacerbated today because hospitals have laid off so many nurses and many units may have only a bare-bones nursing staff.)

Hospitals can deal with these fluctuations in several ways. They can use on-call nurses who work in the hospital on a permanent basis and are paid extra to come in when there is an unexpected surge in demand. They can maintain a pool of part-time nurses who fill in when staffing needs increase. Or they can use agency nurses or float nurses, the hospital equivalent of the kind of out-sourcing of maintenance that is being practiced by discount airlines like ValuJet, with such catastrophic consequences for passengers.

A hospital calls a nursing agency and the agency sends out a nurse who fills in temporarily. That nurse may work on the unit for one shift, for two or three days, or for a month. The nurse may move from hospital to hospital. She may be a traveling nurse who moves from city to city. Some are nurses from foreign countries. Or the hospital floats a nurse from one unit — say a general medical floor — onto another unit — like an ICU.

Many agencies are reputable and screen the qualifications of the nurses they employ. Many agency and float nurses are well educated and experienced. But even the best-educated, most-experienced agency or float nurse can represent a danger to patients. The nurse may not be expert in the patients, diseases, medications, equipment on the unit. Even if the nurse's expertise and the unit she's assigned to match — a cardiology ICU nurse works on a cardiac ICU — she will be at a disadvantage.

That's because high-quality care isn't only a matter of knowing diseases and their treatments, it's a matter of teamwork. To be effective, a nurse needs to know how a particular unit in a particular hospital cares for its particular group of patients. Which drugs, tests, and procedures does it use? Where does it keep its medications and supplies? What kind of working relationships have doctors, nurses, social workers, physical therapists, and other staff forged over the years? If the nurse is a stranger to the system, who will value her judgment if she has a legitimate concern about a patient's treatment?

Because they don't have to spend 80 percent of their energy figuring out how to answer these questions, nurses like Jeannie, Nancy, and Ellen, who have helped define a unit's culture of care, know how to work the system and effectively care for and be advocates for patients. That is not true of a nurse who parachutes into one unit in a hospital on one day and moves on the next.

This use of unlicensed personnel, temporary and floating staff — which is a cornerstone of what hospitals call "patient-centered" or "patient-focused care" — is fast destroying the innovation of primary nursing. Patient-focused care is a concept designed by management consultants — such as the pioneer in the field, Booz-Allen & Hamilton, or American Practice Management — to cut labor costs, streamline the process of patient care, and increase competitiveness. It attempts to move the patient less throughout the hospital and move more services to the patient, and to decrease the number of people — nutritionists, technicians, housekeepers, transporters — the patient sees during a typical day. Consultants also promise nurses that they will be relieved of many nonnursing tasks, such as clerical duties and housework — that nurses are often asked to perform.

To do this, management consultants come into the hospital and totally "reengineer" or "restructure" the process of care. They put nursing under a microscope and try to deconstruct the tapestry of care into a series of tasks, deciding which of these can be farmed out to lower-skilled and thus lower-cost employees. They may also target every other discipline in the hospital through what is called "cross-training" or "multi-skilling." In the hospital, disciplines like social work, nursing, lab-technology, physical therapy — even housekeeping, security, and transport — may no longer have exclusive claim on the work traditionally done in that field. Instead, patient-focused care creates a generic health care worker who is dual- or triple-skilled. Thus we have a housekeeper who also does nursing and transport, an x-ray technician who also doubles as a nurse, and a housekeeper or a security guard who does nursing.

On the face of it, patient-focused care — with its patient-friendly rationale — sounds like a wonderful idea. Finally, the impersonal doctor or hospital administrator or insurance company–driven care of the past is emphasizing what should have been emphasized all along — the patient. The problem is, how will the patient fare when expertise has been eliminated from the health care system? How, in particular, will the patient fare when he or she is being taken care of by people who may be enormously well-intentioned but who do not have the knowledge to distinguish the trivial from the potentially tragic and intervene early to prevent catastrophe? How will the patient fare when nurses with the skill of involvement — the skill to reach beyond the patient's disease and into his or her life — are replaced by workers who may have little skill at all?

When one looks under the surface of patient-focused care, what the patient actually confronts is a workforce that knows a little bit about a number of things but has no expertise in any one field. In the highly complex world of health care, this smattering of knowledge can be a very dangerous thing. Indeed, when one examines the concept more carefully, one quickly sees that there is little that is "new" about this reorganization of nursing. "Expanding the nurse" through the use of lower-skilled, cross-trained, or temporary workers and turning the dwindling number of RNs into middle-management supervisors is simply a modern repackaging of the team or functional nursing models. These are precisely the models that produced the "fragmented, impersonal" care and the demoralized nursing staff Joyce Clifford found when she arrived at the Beth Israel in the early 1970s.

In spite of this, hospitals adamantly insist that nursing layoffs are both necessary and safe. Hospitals argue that they are only responding to lower patient-occupancy rates. In fact, the American Hospital Association and one of its subsidiary groups, the American Organization of Nurse Executives, say that the number of RNs employed in hospitals has increased by 2 percent over the past decade.

Prominent analysts of health care employment contend that this argument is flawed because it considers only total number of nurses, fails to factor in the intensity of patient needs, the new work nurses are asked to do in our restructured health care system, and population growth, especially the increase in the elderly, who use a greater share of health services. "The AHA data on RN employment are not particularly useful," says Margaret Peisert, Health Care Workforce Project Director of the Service Employees International Union. "The American Hospital Association only collects aggregate data on the number of nurses in hospitals. Their figures mix together all the nurses on their payroll. These nurses may be working on floors providing direct care to patients. They may be supervising aides and not providing direct care. They may be in ambulatory care clinics, providing care in the home, or in labs or a nursing home subsidiary of the hospitals. They may be nurse managers or working in utilization review, fighting with insurance companies."

Hospitals, Peisert and others say, have consistently refused to collect data that more carefully pinpoint where nurses are actually working. "We simply don't know how many RNs are working in acute care, directly caring for patients, as opposed to elsewhere in the hospital," Peisert continues. "When we say very specifically there are not enough registered nurses at the bedside caring for acutely ill patients, the AHA responds, 'That's not true, the aggregate numbers of RNs are actually increasing.' But their figures don't address the argument."

Interestingly, in the early 90s, the American Hospital Association stopped collecting and publishing detailed reports on the use of about fifteen allied health professions, including nursing, in hospitals. Significantly, these reports specifically asked about shortages of such personnel. Bill Irwin, public relations spokesman for the AHA, says that he does not know why the association stopped producing those reports, but, he adds, "all the people who did those reports were let go."

Hospitals in America routinely gather statistics on mortality; adverse incidents (medication errors and patient injuries); total complication rates like bedsores, and hospital-acquired infections (wound infections, urinary tract infections, and pneumonias); use of physical and chemical restraints on patients; staffing levels and staff qualifications; and information on the number of times staff are asked to take an unsafe patient assignment. All of these data reflect the importance of nursing care. However, this information is regarded as proprietary and is almost never made public. And it is not systematically used in studies correlating the impact of staffing levels on patient care outcomes.

If the AHA is really interested in finding out how restructuring is affecting patient care, Peisert and others say, it should collect data in a useful manner and correlate staffing with patient outcomes. "In other countries, the impact of staffing on patient care is treated seriously in the scientific world. Adequacy of staffing, short-staffing, nurses' workload — all of this is treated as a variable in outcome studies in countries like Germany, England, and Canada. This is not an issue that is kept in the closet, as it is in the United States," Peisert concludes.

Many health care experts also insist that hospital's refutation of staff nurses' concerns overlooks the relevant factor of increased patient acuity. "You can't say that a twenty or thirty percent decrease in the length of stay of patients in hospitals leads to a twenty or thirty percent drop in the need for hospital personnel," says Dr. David Himmelstein, a leading health policy expert, associate professor at Harvard Medical School, and staff physician at Cambridge Hospital, in Cambridge, Massachusetts. "The first few days of hospitalization require the most work from nurses. That's when patients are sickest. Moreover, it also takes time and effort to get to know people. So when you chop off the last two days of an eight-day stay, you're cutting off the days when the nursing care would be relatively light. And if the result is that a patient comes back to the hospital, a whole new set of nurses has to again get to know them and care for them when they're again very sick."

Similarly, many of those who insist that there are enough nurses at the bedside do not consider some of the new burdens nurses are asked to bear today. Nurses are not only asked to care for patients who are in the hospital. They are also being asked to give advice to patients once they have been discharged — often in an unstable condition. As one nurse who works with mothers who have just given birth at a major teaching hospital explains, "When we have to send patients home this early [24 hours after giving birth], we tell them that they can call the nurses' station anytime day or night if they have a question. But the problem is, when they call they have a lot of questions that take a lot of time to answer. And we really can't take the time. We're already short-staffed and the hospital doesn't add extra staff to man the phones."

"When we consider staffing requirements, we need to consider more than intensity of patient needs," says Charlene Harrington, professor and chair of the Department of Social and Behavioral Sciences at the University of California, San Francisco, School of Nursing. "Admissions, discharges, and transfers need to be taken into account in workload calculations. This is a measure of the activity on a unit. Each of these procedures has a routine and requires a lot of staff time which is over and above the time nurses put into regular patient care duties."

Harrington adds that the complexity of nurses' work must also be factored into staffing calculations. "A nurse on a critical care unit works with more technology than a nurse on a medical floor or in a skilled nursing facility." Their work, Harrington argued, cannot be equated.

Then there is the question of population growth. "You can't just look at the gross number of nurses in a vacuum," says Judith Shindul-Rothschild. "You have to consider the need for their services. One important way of assessing this is to look at Department of Labor data that look at trends in manpower and analyze how many people there are in all occupational categories per one hundred thousand population. If you compare the RNs per one hundred thousand population in 1993 to that in 1994, in every single state there was a decline. In some areas, like New England, the declines were some of the steepest in the country. There is no state where we saw an increase in RNs. In other words, the number of registered nurses is not keeping pace with population growth."

The consequences of nursing layoffs and replacement by aides can be significant. As pointed out in an important article in the journal *Medical Care* entitled "Hospital and Patient Characteristics Associated with Death after Surgery: A Study of Adverse Occurrences and Failure to Rescue," if an adverse event occurs during or after treatment, nurses are some of the prime rescuers in the health care system. If they are not there, a patient in trouble may not be rescued. Consider the problem of replacing skilled nurses with techs. These nurse substitutes are not supposed to work on their own. Rather they are told to report any significant changes in a patient's condition to the nurse who supervises their work. To determine which change in a patient's status is significant and which is not, however, requires clinical judgment — judgment developed through academic training and years on the job. Because the most well-intentioned aides may lack both, they often overlook developments that appear, to them, to be meaningless or trivial.

"Nursing is not a matter of reading machines and coming up with the right numbers," Jeannie Chaisson reminds us. "It's a matter of interpreting those numbers and knowing what they mean. Some techs may take adequate training courses and will be able to draw blood, take vital signs, and read an EKG [electrocardiogram]. But they don't know how to tell me what rhythm the patient is in. They don't know whether the changes are ischemic and what the medical management should be from here on in. They don't know what to tell the physician when they call them to come in and evaluate [a patient], because they're not a nurse. In fact, they won't even know that you often check a patient's vital signs because of how the patient looks, how their color is, what their baseline is, and what you know about their history. This is how you prevent major problems, because the numbers don't crash until the end."

Jane Storrs, a nurse in Washington state, cites two illustrative examples. In one case, a patient who had had a head injury years before came to the hospital after a suicide attempt. He had taken three hundred aspirins. After spending twenty-four hours on another floor, he was admitted to Storrs's unit. Twenty-four hours into his stay, Storrs was talking to him about some medicine he was supposed to take but which the pharmacy had not yet delivered. Had he taken those particular pills before, she asked.

Oh, yes, he replied absently. I think I have some in there, he said, pointing to the top drawer of his bedside table. Storrs opened the drawer and found a plastic hospital bag filled with five hundred Tylenol, and ten bottles of prescription medicine. An aide who unpacked his things had left these medications within reach of a man who, forty-eight hours earlier, had tried to kill himself with an overdose of pills.

During that same week, Storrs was caring for other patients with a clinical nursing assistant (CNA) who is, she said, a very conscientious worker. She simply has little health care background. The aide was trained to check diabetic patients' blood sugar levels to determine whether a diabetic had low blood sugar and was thus at risk to go into a diabetic coma.

The CNA did such a check on one of Storrs's patients and found that the woman had, in fact, very low blood sugar. The unit then became very busy and the CNA neglected to inform Storrs of this finding. Some time later, she bumped into Storrs and told her about the patient's blood sugar reading, adding nonchalantly, "But it's all right. It's not bothering her. She's sleeping."

The patient was not sleeping. She was gradually going into a diabetic coma.

"These aides are very well-intentioned. But the issue isn't good intentions," Storrs says adamantly. "It's education. They don't have it."

Roy Bennett, a nurse at a major Ohio medical center, recounts one of his recent experiences with unskilled nurse substitutes. Bennett was caring for a woman who was undergoing a bone marrow transplant for cancer. She was immunosuppressed and in reverse isolation in a room with the door closed. At this point in her treatment, she was receiving platelets. Because there is a high risk of an adverse reaction to such blood products, and her condition could change rapidly, Bennett was checking on her status every thirty minutes. It had been about fifteen minutes since Bennett last verified that this patient was stable when he ran into a housekeeper, who was carrying a stack of four blankets toward the patient's room. Seeing her load, Bennett was immediately worried.

What was going on, Bennett asked the housekeeper.

She told him that the patient had complained of being cold. In trying to respond to what she — and the patient — perceived to be the patient's needs, she rushed off to do what any ordinary person would do — find some extra blankets.

The problem was that this patient did not need room service–like blanket delivery, but knowledgeable caring. "What the patient was experiencing was not the kind of chill a healthy person experiences," Bennett recalls. "She was experiencing an adverse reaction to blood products. She needed a nurse's immediate action — to stop the blood products, infuse normal saline, and call the physician — to avert a catastrophe. The housekeeper should have called me in but she didn't know enough to do that."

Bennett doesn't blame the housekeeper for trying to help the patient. He does, however, fault his hospital administration for failing to understand what should be obvious. "If you have untrained people at the bedside responding to what they perceive to be patients' needs, you're going to miss things that could be very important to the patient's welfare."

Perhaps one of the most chilling comments comes from one of the workers who have been cross-trained to care for patients in a long-term-care facility. In 1996, a security guard at a long-term-care hospital read an article on avoiding harm in the hospital written by Timothy McCall. In desperation, he reached out to McCall with his concerns about health care. "I am an employee of a 95 bed, long-term care facility," he wrote. "My position is that of security guard. Ninety-five percent of my job consists of maintenance, housekeeping, admitting persons into clinical labs to pick up and leave specimens. Now a class, 45 minutes, is being given so employees can feed, give bedpans and move patients. My expertise is in law enforcement and security (25 years). I am not trained or licensed in patient care, maintenance, lab work etc. I am a licensed security officer.

"This scares me. Having untrained unlicensed persons performing jobs in my opinion is dangerous."

Of this trend, Jeannie Chaisson comments acerbically, "If you have a tech that is skilled enough to do the kind of monitoring and evaluation and teaching that are necessary in an acute care hospital, then you should give them a degree and call them a nurse."

In all of the above cases, nurses were able to intervene in time to save the lives or health of the patients involved. But not all patients are so lucky. In a period of just a few months in 1995, the nation's newspapers reported that at Tampa's University Community Hospital a surgeon amputated the wrong foot and his colleague did an arthroscopy on the wrong knee of another. In the same hospital, an aide accidentally disconnected a patient from a ventilator, with fatal consequences. In Michigan, a woman lost the wrong breast in a mastectomy, while in Baltimore, a man had his prostate removed unnecessarily. In a San Francisco hospital, a patient was forced to dial 911 for help because as he lay hemorrhaging, his cries for assistance went unheeded due to short-staffing.

In a major New York City hospital, the administration discontinued its six operating room head nurse positions. These nurses, among other things, supervised the cleaning staff. The equipment, like the heart and lung machine used in cardiac bypass surgery, is not always properly cleaned between uses. In some quarters for which patients' postsurgical infection rates are calculated, those rates have almost doubled.

At the Dana-Farber Cancer Institute in Boston, two patients were given four times the dose of chemotherapy prescribed in an experimental treatment protocol. Betsy Lehman, a health columnist at the *Boston Globe* and thus a well-informed health care consumer, died, and the other suffered severe heart damage.

And just as I was completing this book, an inexperienced agency nurse was assigned to care for one of the sickest patients in the Brigham and Women's Hospital — a patient in one of its intensive care units. The nurse delivered potassium chloride to the patient too quickly and he died.

These errors were all attributed, at least in part, to problems with nursing staffing or administration. When investigators from the federal Health Care Financing Administration (HCFA) and the Florida Agency for Health Care Administration's Tampa office inspected University Community Hospital, in Tampa, they found that the hospital was pushing too many patients through a poorly staffed operating room. It had too few nurses overseeing patient preparation in the operating room and, on some floors, too few nurses — plus too many poorly trained and inadequately supervised nurse replacements — giving patient care.

When Richard Knox, a health reporter at the *Boston Globe*, and a representative of the state's Department of Health probed the Lehman case, both investigators concluded that disarray in the hospital's nursing department was a contributing factor in the overdose that killed Lehman. Dana-Farber failed to provide patients with their last line of defense against medical errors — nurses who check a doctor's order against the dosage specified in the experimental protocol before administering anything to patients. At the Farber, RNs had been removed from this fail-safe loop. No clinical nurse specialists were available to educate staff nurses about the shifting array of experimental protocols they were expected to administer and monitor. Nurses did not have easy access to experimental protocols so that they could read and check on them. The hospital had no director of nursing at the time and no strong management team. Nurses who had problems and concerns had nowhere to go with them.

Kaiser in San Diego recently gave a $400,000 settlement to a woman who sued the HMO after her husband died of internal bleeding. The suit had contended that staff cuts made it impossible for nurses to do their jobs. And another patient's family is suing Cincinnati's Christ Hospital on similar grounds, after the patient died from an infection after surgery.

These more anecdotal accounts are increasingly reflected in the findings of research studies. A study of 281 hospitals nationwide conducted by the consultant E. P. Murphy found that hospitals that had reduced their staff by 8 percent or more were four hundred times more likely to have increases in patient illness or mortality.

Lucien Leape, professor of health care policy at the Harvard School of Public Health, has long studied errors in medicine. In one study, he estimated that 180,000 patients die annually because of injuries from medical treatment. Leape believes that replacing nurses with unskilled aides and increasing their patient loads will increase medical errors. "Unfortunately, I'm not aware of any studies done proving that decreasing the nurse-to-patient ratio, or "dumbing down," as it's called — what happens when nurses' roles are taken over by lesser-trained people — is linked to increases in more errors or patient injuries. But based on all the evidence from other professions, this trend almost certainly has caused or will cause errors."

Leape says that studies clearly document that errors result from overwork, fatigue, too many things to do in too little time, and stress, all of which nurses report today. Because downsizing is occurring at a period when hospitalized patients are sicker than ever, Leape is especially concerned. "At a time when we need more intensive care and more skill and efficiency in hospitals, intensity of nursing care is being cut back. From a purely theoretical standpoint, this makes no sense. We are decreasing the quality of our nursing care when we are increasing severity. This has got to be a prescription for disaster."

In Shindul-Rothschild's 1996 study, 55 percent of the nurses reported an increase in patient and family complaints. Perhaps the most alarming, 57 percent of these nurses — nurses who had on average been working for sixteen years as RNs — said that the quality of nursing care delivered in their institutions did not meet their professional standards, and 36 percent said they would not recommend that a family member receive care in their institution. "Because they are no longer able to provide patients the care they need, more nurses are becoming demoralized and stating that they are likely to leave the profession than we've seen in almost twenty years," says Shindul-Rothschild.

Nurses are not the only ones worried about the kind of care patients are getting in hospitals today. Many family members interviewed for this book expressed concern about leaving their loved ones in short-staffed hospital units. If they can afford it, some hire private duty nurses to supplement staff nursing care. Others said they — or friends of the patient — had to take time off from work or spend long hours at the bedside in the evenings and on weekends because patients were not getting enough individual attention. Of course, when friends and relatives assume this burden, it invariably falls on female shoulders.

In the beginning of this book, we saw how nursing administrators committed to giving registered nurses the time, knowledge, and institutional support necessary to knowledgeable caring can help to enhance patient care. Unfortunately, many of the nurse administrators who tried to transform nursing from the top are losing their ability — and sometimes the will — to fight internal hospital attacks on their profession. Restructuring is silencing the voice nursing had slowly gained in hospital management. Forty-five percent of those who replied to the Shindul-Rothschild study said they were seeing a reduction in nurse managers, and 38 percent said they had lost their nurse executive and that she or he had not been replaced.

Many hospitals, like the Brigham and Women's, the Massachusetts General, the Mount Auburn, Children's, and the Deaconess now call nursing "patient care services." What were once VPs of nursing are now senior vice presidents of patient care services. (Since the Deaconess-BI merger, the former chief nurse executive of the Deaconess is now vice president for clinical quality.) "Pretty soon," says Trish Gibbons, who is now chief clinical officer of Visiting Nurse Services of Southern Maine, "they'll simply say, Well, why does the head of patient care services have to be a nurse? Why can't he or she be a pharmacist, or a social worker, or even a physician?"

Because of her disagreement with corporate policies, Trish Gibbons, who helped implement primary nursing at the Beth Israel, resigned as chairperson of the nursing department at Tufts New England Medical Center (NEMC) in the summer of 1994. She was the first nursing leader and high-level female executive at NEMC to have a doctorate and offices in the hospital's executive suite. After her departure, the nurse executive was no longer required to have a Ph.D., and her office was removed from the executive suite. (The male physician leaders of the hospital, of course, remained in their plush executive offices.) Some doctors at NEMC seem to believe that Gibbons's departure signals a return to the era of the nurse as physician's handmaiden. "Well, I guess now that Dr. Gibbons is gone, you'll have to take your marching orders from medicine," one physician informed an NEMC nurse shortly after Gibbons left.

Although she has a master's degree in nursing administration, Nancy Rumplik is still working as a clinician in the Hematology / Oncology Clinic. Between the time she entered her master's program and when she graduated, the health care system changed so dramatically that she now shies away from a career in nursing administration. "While I was doing my practice training in management at Children's Hospital, both of the nurses I worked with lost their jobs as managers. I also found that they had responsibilities that had never been included in the nurse manager role before. They were now doing the budgeting for the entire unit. It had become so businesslike that you needed an MBA instead of nursing expertise."

Nurses with years of experience caring for the sick, like Nancy Rumplik, may no longer be managing their colleagues. Just as MBAs and insurance company clerks are now dictating matters of clinical care to physicians, some hospitals are hiring a new breed of "nurse" manager — the MBA who understands the realities of the quarterly profit statement better than far more urgent realities of illness and who seems unable to reconcile the two. The nurse managers who remain on the job, Jeannie Chaisson says, are being turned into the nursing equivalent of the MBA. "Increasingly nurse managers are 'care managers.' Their job is to move patients through the system, not help advance nursing practice."

With this approach comes the very real danger that the kinds of care, education, and connection nurses like Jeannie Chaisson, Nancy Rumplik, and Ellen Kitchen work so hard to give to their patients is simply off the managerial charts. Managers trained to ask how, not why, to consider only what they can quantify and measure, tend to discount and dismiss what it is that actually puts the health and care into our health care system. This is of course, trust, comfort, security, being with rather than doing for in relationships where knowledge is gained through the construction and cultivation of human relationships. In managerial terms, what we have seen Nancy, Jeannie, and Ellen live through with patients is reduced to a series of inputs measured instrumentally in terms of concrete outcomes — at best morbidity and mortality, at worst the crudest calculation of cost savings absent considerations of the quality of care. While it is essential to scientifically analyze the results of nursing care, measures must be sensitive enough to capture what caring means to and does for patients as individuals and the health care system as a whole.

An eloquent critique of this kind of managerialism comes from two British physicians, Julian Tudor Hart and Paul Dieppe. In the medical journal the *Lancet*, they wrote: "The effects of downgrading and neglect of caring by research theory have been magnified by market incentives. Most health service managers do not wish to downgrade caring any more than clinicians, but they are compelled to seek efficiency in terms that effectively ignore what is difficult to measure: the process." But the authors warned, "without caring, real health outputs fall, despite increased and more efficient output of process."

*   *   *

In 1993, the kinds of concerns nurses have voiced over the rapid and dramatic transformation of their profession reached Congress. After studying the issue of hospital staffing in late 1992, the Service Employees International Union (SEIU) testified before Congress on conditions of nursing care in nursing homes and hospitals in the United States. With the help of Senator Edward Kennedy (D-Mass.) and Congressman Henry Waxman (D-Calif.), the union was able to convince Congress that the issue should be studied further. In February 1993, Congress directed the secretary of the Department of Health and Human Services (HHS) to conduct an independent study of the issue of staffing and quality care. The department's Division of Nursing assigned this task to the Institute of Medicine (IOM), which the National Academy of Sciences has chartered to examine health policy issues.

Staff nurses and their unions had hoped that the IOM would not respond as many managers do when confronted with human experience — disdain it as "anecdotal." Because shifts in hospital nursing staffing were so rapid and so recent, they knew that little current research had evaluated their impact. Thus they hoped that the committee would conduct its own primary research on the subject. They also hoped that the committee would make strong recommendations to Congress, asking legislators to mandate better hospital reporting, better government oversight, and strong provisions to assure safe and adequate staffing.

From the beginning, those hopes were disappointed. The IOM's first move was to appoint a controversial figure to chair the committee. This was Carolyne K. Davis. Davis was Ronald Reagan's head of the Health Care Financing Administration and currently works as a consultant for Ernst and Young, an accounting firm with a major management consulting group. In that capacity, she earns a great deal of her income from consulting fees from Beverly Enterprises — one of the nation's largest for-profit nursing home chains. In a letter protesting this appointment and asking that Davis recuse herself as chair, John Sweeney, then president of the SEIU and now president of the AFL-CIO, pointed out that this appointment represented a clear conflict of interest. The IOM declined to cancel the appointment.

Others on the sixteen-member committee shared similar connections to the hospital and nursing home industry. There were no union representatives on the committee, nor any representatives of any other professional nursing organization.

The report's conclusions were a great disappointment to many in the nursing community. In perhaps the most revealing statement in the entire report, the committee said that "restructuring of inpatient services in hospitals, accompanied by a changing mix of nursing personnel, is an inevitable consequence of the demands by society, through the payers of care, to control the costs of health services." Thus, the committee asserted that "society" and an elite group of employers who pay for health care are one and the same. And in an even more circuitous piece of logic, they said that this "society," to whom the real work of nursing has been largely invisible, has somehow decided that nurses are one of the major cost escalators in the health care system.

It is perhaps not surprising, then, that the committee conducted no primary research, tended to devalue the nurses' and nursing organizations' reports of declining quality of care as "anecdotal," and concluded that they could find no evidence of an adverse impact on patients. The committee said it was appalled by the fact that not enough contemporary research had been done on the changes in hospitals but did not suggest that hospitals, in turn, be required to alter their patterns of reporting on nursing staffing and conduct studies that correlate staffing to quality care outcomes.

The committee did not challenge the use of unlicensed personnel to provide direct patient care. Instead, it recommended that hospitals test and certify these nurse replacements and expand their training. Although the report documented how little training hospitals have bothered to give those now entrusted with patients' lives and health, the committee did not recommend that this testing and certification process be mandatory or regulated by either federal, state, or municipal government. The most positive aspect of the report was its recommendation that by the year 2000 there should be twenty-four-hour registered nurse coverage in nursing homes and that more advanced practice nurses be utilized in hospitals.

Reading the IOM report, one is struck by the circular quality of its deliberations. When hospitals and insurers initiate changes like those I have described, they clearly have little incentive to objectively analyze their impact on patients. Few government agencies conduct similar research. When patient care is jeopardized, we are thus left with anecdotal reports. But these are then dismissed as unscientific, and it is suggested that more research be initiated. Given the industry's lack of cooperation and government's lack of oversight, how will those studies be financed and conducted? Moreover, research that documents deaths and injuries inevitably does so after they have occurred. That's why nurses petitioned Congress in the first place, to prevent more deaths and injuries.

Many staff nurses feel that the IOM's conclusions reflect a widespread phenomenon — a betrayal of direct caregivers by some of the nursing academics and administrators who long ago left the bedside. They often claim that researchers are hiding behind abstractions and statistics and are not, in fact, exploring the day-to-day experiences of caregivers and those they care for in the nation's hospitals. It is difficult not to sympathize with this perception. Some of the nursing researchers and administrators I have spoken with have publicly dismissed staff nurses' concerns while privately bemoaning what is going on in hospitals in particular and health care in general. One nurse researcher I interviewed initially told me she is not nearly as concerned about quality patient care issues as staff nurses whose reports she minimized because they were "anecdotal." Then she provided me with an anecdote of her own. Both her parents had been hospitalized over the past several years in a major urban area that has experienced considerable hospital downsizing. Because of concerns for their safety, the family hired private duty nurses and aides to be with their loved ones twenty-four hours a day. Apparently, her sense of urgency about the patient care environment occurred only when "anecdotal information" could negatively effect her own immediate family.

Until nurses' complaints are taken more seriously and studies catch up with reality, we are left with earlier research studies attesting to the connection between expertise in caring and quality outcomes, as well as studies conducted in other countries.

- In 1986, Scott, Forrest, and Brown reported on work that spanned a decade and a large number of hospitals. They found that when nursing staff is better qualified, quality of care is also better and mortality and lengths of stay are lower.

- In 1986 and 1989, studies by Knaus et al. and Mitchell et al. documented that RN staffing levels, and positive nurse-physician communication were *the* factors that bore the most significant impact on mortality in critical care units.
- In 1989, a major study by Hartz et al., published in the *New England Journal of Medicine*, found that "hospitals with a higher percentage of R.N.s and higher nurse to patient ratio had lower adjusted mortality rates. Hospitals that had higher R.N. to patient ratios had 6.3 fewer deaths per 1000 than those with lower R.N. to patient ratios."
- In 1994, Linda Aiken and her colleagues at the University of Pennsylvania School of Nursing again investigated the relationship between nursing excellence and patient mortality. Magnet hospitals that "empower nurses to use their professional skills" and that implement models which "result in more autonomy, control and status for nurses" and that encourage "comparatively good relationships between nurses and physicians" had a 7.7 percent lower mortality rate (9 fewer deaths per 1,000) than hospitals that did not place a similar emphasis on the quality of nursing care.

In November 1995, the journal *Critical Care Medicine* printed a study conducted in Switzerland. It documented the correlation between high RN-to-patient ratios and qualifications of RNs in weaning some of the sickest intensive care unit patients from mechanical respirators. Patients with severe respiratory disease were able to forego respirators far earlier when expert nurses were involved in their care, researchers showed. They were thus able to leave the hospital earlier. "The results of the present study," its physician authors reported, "show a clear-cut relationship between the duration of weaning in severe chronic obstructive pulmonary disease patients and an important, albeit rarely considered factor, the ratio of the effective and ideal ICU nurse workforce."

Because of nursing's central importance to really cost effective care, nurses like Jeannie Chaisson are not the only ones who are protesting about nursing cuts and the attendant decline in quality. More physicians are trying to educate their patients about nursing care privately and are speaking out more publicly to protest its erosion in their hospitals.

At John L. Doyne Hospital, in Milwaukee, Wisconsin, George B.

Haasler, chief of general thoracic surgery at the Medical College of Wisconsin, expressed grave concern about the replacement of RNs with nursing assistants on his service. At Marin General Hospital, located in the richest county in northern California, the head of neurosurgery, Lawrence H. Arnstein, protested the fact that the hospital had cut up to 50 percent of its medical and surgical nursing staff and had shifted many nursing duties to unlicensed aides. In a memo to the hospital's administration in 1995, the doctor reported on a meeting of the neurosurgical section. He wrote: "Each member had a lengthy litany of individual experiences dealing with patient care, errors in inappropriate treatment, dangerous events, and lack of understanding of the problems that seemed almost universal . . . and a feeling of increasing patient discontent which seems to be spreading. Even in these early stages [of cost cutting] it is clear and apparent that the current Marin General effort is a dismal failure. This produces," the memo predicted, "a prospect for the future which is frightening."

John Merritt O'Donnell, chairman of the Department of Surgical Intensive Care at the Lahey Clinic, outside Boston, has voiced similar concern. "One aspect of patient care that has been noticeably affected by nursing cutbacks is the quality of care provided in critical care units," O'Donnell says. "In medical and surgical intensive care units, nurses constantly reevaluate patients and recognize the most subtle changes in vital signs, mental status, and sophisticated monitors that may herald a catastrophic event. Their role has become even more crucial recently because the dramatic reduction in residency training programs has diminished the number of interns and residents previously providing twenty-four-hour-a-day in-hospital coverage. Physicians now, more than ever, rely on nursing assessments and recommendations when making diagnostic and therapeutic decisions on their patients, especially during the night."

O'Donnell concludes that "cutting labor costs by decreasing the nursing workforce is irrational and naive. There are certainly deserving targets for cuts — physician spending, pharmaceuticals, hospital middle management, and insurance. But don't cut nursing care."

Instead of taking this approach, hospital administrators and insurers are perpetuating a decades-long trend that wastes precious health care dollars on the sector of the system that does the least for patients — administration. According to a 1996 study by Steffie Woolhandler and David Himmelstein, associate professors at Harvard Medical School, if any sector in health care is growing, it is not patient care, but rather administration. Between 1968 and 1993, administrative and clerical staff grew by 692 percent — or a sevenfold increase. In 1968, administrative and clerical occupations comprised 18.1 percent of health care full-time equivalents (FTEs), and in 1993 the figure was 27.1 percent. In 1968, nursing personnel comprised 40.6 percent of FTEs, and in 1993, that figure had declined to 36.3 percent.

"In 1993, the study reports, "administration accounted for 57 percent of medical job growth and all of the growth in hospital employment." An even more startling figure highlights this peculiar imbalance in our health care system. In 1970, there were on average 1,298,000 people in America's hospitals on any given day. In 1993, that number had declined to 783,000. On an average day in 1993, there were more than 1,300,000 people in hospitals involved in administration and clerical jobs. While many nurses are struggling trying to provide care for five or even ten patients, there may be almost two people per patient "managing" their care or their paperwork.

These figures reflect the same kinds of shifts that Linda Aiken, a highly respected health policy expert who is a professor of nursing at the University of Pennsylvania School of Nursing and director of its Center for Health Services and Policy Research, has recently highlighted. "The major result of all this restructuring and reengineering has been to ration clinical services of all kinds," Aiken reports. "What this means is that when you look at the data on the numbers of RNs in hospitals, they are there in greater numbers. But when you take into account how sick the patients are, there are the same number of RNs that there were a decade ago, only they are taking care of sicker and sicker patients. And they have less help, not more, taking care of these patients because the overall number of nursing personnel — this includes RNs, LPNs, and aides — has declined. There is a seven percent decline in the total number of nursing personnel nationally over the last decade. This coincides within an 11 percent increase in total hospital personnel and an astonishing 46.5 percent increase in administrative personnel — higher-level billing department staff, advertising and marketing staff, and supervisors, executives, and CEOs.

"This shows," Aiken states emphatically, "that over the past decade, nursing has borne the brunt of hospital restructuring."

What is more alarming, Aiken says, is that hospitals are undertaking even further reductions in nursing personnel. "Before further reductions are undertaken, hospitals should set as a first priority examination of their expenditures of nonclinical personnel, and they should look at how spending can be reduced on the nonclinical side of hospitals."

Jeannie Chaisson hopes this will happen before it is too late. "At work, we were joking over the weekend that since insurers no longer want to pay for care and are only concerned about profit, maybe we won't provide hot meals anymore. If people want hot food, they can order take-out. Pretty soon we won't even give patients a mattress or sheets and pillowcases. We'll give them wire springs and they can provide mattress and linens themselves. And of course, families will have to take care of their own loved ones because there won't be any more nurses there to do it. If you want to see what we'll have then, just take a look at a Third World country. Is that what we want from our health care system?"

Preserving the Tapestry of Care

Each year in May, a week is set aside to celebrate American nurses. Planned to coincide with the anniversary of Florence Nightingale's birthday, May 12, it has become the occasion for a variety of commemorative events sponsored by hospitals, professional associations, or nursing unions. Over the past several years, however, many nurses feel there is little to rejoice about during Nurses' Week. In many cases, the annual event has been marked by protests rather than celebrations.

In this spirit of protest, about four hundred nurses from the Massachusetts Nurses Association (MNA) assembled at the State House in Boston in May 1996. While a camera crew from *Nightline* filmed the gathering, staff nurses, nurse researchers, Congressman Barney Frank, and a representative of the Massachusetts Medical Society spoke out in favor of a number of bills the MNA had drafted. The legislative package, entitled "Nursing's Agenda for Quality Care," included a bill that would create a standard operating definition of safe staffing in Massachusetts hospitals; one that would mandate that hospitals collect and publicly report data correlating a variety of health indicators with availability of quality nursing care; and a bill that would allow patients the right to know the qualifications of those caring for them (whether a "patient care technician" was, in fact, a real nurse or simply an aide).

At the same time, visitors driving on the highway in Albany, New York, were greeted by the sight of a huge fuchsia billboard with bold white-and-yellow lettering asking the following question: "Must Patients Ask for a Real Nurse?" The billboard, strategically placed on the exit that leads directly to the state capitol, was part of the New York State Nurses Association campaign to educate New Yorkers about the threats to nursing care in the state.

For the past several years, nursing organizations, unions, and professional associations all across the country have engaged in similar activities. In 1994, for example, the American Nurses Association (ANA) launched a three-year public education campaign centered around the theme "Every Patient Deserves a Nurse." The ANA has distributed over five hundred thousand copies of a brochure informing patients about their right to quality nursing care in hospitals. It explains the role that nurses play in hospitals and suggests questions patients should ask before being hospitalized, during a hospital stay, and after discharge.

The ANA has also developed a "Nursing Care Report Card" for acute care hospitals. Because nursing's contributions to health care are so often invisible, the ANA wants to correlate staffing levels with data about patient satisfaction, pain management, skin condition, total nursing care hours per patient, hospital-acquired infections, and patient injury rates. The ANA has been active in lobbying at the state and national levels against Medicare and Medicaid cuts, reductions in minimum staffing levels, and other threats to public health and patient care.

In April 1996, the ANA drafted legislation that has been introduced in the U.S. Congress called the Patient Safety Act of 1996. The bill requires that hospitals make public information about staffing levels, staff mix, and patient outcome. It mandates whistleblower protection for nurses who speak out publicly about threats to patient safety. In the case of hospital mergers and acquisitions, it asks the Department of Health and Human Services to assess their impact on the health care of the community involved in terms of quality of care.

In 1994 and 1995, the California Nurses Association (CNA) initiated a "Patient Watch" campaign. As part of this campaign, CNA took out advertisements in the pages of the *New York Times, Los Angeles Times, San Francisco Chronicle*, and other newspapers. The first of these ads displayed a picture of an acutely ill patient. "It's 3 A.M.," the headline read. "Who will come when you need help?"

"Hospitals and HMO's are cutting care to make record profits," the ad continued. "Patients are paying the price. Just ask any registered nurse who provides direct care."

The CNA ads are part of an ongoing attempt to reach out to patients and their families to encourage them to demand legislative and regulatory action to protect patient care and safety. Working with other health care and consumer groups, the CNA also filed a class action lawsuit accusing Alta Bates Hospital in Berkeley, California, of consumer fraud in its own advertising. Alta Bates has claimed that its corporate redesign will improve patient care. The CNA suit argues that the opposite is true. It also charges that the hospital has systematically misrepresented its financial condition and denied nurses the right to speak out as patient advocates. Alta Bates denies these charges.

In 1996, the CNA, along with the California-based Consumers for Quality Care, developed a state referendum initiative for the November '96 ballot called "The Patient Protection Act" that has been supported by Ralph Nader. If passed, the measure would closely regulate the behavior of managed care organizations in the state that has the most HMO enrollees in the entire nation. Among its provisions, it would require safe staffing in all health care facilities; prohibit HMOs from offering financial incentives to either nurses or doctors to encourage them to deny patients needed care; require HMOs and hospitals to release information to patients about their own care; and prohibit the HMO gag clauses that now restrain doctors and nurses from fully discussing their diagnoses, financial incentives to withhold care, and treatment options with patients. The referendum would also mandate that appropriately qualified providers examine patients before care is denied. It would tax health care mergers and acquisitions and sales of assets, as well as CEO compensation above $2 million, and use those funds to pay for care for the poor, and to pay the costs of enforcing the act itself. It would also establish a consumer watchdog agency to monitor HMO practices, bar use of mandatory arbitration in malpractice disputes, and prohibit disclosure of medical records without patient consent.

The campaign attracted widespread attention — particularly because of its dramatic depiction of the stories of people who said they had been harmed by HMOs. Throughout the months of September and October — up until the day of the election — the campaign sent out a report on what it called an "HMO casualty of the day" to the media, politicians, and activists. These testimonies often highlighted the impact of the denial of nursing care on those who need it. Because California has dealt with corporate health care and its version of managed care for far longer than the rest of the country, many observers view this campaign as a precursor of similar battles to come in other states as for-profit health care burgeons.

The Service Employees International Union has sponsored a similar initiative in California called the Health Care Patient Protection Act. This contains provisions similar to those in the CNA-sponsored referendum but does not include taxes on the health care industry, the consumer watchdog agency, the issue of malpractice, or disclosure of patients' medical records.

The New York State Nurses Association (NYSNA) has devoted a million and a half dollars to its health care education drive. The NYSNA produced posters that were displayed at bus shelters near hospitals, in subway stations, and on commuter railway trains. Their message: "Ask for a Real Nurse, Ask for an RN." In addition to the main campaign, other ads, like one in the *New York Times*, specifically targeted hospitals like Mt. Sinai Medical Center that are replacing registered nurses with aides. This particular ad informed patients that Mt. Sinai planned to replace as much as 40 percent of its entire RN workforce. "Our members want to protect the three most important things in their professional lives: their patients, their jobs, and their practice," the ad declared. "That is why we are alerting the public to this health care menace." The association has also helped to draft and lobby for legislation to protect patients from the excesses of an unregulated managed care industry.

In New Jersey, the Hospital Professionals and Allied Employees (HPAE), an RN union affiliated with the American Federation of Teachers, helped secure passage of the much-publicized New Jersey bill curtailing drive-through deliveries. Members of the HPAE have also created a new organization, Nurses for Quality Care. This group is encouraging all New Jersey nurses — whether union members or not — to speak out to legislators and the public about conditions in their hospitals. And in Seattle, Washington, nurses in District

1199NW of the Service Employees International Union have conducted their own informal research to try to uncover what is really happening to their patients. Nurses from Providence Medical Center, a hospital that had engaged in restructuring, stood outside the hospital distributing patient care surveys asking patients to tell them what they thought of the care they had received. A hundred and twenty written surveys were returned by mail and in person. Although many patients were generally satisfied with the care they received in outpatient settings as well as on the critical care floors, patients on general medical, surgical, and oncology floors reported that nurses were under a lot of pressure and didn't have time to give patients the attention they needed. The union publicized the results in a survey report form that was given out at the hospital and mailed to its board of trustees and given to local legislators. The hospital argues it gives high-quality care.

In the Washington state legislature, the union also proposed and successfully lobbied for whistle-blower legislation that protects consumers and health workers who expose quality care problems. These activities are part of a larger national SEIU effort to protect patient care. Nationally the union is working in coalition with other unions and consumer organizations like the Washington, D.C.–based Consumers for Quality Health Care to develop national legislation that will protect patients under managed care. In an ongoing battle against HMOs that cut costs by cutting caregivers, it is approaching large union purchasers of health care to set up criteria for quality and for fair treatment of health care workers.

In Boston in September 1996, twelve hundred nurses from the Brigham and Women's Hospital voted to strike if the hospital failed to include language in their contract giving nurses the power to decide if and when they would delegate to unlicensed aides. The hospital had balked at this demand. But the nurses took their case to the media and the public. They leafleted and picketed outside the hospital to alert patients and the public about what they considered this threat to patient care.

After a marathon bargaining session that began on September 19 and ended in the early morning hours of September 20, the nurses had won this contract provision.

These examples represent only a small fraction of the kinds of activities that nurses are engaged in today. Most of the nurses who have spoken out publicly against staffing cutbacks and the excesses of managed care are staff nurses — the majority of them union members. Echoing hospital administration, some press reports have suggested that complaints are being voiced by only a small number of self-interested nurses more worried about their jobs and pay than patient care.

Unionized nurses — who represent less than 12 percent of all RNs — have become hospital restructuring critics in disproportionate numbers because they have greater legal protection against employer retaliation. Nurses not covered by union contracts have little effective recourse if they are fired for challenging management on patient care issues. This is exactly what happened to Cheryl Churchill, an obstetrical nurse at McDonough District Hospital in Macomb, Illinois, when she complained that an improperly implemented nurse cross-training program was endangering obstetrical patients at her public hospital. She was fired in 1987 and her wrongful discharge case was initially thrown out of court. She has had to pursue her claim — that her First Amendment freedom-of-speech rights were violated — all the way to the Supreme Court. Ruling on a narrow constitutional issue, the Supreme Court justices sent the case back to a lower court to determine whether her criticism was protected free speech. This process has taken years and is still not resolved. At this writing, Churchill has not been reinstated in her job.

Two nurses represented by the CNA at Alta Bates Hospital in Berkeley were disciplined after speaking to the press about their concerns, and one was later fired. When many nurses, like the ones interviewed for this book, have spoken out in public to defend their patients, hospital administrators have called them on the carpet, interrogated them about their statements, and either explicitly or implicitly threatened their employment.

Because of the actions of courageous nurses, doctors, and patients all over the country, patients are rebelling against many of the insurance company practices that deny them care. As stated above, in Maryland, New Jersey, and Massachusetts, coalitions of women's health activists, female patients, nurses, and physicians have successfully challenged insurance company policies — known as "the OB Express" or "drive-through delivery" — that force maternity patients out of the hospital twelve to twenty-four hours after their babies are born. Advocates of longer hospital stays are not seeking expensive, unnecessary treatment. What they want is appropriate medical monitoring and the evaluation, caregiving, and education that nurses provide newborns and their mothers. Similarly, they are seeking follow-up care at home delivered by nurses who have the obstetrical and pediatric experience necessary to protect both mother and child.

More patients and their families may need to get involved to ensure that nurses are available to care for them. In order to preserve the tapestry of care, they need to know more about the qualifications of those caring for them. "People don't take a car to the garage unless they have certified mechanics," Jeannie Chaisson observes. "They want evidence of their training and certification well displayed. Why, then, do they leave their grandmother in a hospital with someone who isn't qualified to care for her? Patients and family members need to ask themselves: Who do you want at the bedside when you're in the hospital?"

For Jeannie, the right answer is simple. "If I get sick, I want hundreds of degrees, years of experience. I don't want someone who graduated from high school and got a two-weeks training course to decide when I'm stable."

One part of the solution to the nursing crisis is for patients to scrutinize more carefully the care they receive. It is ironic that the very same patients who are starting to educate themselves about how to find the right doctor and who are also asking more informed questions about drugs, tests, and procedures often fail to inquire about the number and qualifications of the nurses who will be caring for them in the hospital, a skilled nursing or rehabilitation hospital, nursing home, or at home.

Just as patients are learning to ask whether a physician is board certified or has financial incentives not to refer them to a specialist, they can ask similar questions about nursing care. When a physician or surgeon recommends hospitalization for any reason, questions about how an operating and recovery room are staffed — with registered nurses or aides — are extremely relevant. A hospital's nurse-to-patient ratio on medical and surgical floors — one nurse to four patients or one to twelve patients on the day shift — will determine the course of one's recovery. Patients will want to know if a hospital uses large numbers of little-trained aides, cross-trained workers, float, or per diem agency nurses. When a patient or family member sees a "nurse" wearing a badge identifying him or her as a "patient care associate," "patient-care technician" or "multiskilled caregiver," it's important to know who these staff really are. Are they registered nurses, licensed practical nurses, aides, or workers who have been "cross-trained?" If they are not nurses, it is hardly unreasonable if a patient balks when they try to give the kind of hands-on care, monitoring, and education that only a registered nurse can perform safely.

When hospitals and HMOs try to deprive patients of nursing care through early discharge policies, similar information about the staffing of any nursing home or "subacute" facility to which they are transferred is essential. These facilities are fast becoming the acute care hospitals of the late twentieth century, and no patient should assume that these facilities have adequate quantity and quality of staff. Patients may feel that they do not have a choice when they are assigned to be discharged to such settings. But we have seen how informed consumers, asking the right questions, can both get what they want out of the system and begin to change the system itself.

Similarly, home care agencies need the same scrutiny. Patients are being discharged to the home with serious medical conditions and complex treatments. Patients will never get the care they need and families will falter under the burden of their care if a home care agency is staffed predominantly with aides or with new nursing school graduates who lack the kind of educational resources available to them in the hospital. Moreover, many patients need specialized nursing care. A pediatric nurse does not necessarily know how to deal with the problems of an oncology patient. An orthopedic nurse who has cared only for adults may not be familiar with the problems of newborn babies and their mothers. What patients need are experienced RNs, including nurse practitioners and sometimes nurses who specialize in the care of particular diseases and conditions, caring for them, supporting their families, and giving them necessary education in the home.

If patients do not get this kind of care in the hospital, nursing home, or home, then it may be time to complain. Complaints should not scapegoat individual nurses for their alleged failures to care but should highlight the larger problem: hospitals and other institutions are not employing enough nurses to provide quality patient care. If nurses are not there to answer the buzzer; if nurses are not available to help a patient go to the bathroom, walk, or learn about self-care; if care is fragmented and depersonalized, letters and phone calls to hospital or health plan administrators as well as to the employers who select health plans for their employees are called for.

Patients may want to contact state and federal regulators and officials. State departments of insurance, health, or social services, and legislative health care committees are a good place to start. And greater public support for legislative initiatives like those proposed by nursing organizations and lobbied for by many medical associations is certainly important. Many states mandate by law staffing ratios for the number of healthy children a family day care provider can care for and for the number of healthy students a teacher can teach in a public school classroom. Legislators may even mandate how many firefighters must be on a fire truck. But when it comes to how many of the sickest, most vulnerable human beings one nurse can care for, the sky seems to be the limit.

More doctors should also take a far more active role in defending the kind of caregiving that is essential to their patients' curing, healing, coping, and even survival. When physicians recommend that patients undergo a procedure or treatment, patients assume that the physician is not only assuring the quality of his or her services, but also those provided by any health care institution involved. Today, however, physicians cannot always speak for the care provided by the institutions in which they work. And they certainly cannot vouchsafe the care delivered in the dizzying array of nursing homes and "subacute facilities" to which their patients may be sent during the process of recovery. If physicians are to follow the central tenet of the Hippocratic oath — "Do no harm" — they have a moral responsibility to understand the importance of nursing care and to act both within their institutions and in the public arena to make sure their patients can benefit from it.

It's also time to reconsider the wisdom of the current drive for shortened length of hospital stays and increased reliance on nursing homes and other so-called subacute facilities and ambulatory clinics as the preferred new setting for health care delivery. As Uwe Reinhardt has argued, "The centerpiece of this nation's cost control strategy — a single-minded and unceasing quest to reduce the number of hospital inpatient days per capita — may actually have been counterproductive. In all likelihood, that strategy has served to drive up total national health spending."

It's important for the public to understand that hospitals are not necessarily expensive places in which to recover from sickness. They are only expensive on the most acute inpatient days when many tests and services are provided. They are not particularly expensive — indeed may even be less expensive than subacute facilities and nursing homes — when the patient is recovering and needs more nursing care and fewer medical tests and treatments.

Of course, hospitals can be unhealthy and unpleasant places to be. It is sometimes better to be cared for at home. But the decision about length of hospital stay should be made by patients, nurses, and doctors. That decision should be based solely on the condition of the patient and his or her home environment. If a patient is not acutely ill; if the home is clean and safe; if insurance provides adequate home care by expert nurses; if family members are available to supplement that nursing care; then patients can be safely discharged from a hospital while recovering.

But today, decisions about hospital discharge routinely put the condition of particular patients who live in a particular context last and insurers' and employers' need for profit first. That must change — not just for mothers and their newborn babies, but for all patients. Not only does radically reducing hospital stays make no quality sense, it also makes little economic sense. In the short term, hospitals should curtail their "perverse pricing" practices and price more accurately. This would discourage some of the worst HMO abuses that are occurring today. In the long term, far greater savings could be wrested under a universal health care system that gives hospitals annual budgets. In other countries, this has encouraged wiser use of resources.

The Institute of Medicine study demonstrates that a rigorous research agenda is also needed. When nurses and doctors complain about declining quality of care, hospitals, HMOs, and elite panels of experts often respond that their concerns are not substantiated by research. Before we act on your complaints, the experts say, you have to prove that you are right, that hospitals are unsafe today. But the burden of proof should be borne by those institutions that are making revolutionary changes. *They* should prove that the changes they are implementing are safe — before those changes are made. They seem unwilling to do this. They are instituting a grand untested experiment. And they are making it difficult to conduct research — even after the fact — that assesses the impact of this experiment.

It is essential that government and foundations fund research studies that correlate the impact of understaffing, use of aides, and transfers to subacute facilities with patient outcomes. To undergird policy and political decisions we also need to chart the experiences of patients discharged after ambulatory surgery or discharged to the home from the hospital while acutely ill. Are their pain and other symptoms being adequately managed? Are they eating, walking, bathing, and safely carrying out the other activities of daily living? Do they understand the medication regimens they are on and how to use the complex medical technology they may need to manipulate in the home? And how are their family caregivers, who must now act as professional nurses, bearing up under this new burden?

Hospitals should also report data in a way that tells us where nurses actually work and what kinds of patients they actually care for. Despite hospital and HMO opposition, all of the data that hospitals and HMOs collect should be made public and available to health care researchers. The research studies that result from an analysis of this kind of data — not assertions and assumptions — should guide health policy.

Until such research is available, political representatives should pay far greater attention to the complaints of patients and caregivers. These complaints — that care is being managed right out of the health care system — have turned from a trickle to a torrent. What they indicate is that no one can escape the erosion of nursing care. Affluent Americans may believe that they can buy their way out of some of the worst excesses of managed care. If they can afford it, they can still pay to see the doctor of their choice and consult with a specialist of their choice. They can pay for an emergency room visit or to have a procedure or drug a managed care company may not approve.

But it does little good to pay a well-trained surgeon to perform a bypass operation if the skilled nurses necessary to help patients recover from such surgery are no longer at the bedside. It is extremely dangerous to receive a high-tech bone marrow transplant if skilled oncology nurses are no longer available to monitor the impact of such highly toxic treatment and help temper its side effects. And if the nurses whose expertise and experience allow them to collaborate with, educate, and challenge physicians are driven out of the profession, our entire health care system will suffer.

No amount of money can save sick people from the well-intentioned ministrations of those with little skill and educated judgment. Nor will another oft-proposed panacea — hiring private-duty nurses to care for hospitalized patients — protect the sick and vulnerable no matter how well-to-do. Private duty nursing is a poorly remunerated field that may not attract the best nurses. Unlike hospital or home health care nurses, whose qualifications are guaranteed by the hospital or agency they work for, private duty nurses may lack the skill and knowledge and system savvy of nurses who work in hospitals. They may not specialize in the particular medical problem from which the patient suffers, and they often do not know the routine and practice patterns of the unit's nursing and medical staff. Because they are not part of the unit's permanent health care team and culture of care, their patients may suffer.

We can no longer afford the attitude described by Julian Tudor Hart and Paul Dieppe in the previous chapter. As those authors point out, many bottom line–driven health care administrators, legislators, and health policy planners seem to think that health care institutions can afford to focus on "technological procedures, pharmacological interventions . . . and reducing labor costs" because "human support" will somehow survive on its own. These authors remind us that caregiving and caregivers must also be nourished to survive. Ironically, many of the very same people who insist that CEOs, high-level executives, biomedical researchers, and physicians should reap greater and greater rewards so they can attract the best and brightest, continue to insist that caregivers should soldier on and make do with less and less. But if hospitals and other health care institutions become focused only on the bottom line, caring will not automatically take care of itself. Women will not continue to care for us no matter how poorly they are treated. Expert caregiving skills will not be passed on to a next generation of nurses if the preceding generation is pushed out of the workplace. The art and science of caregiving do not flourish in adversity. They flourish in the same kind of resource- and respect-rich environment that has nurtured medicine for over a century and that should finally nurture nursing as well.

Our health care crisis is not only about money. It's also about quality of care. Patients should also be able to have the option of receiving primary care or other services from a nurse practitioner. Services from nurse practitioners or nurse midwives should be routinely available and reimbursed by all providers of health insurance. Given the aging of the population, medical practices that care for elderly patients as well as the new life care communities increasingly serving the affluent elderly should also offer the services of geriatric nurse practitioners like Ellen Kitchen. Patients and families should also demand that such services be made available just as in the late sixties and seventies they demanded — and got — access to and reimbursement for the services of nurse midwives. And if patients are to die in comfort and with dignity, it is essential for them to understand the role nurses play in the dying process. The entire discussion about how we die has been hijacked by the issue of physician-assisted suicide. But we have seen how nurses help patients navigate the dying process. Rather than focusing almost exclusively on the issue of how doctors can help patients end their lives, is it not time that we talked about what we can do for patients — that is, provide them with the kind of palliative care services that nurses and physicians, working in true collaboration, can deliver? What patients and their families should be demanding from the medical system is that their doctors learn how to care for them. To do this, nurses could be some of their teachers.

To ensure this kind of quality of care in all settings, patients and consumers should thus be far more concerned about the parlous state of nurse-physician relationships and about the public image of nursing. As we have seen — and as research studies have documented — collaboration between the two largest health care professions is crucial to patient care. Anyone who uses the health care system should be concerned about the quality of communication between doctors and nurses and the imbalance of power between medicine and nursing. If nurses and physicians do not effectively and consistently communicate and collaborate, if they do not teach one another and learn together, patients will also suffer.

Medical schools and the teaching hospitals that train physicians, nurses, and other health care professionals need to do far more to encourage genuine nurse-physician collaboration. Making medical education more humane by reducing the number of hours — and thus the chronic sleep deprivation — required of residents is a key component of collaborative doctor-nurse relationships. Nurses in all hospitals should also be given more latitude in matters of patient care than many currently enjoy.

"If doctors wrote orders that allowed nurses to adjust medications within wider parameters, they would not have to bother doctors so frequently in the middle of the night," suggests oncologist Glenn Bubley. "Nurses," he continues, "should be treated as full members of the health care team." This means that they should round with the team in the morning and be full participants — not outliers — in these discussions about patient care. "Instead of leading off with the intern reporting on the patient, the nurse should really lead off the discussion on morning rounds," Bubley contends. "She's after all the one who knows more about the patient than anybody. If she is truly included in discussions about patient care, she would know more about the plan of care and wouldn't have the sense that she is flying alone by the seat of her pants in the middle of the night. That way she wouldn't have to call the doctor as much."

Both educational and clinical institutions must treat nurse / physician relations and communication as a moral and ethical issue. Physicians-in-training should learn what it is nurses do and in which areas they are expert. The Beth Israel nurse-for-a-day in the surgical clerkship of the Harvard Medical School is an important step on this path. At this writing, the medical school is planning to incorporate a session on nursing into the third-year coursework required of all medical students. Every medical student should be required to follow a nurse for a day in the course of his or her training. And nursing students should do the same — following a doctor for a day. When they enter hospitals, hospitals should give interns guidelines about how to deal respectfully and collaboratively with nurses. Indeed, nursing and medical schools should encourage nurses and doctors-in-training to undertake some part of their coursework together.

After her experience at Columbia University College of Physicians and Surgeons, internist Rita Charon argues that "it's naive to think that a few, short, simple interventions — like combining nursing and medical school students for the odd lecture or discussion group — will reverse their old, deep antagonism. We faculty in medical and nursing schools need to make deep, serious, professional commitments to real egalitarian respectful relationships in the care of the patient. We can do it," Charon insists. "We can overcome the antagonisms when the care of the patient is the center of our work."

Thus, hospitals, clinics, nursing homes, and other health care institutions should teach nurses and physicians to view each other as members of a health care matrix rather than as a militarized hierarchy. Whether they are professionals-in-training or fully licensed providers, systematic communication between these groups — like that routinely conducted in the Beth Israel Home Care Department and recently initiated in the Hematology/Oncology Clinic — would be institutionalized on all units and levels.

Physicians may complain that they have little time in their busy schedules for yet another series of meetings and discussions. These objections, while understandable, cannot stand in the way of achieving a healthier integration of medicine and nursing in the health care system. We simply can no longer afford the dysfunctional, traditional-family model that dominates medical institutions. Change must become a priority.

Collaboration would not only help patients and their nurses, it would immeasurably improve the working environment for doctors. Alliances between the two disciplines are essential today as both professions fight off challenges to their clinical judgment in an era of corporate-driven health care. The great irony of corporate-driven managed care is that physicians, who once had the kind of clinical autonomy and respect many segments of organized medicine denied to nurses, are now suffering some of the same problems that have long plagued nursing. Insurance company executives and their utilization review personnel are now trying to tell doctors how to do their job and are intruding into the doctor-patient relationship. Sometimes the person doing that intruding is a nurse. In yet another perverse irony of the new system, managed care companies hire nurses to sit at video display terminals and — following clinical rules determined by bottom line–oriented corporate policies — dictate to physicians. To some nurses, it may appear that nursing has finally gotten some power over medicine. But this power is ephemeral, because the nurse is actually acting as the instrument of the corporation.

The only way nurses will really attain the kind of power that they are due is when doctors, nurses, and patients join together to create a model of health care based on the imperatives of caregiving rather than of profit making. The wholesale denial of care so prevalent in market-driven health care is not the avenue to cost-effective care. If doctors and nurses devote themselves to a sustained conversation that also includes patients and other providers, they can combine their insights and expertise to defining sensible, effective care for individual patients.

Of course, nurses will never attain this kind of power if their public image does not improve. And to do this, the media and the public will have to become aware of the way in which most hospitals silence nurses and encourage hospitals to promote the achievements of *all* professionals. The Beth Israel is unusual because its public relations department has actively tried to educate the public about the work of nurses. Today, most hospital public relations departments promote only medicine and biomedical innovation. Few make any effort to promote nurses' work. Sometimes they actively discourage nurses from talking to the media or may refuse to publicize their innovations and expertise.

An emergency room nurse at a major northeastern hospital told me a typical tale. During the period when Nancy Rumplik was so worried about the battering of Deborah Celli, this nurse and her colleagues were also trying to deal with women who were the victims of domestic violence. The state had mandated that emergency departments establish policies and procedures for caring for victims of domestic violence. The nurse and her committee designed training for all the nurses in the emergency room as well as for any physicians or volunteers who wanted to attend. To facilitate this process, the nurses in the ER asked the hospital — one of the richest in the nation — to allocate resources so that social workers could be on-call to assist nurses in dealing with battered women. "These women," the nurse said, "need special help. While we're helping to treat their injuries, we need help getting them shelter, finding resources in the community and planning for their safety."

The hospital resisted. Administrators insisted that the ER did not, in fact, care for a great many battered women and thus didn't need to provide special social work assistance to deal with them. Over a period of weeks, the nurse conducted a chart review to prove just how many victims of domestic violence came through the ER doors. She insisted that she would not train nurses in policies and procedures if she did not have the minimal resources needed to deal effectively with this group of patients. The hospital continued to balk at her request. "We allocate a lot of resources to medicine in trauma care," she said, "but somehow they couldn't find the small amount for social work coverage on nights and weekends."

After the nurse continued to fight for this program, the hospital finally relented. When the program was up, running, and successful, local newspapers found out about it and called the hospital public relations department to arrange interviews for a story. Rather than allow this nurse — or any of her colleagues — to speak directly to the media, the hospital insisted she brief an administrator and he in turn would speak to the press. When the nurse protested and insisted she should be the one to talk with the press, since it was her program, she was denied the opportunity. "I would get a phone call from an administrator and I would have to sit there while he was talking to the press on the phone. I could be trusted to develop this program, to train the staff, to care for the patients, and do all the follow-up, but I could not be trusted to talk to the media about the program I had developed and implemented. This is one of the doc Meccas of the universe, and they will never highlight nurses," she concluded.

This nurse explained that nurses are also given second-class treatment in internal hospital communications. "When hospital publications talk about doctors' work, they talk about their educational background, their professional affiliations and involvements. When they briefly mention a nurse's accomplishments, they never say where she went to college, what professional organizations she's involved in, or what roles she takes on outside the hospital."

Other hospitals seem to be equally nervous about letting nurses out in public alone. Several years ago, for example, a public relations staffer at the Massachusetts General Hospital asked me for suggestions about how her department might better promote nurses.

I asked her if her office had a list of physicians' names that were consulted when a reporter called seeking a medical expert.

Of course, she answered.

Did they have a similar list of nurses' names, I asked.

No, she replied. Then she thought for a moment and announced that her department could compile such a list. When a reporter called, they could present the name of a physician and pair him or her with a nurse. I applauded her idea, and then added, "Nurses are perfectly capable of speaking to the press unescorted. In many instances, nurses know more than physicians about a particular area of health care."

She paused and then blurted out, "Oh, we could never promote *that idea!*"

That idea is, however, one that the public and press needs to hear. Hospital administrators should be committed to helping patients understand that they exist not only to provide medical care but to provide expert nursing care.

Hospitals are repositories of thousands of stories about the value of nursing care. Yet these stories are some of the best-kept secrets in America. Not only because hospitals refuse to tell them, but because reporters tend to ignore them. When the mass media define health care as "medical care," nurses and their innovations in care, treatment, and research or insights about health care restructuring and policy are inevitably left out of coverage.

The idea that doctors — and, of course, health plans or insurers — are the only major players in that debate is so pervasive that it even suffuses the work of some of the most articulate critics of the medical status quo. Health policy experts, even some of the more humanistic physicians who have tried to convince their physician colleagues to be more attentive to patient needs and caregiving issues, tend to forget the power and importance of nursing. Focusing on the problems or promise of physician care, they neglect contributions of those nurses who have refined more relational models of patient care.

The almost total invisibility of nurses in the media and policy debates reinforces the public perception that nurses do little more than dispense pills, empty bedpans, and distribute comforting pats on the head. This picture must change. It has changed somewhat for nurse practitioners. While patients, members of the media, and health care policymakers tend to ignore or fail to understand the importance of bedside nursing, they may readily embrace nurse practitioners because their work so resembles that of doctors' — especially the old-fashioned kind, fondly remembered for their home visits. Nurse practitioners take histories, use diagnostic tests, and can prescribe medication. The public increasingly supports greater autonomy for these nurses and more equal relationships with doctors because, unlike bedside nurses, NPs are viewed as "important" health care providers. The danger of this view is that it ignores the importance of the far greater number of nurses who work in traditional settings.

According greater respect to nurses means according respect to all nurses. Journalists could help the public better understand the realities of health and illness and the complexity of health care if they expanded their list of sources to include nurses. To do this, they will, however, have to understand the ways in which many hospitals silence nurses, and insist that nurses play a greater role in their reporting of health care.

The struggle for an accurate public depiction of nurses' work is not just a public health issue, it is also a women's issue. Everyone interested in the progress of women has a stake in the successful defense of the largest female profession in the country. When hospitals insist that nurses be seen but not heard; care for the sick day in and day out but get no public recognition for it; when physicians feel they are too busy to systematically communicate with nurses; and when medical students continue to be taught that nurses are their handmaidens, the gender implications are unmistakable. These problems will not be remedied by greater numbers of female doctors. They will only be remedied when those women and men interested in greater equality between the sexes value care as much as cure. At least some of the feminist energy devoted to helping women succeed in the medical profession should thus be channeled into the fight nurses are waging to defend patient care, to maintain their professional integrity, and to play a more influential role in health care policy deliberations.

The gender implications facing nursing continue to be both fascinating and troubling. Consider, for example, the significance of asking nurses not to identify themselves as RNs and, along with other so-called lower-level hospital staff, to refer to themselves as some version of "patient care technician." The kind of women's caregiving work that our society has traditionally undervalued is once again trivialized as all those who work in direct patient care are turned into generic health care workers. Only those in the elite "male" profession of medicine are allowed to retain a separate identity and display their distinct professional qualifications. We are returning here to the kind of pernicious stereotypes of a woman is a woman is a woman, a nurse is a nurse is a nurse.

Similarly, there is a fundamental connection between the future of nursing and women's ability to comfortably navigate the passage between workplace and home. Professional nursing has helped make it possible for many women who work outside of the home to continue doing so. Professional nurses are the ones who take care of sick children, spouses, and relatives. Since someone has to care for the acutely ill patients sent home inappropriately, dehospitalization of patients in our society inevitably targets women who will be asked to perform the lion's share of "nursing" in the home or to take time off work to watch over hospitalized patients who do not get adequate nursing care. The same women who now have to care for young children, care for older relatives, and care for the chronically ill are now being asked to care for the acutely ill and the dying in the home and sometimes in the hospital.

Health care has always been a women's issue. Women are the largest percentage of health care workers. The largest profession in health care is nursing. Women are the main family caregivers of the sick. To attack nursing is to attack all women.

Supporting nurses' efforts is more important than ever before because nurses' voices are critical to any effort to control cost and maintain quality. Because of advances in public health, higher standards of living, and progress in science and technology, many of our physical and emotional problems arise from chronic conditions that require care for decades. The so-called "cures" we have developed for these problems and others tend to be expensive interventions that sometimes bring little benefit.

It is clear that Americans use far too much expensive technology and treatment. As noted previously, HMOs are now trying to deny patients many expensive medical treatments and drugs. And this has created a great public outcry. Ironically, however, some of the drugs, tests, consultations, and procedures that HMOs are trying to limit, may, in fact, offer little to patients. Many can be reasonably withheld. The critical question — for patients and for our society — is who benefits from treatment restrictions, how are such decisions made, and what alternatives are offered instead.

This is where nursing's wisdom comes in. Consider Nancy Rumplik, Jeannie Chaisson, Ellen Kitchen, and the hundreds of thousands of other expert nurses in this country.

When Jeannie Chaisson is concerned about patients who are receiving aggressive, heroic treatment, it's not because the cost will affect her bottom line or increase her yearly income. When she encourages her colleagues and terminally ill patients to think critically about treatment options, she also offers an alternative to aggressive high-tech treatment — her presence, her attention, her willingness to help patients and their families navigate their last days of life.

When Nancy Rumplik and her colleagues raise objections to repeated cycles of chemotherapy, invasive diagnostic tests, or high-tech treatments that will needlessly prolong death, their prescription is not abandonment. It is the kind of palliative care that directly addresses patients' pain and suffering and the needs of their families both before and after a loved one dies. When one of her vulnerable patients is discharged from the hospital, Ellen Kitchen does not visit them less, but intensifies her efforts to monitor their condition and provide social and emotional support.

In more and more managed care settings, some nurses whose jobs have been spared are indeed assigned a larger role. But it is nothing like the roles played by Nancy, Jeannie, and Ellen. Today nurses are increasingly deployed as gatekeepers and utilization reviewers who make judgments largely based on financial criteria. Or nurses are turned into "case managers" who are asked to manage patients' cases without any meaningful patient contact.

This is not the role nurses should play in our health care system. We should be building on nurses' knowledge of relationship, their skilled intuition and involvement, not obliterating these contributions to patient care. A true commitment to health maintenance and disease prevention, and to helping patients and families take care of themselves and each other, necessarily involves giving nurses the time to get to know patients and help them overcome their problems before, during, and after medical events.

Like many, I believe we must replace our current system of wasteful, fragmented, impersonal care with a well-funded one that involves the genuine management of care. But nurses, doctors, patients, and their families — in collaboration with others in health care — must manage this care. And to find the money to finance it, we should not cut nursing staff and eliminate nursing expertise, but rather should target the real health care cost escalators — the exorbitant salaries of hospital administrators and insurance executives, the incomes of high-priced medical specialists, the outrageously inflated cost of drugs and medical equipment, the construction of unnecessary hospital facilities and purchase of redundant technology, and wasteful health plan and hospital advertising and marketing. The cost of administering and marketing America's fifteen hundred private health insurance plans now consumes over $45 billion a year or about 15 percent of our insurance premiums. And savings wrested from the system are not set aside to increase access to the uninsured or to refine and develop innovations in direct care but go instead to hospital and insurance company executives, shareholders, and employers who purchase insurance.

Although this book is not intended to be a polemic on behalf of any particular health care reform proposal, it is clear that America must deal once and for all with an utterly irrational health care financing system that allows private interests to make billions in profits from the pain and suffering of their fellow citizens. America is the only country in the industrialized world that does not provide tax-supported universal health care coverage in some form. It is no accident that countries with such systems — like Canada, Australia, and the Scandinavian nations — have 30 to 40 percent more nurses per thousand population than the United States. The choice is becoming increasingly stark. Either we spend our health care dollars on private insurance and for-profit health care or we spend money on enhancing quality care at the bedside.

To protect that kind of care, we must recognize and reward one of our most valuable health care resources. Nurses like Nancy Rumplik, Jeannie Chaisson, and Ellen Kitchen teach us the true meaning of life support. They teach us not only the value of cure but of care. They teach us about the possibilities of modern medicine and about its limitations. To listen to nurses, as we must do today, is to understand the essence of health care. To defend nursing, as we must do today, is to protect not only a particular profession, but to protect ourselves. We look to technology and medicine to prevail over disease and death. But I have become convinced that the only victories we can win over our vulnerability and mortality are those of the human spirit and human community. Nurses and the patient relationships they forge create that kind of community. They not only help us to heal, they embody the more powerful and enduring victory of care.

Afterword to the Cornell Edition

When I began to do research for *Life Support* in the early 1990s, my goal was to help people outside of nursing understand the work that nurses do. As I explain in the preface, I had been utterly oblivious to nurses before 1984, when I went to the hospital to have my first baby. The fact that my father was a famous physician, coupled with a steady diet of Hollywood's medico-centered version of the hospital, had shaped my view of health care work: to me it was a doctor-only affair. Yet, when I became vulnerable enough to need hospital care, I was surprised to discover that nurses were as important, if not more so, as my friend the doctor. After I finished writing the book, my appreciation for our societal blindness about nursing did not diminish. For example, when I gave the manuscript to a friend, she applauded my portrait of nurses' kindness and compassion but warned me that I had made a terrible mistake that I needed to correct before the book was published.

What, I asked.

In my portrait of Nancy Rumplik's work, I explained that the oncology nurse administered and monitored chemotherapy. Nurses don't do that, my friend confidently insisted. Doctors do.

I had to laugh as I informed her, that no, actually they don't. That is the nurses' job. Oh, she said, stunned and a bit abashed. Really, I didn't know that, she confessed sheepishly.

While promoting the book on a radio show, the interviewer—a savvy female talk-show host—told me she too found my description of nurses' caring work perfectly accurate. What she found surprising, she said, was that the nurses I profiled knew so much about medications and diseases. Fortunately, I had my wits about me, and I responded that what was surprising was that she was surprised. How could people imagine that nurses knew so little?

Reflecting on this encounter sometime later, I concluded that perhaps it was not so surprising that this talk-show host was uninformed. It would have been more remarkable if she had known that nurses have medical and technical, as well as caring knowledge, because no one in our society—sometimes not even nurses—seems prepared to illuminate more than the caring side of nursing. That is why I wrote *Life Support*, to bring nursing, in all its dimensions, out of the closet—or the cloister to be exact—where it was in 1996 and where, sadly, many nurses and much of nursing still are today.

Since I wrote *Life Support* a lot has changed for the nurses I followed and the institution in which they worked. Shortly after I finished my observations at the Beth Israel Hospital, it merged with the New England Deaconess Hospital located catty corner across the street. This was the era of merger mania when hospitals felt they had to integrate vertically, horizontally—in any shape or configuration that would allow them to gain more clout with managed care insurers. The merger of the Beth Israel, a gem of a hospital that had developed a culture that placed a high value on nursing, with the New England Deaconess, a hospital that had a reputation as one of Boston's shrines to physician power, is analyzed by the sociologist Dana Beth Weinberg in *Code Green: Money Driven Hospitals and the Dismantling of Nursing*, which explains what happened to the Beth Israel and nursing in much greater detail than I can muster in this short afterword. To briefly summarize, when the two hospitals merged, doctors clashed, the nursing department was dismantled, primary nursing became a thing of the past, and most of the nurses I followed or observed eventually left the hospital or were unceremoniously kicked out. Joyce Clifford was moved upstairs, as it were. Trish Gibbons, who helped Clifford pioneer primary nursing but subsequently worked in other facilities, returned to the hospital to replace Clifford as chief of nursing. One day when she came in to work, she was greeted with a pink slip and escorted to clear out her office and then out of the hospital by a security guard.

The hospital did not only hemorrhage nurses; it hemorrhaged money and almost went bankrupt because of the business strategy that was supposed to strengthen it. Today, it has recovered its financial stability but not its reputation for nursing excellence. The current head of the nursing department does not have chief executive status and has much less power in the merged institution.

Ellen Powers, nurse manager of the hematology oncology service, departed. Marion Phipps was pushed out after more than thirty years of service. Nancy Rumplik remains in the clinic. At this writing she has been at the BI or BI Deaconess for twenty years. She says that she had a difficult time during the merger period and afterward, but things have gotten better. What happened to her unit, however, reflects the diminished power of nursing inside the hospital. Although nurses at the clinic report to a nurse manager, that manager no longer reports to the nursing department and nurse administrators. Instead they report to the ambulatory department—to Ellen Volpe, the Director of Operations for the Ambulatory Department— who is neither a nurse nor a physician.

Jeannie Chaisson stayed on when the hospital merged. As cost cutting seemed to become the hospital's number-one priority, the institution dramatically curtailed her role as educator of and provider of clinical support to nurses. When I observed her work, she worked four days as a clinical specialist and one day as a staff nurse on the unit. With the merger, that ratio was reversed. The hospital felt education of staff was a luxury it could no longer afford, and more and more CNSs lost their jobs. Those who remained were no longer asked to provide the many in-house educational programs that had been the hallmark of the Beth Israel. Jeannie finally decided to leave. There was simply no place for her, she felt, at this newly restructured institution in which education and support for nurses seemed to have been restructured entirely out of the hospital. She now works in home care and hospice.

Although there were many changes at the Beth Israel, including the departure of two of the nurses about whom I write in this book, the essential message of *Life Support* remains unchanged and is, in my view, even more important today than when it first appeared in print in 1997. All over the country, indeed the world, nurses are working too long and too hard with patients who are too sick. I have watched the toll this takes on nurses and patients. Since this book first came out, my mother, father-in-law, and mother-in-law have grown older, become sick, and died. I myself recently had a first-hand experience, and not a particularly happy one, with hospital care. As I lay in my hospital bed waiting for nurses who had too many patients to get to me I kept thinking (to put it quite bluntly), how can anyone screw around with nursing?

How can anyone ask human beings to take care of seven or more postsurgical patients on days and sometimes more on nights? Why on earth do hospital administrators think that things are less busy because it is the middle of the night? My pain did not miraculously recede at the stroke of seven or eight when the day nurses left and the night nurses arrived. The risk of infection does not take a break for the night. Those parts of my body—bowels, bladder, lungs, veins, and arteries—that were sluggish during the morning and afternoon did not suddenly leap into action because it was the evening shift. I came out of emergency surgery sometime after 11 p.m. I was not less sick or in less need of care because it was nearly midnight.

Yes, there are fewer tests and procedures at night, but your nursing needs remain the same or even increase. Plus your emotional terror at being sick, vulnerable, and utterly dependent probably grows worse at night, when the healthy, concerned friends and relatives who visited or called during the daytime are far away, peacefully sleeping while you are lying alone in an alien environment from which all doctors (who barely see you anyway) have disappeared. Only the nurses stand between you and your terrors and the many complications that lie in wait for you.

How can people not get it?

What they do not get is that nursing is not so much about caring and compassion as it is about competence. Nursing is grounded in the competence born of accumulated knowledge. It is this knowledge that allows a nurse to recognize not just what a patient is thinking and feeling but the signs of the different complications and problems that patients cannot themselves anticipate or prevent.

When I initially wrote *Life Support*, I described nursing as a "tapestry of care" and titled the book's first chapter after this concept. If I were writing the book today I would no longer choose that term.

Instead of weaving a "tapestry of care" I think nurses weave a "tapestry of competence." Care is part of that competence. Rather than competence being grounded in care, as nurses so often describe it, I believe that nurses' ability to be attentive, empathic, and compassionate depends on their knowledge and skill—in other words, their mastery of the science of nursing. This, in turn, allows them to imbue their practice with the art of nursing.

I do not believe caring is "heart" work. I believe it is all head work. Even the most intensely intimate and empathic work nurses do with patients stems from the skill and knowledge that is lodged in their brains. How does a nurse know when to ask a difficult question? How does a nurse know when to offer complex information? Even holding a hand and certainly cleaning a butt—two activities that are often used to trivialize or dismiss nursing—require complex cognitive functioning and critical decision making. Many patients do not want to be touched. How does a nurse know which one will tolerate closeness? As for butt wiping, I have learned from personal experience that when we adults soil ourselves, we feel deeply humiliated. One of the important skills a nurse can learn and refine is how to clean up after someone without making them feel mortified and disgusting.

To be able to master what Patricia Benner has called the "skill of involvement" nurses need to first *know* in order to then *feel*. Without their knowledge of cancer, diabetes, geriatrics, wound care, and so many other areas impossible to enumerate, nurses' ignorance and anxiety would overwhelm their ability to be caring and compassionate. Perhaps they would be able to offer a kind word or gesture, but nurses' healing work involves a great deal more than that.

Many people who have read *Life Support* said they consider Nancy Rumplik, Jeannie Chaisson, and Ellen Kitchen to be extraordinary women and nurses who could not possibly be representative of the majority of nurses. These three nurses, some argue, were born to care. Nothing could be farther from the truth. What distinguishes these three nurses is their knowledge and experience. They have all been through many years of schooling and years on the job. They have learned not only in the classroom outside of the hospital but from each other, from their colleagues who are physicians, social workers, and pharmacists, as well as from numerous others both lower and higher in the hospital hierarchy. Yes, they are experts. But their expertise is the product not of devotion but of individual time and energy as well as a heavy dose of institutional support.

The Beth Israel Hospital—when I wrote about it a decade ago—nurtured and advanced that expertise. First of all, the hospital hired well-educated nurses. Second, it recognized that undergraduate education needs to be supplemented by education on the job. Nurses, like doctors, need to learn about the latest theories, medications, treatments, procedures, equipment, and interventions. The clinical nurse specialist job held by Jeannie Chaisson, Marion Phipps, and others was the embodiment of that recognition. Nurses like Rumplik were given tuition reimbursement so they could pursue graduate studies and allowed time off the job to attend off-site conferences and seminars. The hospital also put money—lots of it—into fostering nurse–physician collaboration and teamwork. Nurses were rewarded for moving forward in their education but staying at the bedside. They were not encouraged to get a masters degree or doctorate and move "up" and away. Nancy Rumplik, for example, earned her masters degree in nursing administration and family nursing but still remains doing what she did when I first met her in the early 1990s—only more effectively.

At the Beth Israel, nurses' competence and compassion was also supported by time, which in turn, was grounded in financial resources. The encounters I describe where nurses ferret out and address patient concerns are based not only on their skill but on staffing and thus nurse-to-patient ratios. That term, "nurse-to-patient ratio," was never mentioned during the years I spent observing nurses at the Beth Israel. It did not need to be. Time and adequate ratios were a given, the sea in which these particular fish swam. Just as fish never notice the water through which they navigate, Nancy, Ellen, and Jeannie never mentioned staffing or nurse-to-patient ratios until they began losing that time and those average patient loads (otherwise known as ratios).

When I reconnected in 2007 with Nancy Rumplik to get an update on her professional journey, I asked her about the patient load she carried in the early 1990s. She thought for a moment and then said haltingly, as if the very term did not apply to that period, "I think it was between five and eight." When I asked what happened after the merger, there was no hesitation in her voice. "The load about doubled," she said. "You definitely had less time with patients.

Things were really difficult. We lost a lot of nurses to the Farber [the Dana Farber Cancer Institute adjacent to the BI]. But I felt if I hung in there, things would eventually change."

Nancy says they have. Even though patients are much sicker now and the treatments they undergo are more arduous, her patient load has not gone back to what it was in the early nineties. Today, Nancy said, she cares for between eight and ten patients, sometimes twelve. "This means you have to be a lot quicker in your assessments, and you have less time with patients," she said.

What we learn in this book is that nurses' ability to exhibit their knowledge and compassion is not determined only by their own mastery of the skills it takes to be a nurse but on the concrete conditions of their job. If we want more care from people like Nancy, Jeannie, and Ellen, we have to provide them with the right conditions.

Another lesson of this book is that it takes years of experience on the job to produce the kind of expertise that Nancy, Jeannie, and Ellen brought to their patients. These nurses were not new graduates of nursing school. When I observed their work they had each been a nurse for a decade or longer. Not every nurse who works for ten years or more becomes the kind of nurse I describe in this book. But without that many years on the job, it is very difficult to demonstrate the kind of expertise these nurses bring to patient care.

That is why I am so concerned about nursing today. So many of the newly graduated nurses I meet view the hospital bedside as a kind of pit stop, a place to gain a few years of experience before moving on to work in administration, as a nurse practitioner, or in other advanced-practice jobs. I recently spent two weeks interviewing about thirty nurses for a project I was doing at a major teaching hospital. About eight of these nurses were new grads and had between one-and-a-half and five years' experience on the wards. I learned that all of these recent graduates were either in graduate school or applying to graduate school. Many were planning to become nurse practitioners who worked in the hospital replacing resident physicians. This has become a trend in the nurse-practitioner movement. Because of new limits on resident hours promulgated by the Accreditation Council for Graduate Medical Education (ACGME), residents can no longer work one-hundred-hour weeks. Faced with fewer residents in the hospitals, hospitals are hiring nurse practitioners to replace them. These NPs work for doctors or for medicine. When I asked these young men and women if they would be practicing nursing, they responded that no, they would be practicing medicine. Some said they would infuse their medical practice with a nursing background or philosophy. Some did not mention nursing at all.

I have sat in on the rounds that are now conducted in teaching hospitals in which these many NPs play a leading role. I have been impressed by how little difference there is between NPs as resident replacements and medical residents. In many instances and in my own dealings with some of these NPs, there is simply no evidence that they are using a nursing background. None of the questions they ask or concerns they raise are any different than would be asked by the physicians for whom they are substituting. Will it really help nursing, I wonder, to have nurses as residents? Will it elevate the profile of the staff nurse when someone learns he or she is smart enough to replace a doctor? How does that help? It is like telling a woman, wow, you are so smart you could be a man! That still leaves the idea that woman equals not smart and man equals smart right there on the table.

Clearly nurses need a career ladder. The nurses at the Beth Israel had one, one that allowed them greater challenges and continuous learning. This ladder did not lead them away from the bedside but nurtured their expertise so that the sickest patients were able to benefit from it. To me this is the genius of the Beth Israel model. That model was systematically dismantled in reality, but it lives on in the pages of this book.

As nurses and our society search for a way to transform nursing at the bedside perhaps they should consider and learn from what it took to transform the Beth Isreal, a hospital that had a demoralized nursing staff and a high turnover rate into one that had perhaps the most satisfied nursing staff in the country and almost no turnover of nursing staff. Circumstances may have changed. Patients may cycle in and out of the hospital more quickly. They still need nursing care. We still need nurses—more of them than ever before.

As I said earlier, when I was sick I learned quite personally about the power of nursing. The lessons I learned were sadly mostly negative. They taught me what happens when nurses are too busy and have too many patients. But I have also had some very positive personal encounters with nursing. One of the most impressive occurred when my mother died in a nursing home at age ninety-four, and Jeannie Chaisson took care of her.

By that time, Jeannie had left the Beth Israel and was working in home and hospice care. When my mother suddenly stopped eating and refused to get out of bed, I called Jeannie and asked if she would provide Medicare hospice services for my mother. My mother's doctor, Emily Lowry, and I both decided that there was no point in sending my mother to the hospital for a "work up" to find out what had happened. Maybe it was a stroke, maybe something else. I firmly believe it was an act of will. Although she had lost her memory, I think my mother simply decided that it was her time and she was ready to die. In fact, she told one of the women in the nursing home just the day before that she would not be around much longer. She was going far, far away.

With Emily's help, Jeannie became my mother's hospice nurse. Throughout the nine-day vigil of my mother's death, Jeannie followed the same routine she initiated the first day she came to see her new patient. Although she is a clinical specialist, a so-called advanced practice, elite nurse, she never once put herself above the RNs, LPNs, or nursing home aides who were responsible for my mother's care. She went up to the nurse's desk and checked in with the RN on duty, then she talked to the LPNs and the aides. How was my mother? What were their concerns? How could she help? she asked. The message was clear: They were not there to serve the fancy nurse; she was there as a resource to serve them, the patient, and the patient's family.

When Jeannie visited my mother, she would check her body, looking for signs of an incipient problem, such as a bedsore. Invariably she found that my mother had wet her diapers. Unlike some other nurses who believe that their education has granted them the privilege of not having to soil their hands cleaning a dirty bum or giving a bed bath, Jeannie never called in the aides to clean or change my mother. She did it herself.

On that first day, as I watched her examine my mother's naked body, she asked me where the aides kept their washcloths and basins. I didn't know, but said I would go ask. When I did, the nurses told me the aides would clean my mother. But I knew what Jeannie wanted. I insisted they show me where the supplies were kept, and I brought

Jeannie all the necessary gear. Together, she and I washed and diapered my dying mother. For Jeannie, this was no big deal. For me, it was. But Jeannie helped me overcome my concerns about giving bodily care to a dying loved one. As I helped with what so many people consider to be "dirty work," I once again recognized just how important, and how skilled and mindful, that work really is.

As my mother slipped farther away, Jeannie made sure that her patient would have enough medication to keep her comfortable. Again, working with my mother's doctor, she made sure the necessary morphine was available. When those last hours finally came on a Sunday morning, the nursing home called. My husband and I and our two daughters hurried over. So did Jeannie. As we sat around the bedside, listening to my mother's labored Cheyne-Stokes breathing, Jeannie asked my daughters how they were doing. That weekend, my eldest daughter, Alex, had been in a high school musical, *Anything Goes* by Cole Porter. She told Jeannie about the play, and Jeannie asked her about the songs. Then she skillfully suggested that Alex sing one or two.

It was something I would never have thought of. I was socialized to believe that death is supposed to be solemn event. I would never have encouraged my daughter, or anyone else, to sing show tunes at the bedside of a dying woman. But suddenly, my daughter launched into a Cole Porter medley. Finally, thanks to her nurse, my mother left us as her granddaughter's sweet soprano sang out "I get no kick from champagne, I get a kick out of you."

Notes

Because this book is intended for the general reader, I have not included scholarly notes. Where I quote from nurses and other sources, this information generally comes from interviews I have conducted. When I have indicated the source of written material, further information on that source can be found in the extensive selected bibliography at the end of this volume.

Other sources are indicated below in notes for each chapter.

Chapter 1

Data on restructuring comes from Frank Cerne's article in *Hospitals and Health Networks* as well as from a vast literature on hospital restructuring cited in the notes to chapter 11. Data on the number of nurses in America were gleaned from the American Nurses Association and the Institute of Medicine report cited in the bibliography. Nursing salary information is from the U.S. Department of Health and Human Services, Public Health Service Division of Nursing, Health Resources and Services Administration, and from the Institute of Medicine report. The Massachusetts Nurses Association provided information on the salaries of unionized nurses in the Boston area. Data on hospital CEO salaries are from James P. Farrell and Jose A. Pagoaga's story in the September 5, 1995, issue of *Hospitals and Health Networks*. Information on CEO salaries in HMOs and for-profit hospitals comes from Milt Freudenheim's report in the *New York Times* and from reports in *Modern Healthcare* and from the *Jenks Health and Business Report*.

As I said in the preface, the notion of the tapestry of nursing was articulated in an article written by myself and Ellen Baer for the *American Journal of Nursing*. The study on media coverage of nursing is entitled "Who Counts in News Coverage of

Health Care?" and was conducted by Bernice Buresh, myself, and Nica Bell. The studies I discuss that document the importance of nursing care are those mentioned again at the end of chapter 11 by Aiken; Scott, et al.; and Knaus, et al.

Chapter 2

Information on Florence Nightingale, her life, her participation in the Crimean War, and her contributions to health care comes from Nightingale's own works; the major biography of Nightingale by Cecil Woodham Smith; selected letters in Vicinus and Nergaard; the work of Calabria and Macrae; Bullough, Bullough, and Stanton; and discussions with Joan Lynaugh. Information on the Beth Israel's transformation comes from discussions with Joyce Clifford, Mitchell T. Rabkin, and Trish Gibbons as well as from Clifford and Horvath's book *Advancing Professional Nursing Practice*. Additional information on nursing education and developments in nursing comes from discussions with and papers of Joan Lynaugh and from Barbara Melosh's book *The Physician's Hand* — which should be required reading — on the schisms between nursing leadership and staff nurses. Similarly, Susan M. Reverby's excellent book *Ordered to Care: The Dilemma of American Nursing, 1850–1945* offers another invaluable view of the history of nursing. It is also interesting to compare the history of medicine's educational advancement as outlined by Starr and by Rosenberg with nursing's perennial educational obstacles.

Nancy Rumplik has written eloquently about her nursing philosophy in an unpublished paper she kindly shared with me. She also described her care of the patient Jesse in a paper written with her nursing colleagues entitled "To Satisfy Jesse, We Needed a 36-Hour Day."

Chapter 3

A thorough presentation of the issues of wound care is found in the article cited by Bolton, et al. and in Miller and Delozier's work for the AHCPR.

Information on physician-nurse relationships described in this chapter comes from extensive interviews and long observation as well as from scholarly work such as that of Joanne Ashley and Barbara Melosh. L. Stein's articles "The Doctor-Nurse Game" and "The Doctor-Nurse Game Revisited" are classics in the field. Joan Lynaugh and Barbara Bates's article "The Two Languages of Nursing and Medicine" is not only extremely shrewd and clever, but very illuminating. And Adele Pike's article "Moral Outrage and Moral Discourse in Nurse-Physician Collaboration" presents a more scholarly — and very moving — discussion of nurses' dilemmas when physicians discount their views and insights into patient care. It is interesting — but not surprising — to note that there is a vast literature on the subject of nurse-physician collaboration — or the lack thereof. But with a few notable exceptions — like contributions by Bates and by Stein — most is written by nurses, not physicians.

Chapter 4

Valuable works like Safriet's, Mezey and McGivern's, and Brush and Capuzetti's, discussions with Joan Lynaugh and Ellen Baer, and material from the American Nurses

Association have helped inform my view of nurse practitioners' work. The state medical society advertisement mentioned in this chapter was from CALPAC and documents from the AMA opposing autonomy for advanced practice nurses included a report released by the AMA's House of Delegates interim meeting in New Orleans, December 5–8, 1993, and a "Dear Colleague" letter the AMA sent out to influence-makers dated September 24, 1993, which included a section-by-section critique of the Clinton health plan.

Chapter 5

For an illuminating look at illness from the patient's perspective, there can be no better or more serious volume than Kay Toombs's *The Meaning of Illness.*

The work of Patricia Benner — books like *From Novice to Expert, The Primacy of Caring,* and *Expertise in Nursing Practice* — has been critical to my understanding of nursing. In a paper entitled "The Phenomenology of Nurses' Way of Knowing the Patient," Benner and coresearchers Christine Tanner, Catherine Chesla, and Deborah Gordon argue that this skill is "not a trait or talent of the nurse, or abstract knowledge. . . . The skill of involvement and the skill of seeing salient patient changes are based upon engagement in the clinical situation. Knowledge of particular patient populations is built up with many instances of knowing particular patients. This way of knowing helps fill out one's understanding of common issues, common expectations and common timetables."

Nel Noddings's insights into caregiving have also informed my views. As Noddings observes in an essay entitled "The Caring Professional," "When we care, our consciousness exhibits two fundamental characteristics: First, we are in a receptive mode; we attend nonselectively to the cared for. We are, at least momentarily, engrossed in the other's plans, pains, and hopes, not our own. Second, we feel our motive energy flowing toward the other. We want to help in furthering the plan, relieving the pain, or actualizing the hope. What we actually do to enact our part in the caring relation is contingent on many factors, but these two fundamental characteristics describe our basic consciousness."

Noddings contends that a moral education is what produces caring relationships. This moral education, she says, has four major components — modeling, dialogue, practice, and confirmation. I believe this moral model is evident in the work of all three of these nurses and all expert nurses.

Benner's and Noddings's work is part of a broader literature on caring that has come under a certain amount of criticism from some feminist authors, notably Susan Faludi, Katha Pollitt, and Wendy Kaminer. Anyone interested in a detailed discussion of this subject should look at essays by Gordon, Gordon and Benner, and Alisa Carse in *Caregiving: Readings in Knowledge, Practice, Ethics and Politics* (edited by Gordon, Benner, and Noddings), and at Mary Jeanne Larrabee's book *An Ethics of Care.*

For a more thorough look at the politics of cancer, I would suggest Howard P. Greenwald's excellent book *Who Survives Cancer?* and Robert N. Proctor's *The Cancer Wars.*

Because I did not meet Carol Benoit until after she had her transplant, I have combined another patient's inpatient experience with hers for narrative flow.

Chapter 6

The section on nursing research has been enhanced by discussions with nurse researchers Ruth McCorkle, Kathleen Dracup, and others as well as staff at the National Institute for Nursing Research.

Chapter 7

Karen Buhler-Wilkerson's work on the development of home health care in the U.S. was key in the writing of this chapter, as were the work by Lillian Wald and the Wald biography by Siegel.

Chapter 8

Peggy McGarrahan's book *Transcending AIDS* contains much interesting material on how nurses deal with different kinds of AIDS / HIV patients. Using AIDS as the lens, the book also vividly documents and analyzes the complexity of nursing practice. Work by Nuland; Siebold, Corr and Corr; Cohen; and interviews with many other hospice and palliative care nurses and physicians inform this chapter. Information on the inadequacies of medical training for the end of life came from testimony by Kathleen Foley and from "Caring for the Dying" by the American Board of Internal Medicine. Since this research was done, there has been more work going on at the Beth Israel on trying to provide better care for patients at the end of life. Glenn Bubley and nurses, social workers, and some other physicians in the oncology department are trying to work seriously on this issue. The Beth Israel has merged with the Deaconess Hospital. The Deaconess is to be congratulated for working with the hospice agency HealthCare Dimensions to start the first inpatient palliative care unit in Boston. Bubley's group will be working to help patients enter that program.

Chapter 11

Discussions of the Clinton health plan and HMO behavior come from countless magazine and newspaper articles as well as works by Gordon and McCall; Himmelstein and Woolhandler; Bodenheimer and Grumbach; Fein; Harrington and Estes; Baer, Fagin and Gordon; and Lindorff. Figures on hospital length of stay come from Reinhardt and from the American Hospital Association's *Hospital Statistics: Emerging Trends in Hospitals*. Figures on Kaiser and Sharp come from David Olmos's report in the *Los Angeles Times*, and from Kaiser's business plan. Information on Sharp comes from Sabin Russell and Rebecca Smith's articles in the *San Francisco Chronicle* and *San Jose Mercury News*, from Sharp's *Handbook*, and from *Consumers for Quality Care*. The Lewin VHI study was cited in *Modern Healthcare*'s article "Subacute Care: Old Wine in New Bottles."

Information on what is going on in nursing comes from the American Hospital Association, the American Nurses Association, many professional nursing organizations and unions, and interviews with hundreds of individual nurses from all across the country. Reports in the *American Journal of Nursing*, some of which are cited in the bibliography, provide a critical running commentary on the impact of hospital restructuring and corporate-driven health care reform on patient care.

The discussion of hospital profits comes from *Modern Healthcare* and from a study done by Harvard School of Public Health professor Nancy L. Kane. Other information on mergers and acquisitions and administrative overhead is from the Institute for Health and Socio-Economic Policy and Health Affairs. Estimates of Abramson's profits on the merger between Aetna and U.S. Healthcare and the cost of the care of the uninsured in Massachusetts were made by Himmelstein and Woolhandler. Alan Sager and his colleagues at the Boston University School of Public Health's Access and Affordability Project have written extensively about hospitals' responses to competition under managed care and corporate health care. Arthur Caplan at the University of Pennsylvania's Center for Bioethics has spoken eloquently about ethical problems embodied in corporate health care. And Steve Twedt at the *Pittsburgh Post-Gazette* has done excellent journalistic coverage of this trend.

Much of the literature on patient-focused care is from nursing journals like *Nursing Management*, which have run many articles discussing restructuring. Articles by Baer and Gordon; Krapohl and Larson; Richardson; Porter-O'Grady; Buerhaus; Ball, et al.; Townsend; Weber; and Matheis-Kraft, et al. elaborate on this concept of patient-focused care. Hirschhorn's paper "The Political Economy of Nursing" contains a rather chilling prediction of what will happen to nurses' allegiance under a corporate-driven system.

Selected Bibliography

Aiken, Linda, et al. 1994. "Lower Medicare Mortality Among a Set of Hospitals Known for Good Nursing Care." *Medical Care*. Vol. 32, no. 8.

American Board of Internal Medicine. 1996. "Caring for the Dying: Identification and Promotion of Physician Competency." Philadelphia.

American Hospital Association. 1996. Hospital Statistics: Emerging Trends in Hospitals, 1995–1996 edition. Tables 3A and 3C. Chicago: American Hospital Association.

American Nurses Association. 1994. "Report of Survey Results: The 1994 ANA Lay-offs Survey."

"American Nurses Association Nursing Report Card for Acute Care Settings," prepared by Lewin-VHI, Inc. 1995.

Annas, George J. 1995. "Women and Children First." *New England Journal of Medicine*. December 14.

Aries, Philippe. 1981. *The Hour of Our Death*. New York: Oxford University Press.

Ashley, Joann. 1976. Hospitals, Paternalism, and the Role of the Nurse. New York: Teachers College, Columbia University.

Associated Press. 1996. "Ohio Blues Execs to Net Millions in Deal." *Modern Healthcare*. May 13.

Backer, Barbara A., Hannon, Natalie R., and Russell, Noreen A. 1994. *Death and Dying: Understanding and Care*. New York: Delmar.

Baer, Ellen D., and Gordon, Suzanne. 1994. "The Gender Battle in Nursing." *Boston Globe*. December 28.

Baer, Ellen D., and Gordon, Suzanne. 1994. "Money Managers Are Unraveling the Tapestry of Nursing." *American Journal of Nursing*. October.

Baer, Ellen D., Fagin, Claire M., and Gordon, Suzanne, eds. 1996. *The Abandonment of the Patient: The Impact of Profit-Driven Health Care on the Public.* New York: Springer.

Ball, Cathy, et al. 1991–1992. "Patient-Centered Care: Redesigning Work at Deaconess Hospital." *Quality Letter.* December / January.

Bandman, Elsie L., and Bandman, Bertram. 1988. *Critical Thinking in Nursing.* Norwalk, Connecticut: Appleton and Lange.

Bates, Barbara. 1970. "Doctor and Nurse: Changing Roles and Relations." *New England Journal of Medicine.* July 16.

Bates, Barbara. 1992. *Bargaining for Life: A Social History of Tuberculosis, 1876–1938.* Philadelphia: University of Pennsylvania Press.

Bates, Barbara, and Lynaugh, Joan. 1973. "Laying the Foundations for Medical Nursing Practice." *American Journal of Nursing.* August.

Baumgart, Alice J., and Larsen, Jenniece. 1992. *Canadian Nursing Faces the Future.* Boston: Mosby Year Book.

Bellah, Robert N., et al. 1991. *The Good Society.* New York: Alfred A. Knopf.

Benner, Patricia. 1984. *From Novice to Expert.* Reading, Massachusetts: Addison-Wesley.

Benner, Patricia, Tanner, Christine A., and Chesla, Catherine A. 1996. *Expertise in Nursing Practice.* New York: Springer.

Benner, Patricia, and Wrubel, Judith. 1989. *The Primacy of Caring: Stress and Coping in Health and Illness.* Reading, Massachusetts: Addison-Wesley.

Benson, Herbert, and Stuart, Eileen M. 1992. *The Wellness Book.* New York: Birch Lane Press.

Beresford, Larry. 1993. *The Hospice Handbook.* Boston: Little, Brown.

Berliner, Howard S., Kovner, Christine T., et al. 1994. "The Supply and Demand for Health Workers in New York City, 1995–1997: A Report Prepared for the New York State Department of Health Bureau of Health Resources Development." New York: New School for Social Research.

Binstock, Robert H., and Post, Stephen G. 1991. *Too Old for Health Care?* Baltimore: Johns Hopkins University Press.

Bodenheimer, Thomas S., and Grumbach, Kevin. 1995. *Understanding Health Policy: A Clinical Approach.* Stamford, Connecticut: Appleton and Lange.

Bolton, L. L., Van Rijswijk, Lia, and Shaffer, Franklin A. 1996. "Quality Wound Care Equals Cost-Effective Wound Care: A Clinical Model." *Nursing Management.* July.

Boydston, Jeanne. 1990. *Home and Work: Housework, Wages, and the Ideology of Labor in the Early Republic.* New York: Oxford University Press.

Brady, Judy. 1991. *1 in 3 Women with Cancer Confront an Epidemic.* Pittsburgh: Cleis Press.

Brody, Elaine M. 1990. *Women in the Middle: Their Parent-Care Years.* New York: Springer.

Brown, Michael. 1992. *Nurses.* New York: Ivy Books.

Brush, Barbara L., and Capezuti, Elizabeth A. 1996. "Revisiting 'A Nurse for All Settings': The Nurse Practitioner Movement, 1965–1995." *Journal of the Academy of Nurse Practitioners.* January.

Buerhaus, Peter I. 1992. "Nursing, Competition and Quality." *Nursing Economics.* January–February.

Buhler-Wilkerson, Karen. 1991. "Home Care the American Way: An Historical Analysis." *Home Health Care Services Quarterly.* Vol. 12, no. 3.

Buhler-Wilkerson, Karen. 1993. "Bringing Care to the People: Lillian Wald's Legacy to Public Health Nursing." *American Journal of Public Health.* December.

Bullough, Vern L., Bullough, Bonnie, and Stanton, Marietta P., eds. 1990. *Florence Nightingale and Her Era: A Collection of New Scholarship.* New York: Garland Publishing.

Burda, David. 1993. "Jobs Go First." *Modern Healthcare.* Nov. 1.

Buresh, Bernice, Gordon, Suzanne, and Bell, Nica. 1991. "Who Counts in News Coverage of Health Care?" *Nursing Outlook.* September / October.

Calabria, Michael D. and Macrae, Janet A., eds. 1994. *Suggestions for Thought by Florence Nightingale.* Philadelphia: University of Pennsylvania Press.

Callahan, Daniel. 1990. *What Kind of Life: The Limits of Medical Progress.* New York: Simon and Schuster.

Campbell-Heider, Nancy, and Pollock, Donald. 1987. "Barriers to Nurse-Physician Collegiality: An Anthropological Perspective." *Social Science Medicine.* Vol. 25, no. 5.

Cassell, Eric J. 1991. *The Nature of Suffering and the Goals of Medicine.* New York: Oxford University Press.

Cerne, Frank. 1994. "The Fading Stand-Alone Hospital." *Hospitals and Health Networks.* June 20.

Chinn, Peggy L., and Kramer, Maeona K. 1991. *Theory and Nursing: A Systematic Approach.* Boston: Mosby Year Book.

Clifford, Joyce C., and Horvath, Kathy J. 1990. *Advancing Professional Nursing Practice: Innovations at Boston's Beth Israel Hospital.* New York: Springer.

Cohen, Kenneth P. 1979. *Hospice.* Germantown: Aspen Systems Corporation.

Cook, Robert. 1993. *Fatal Cure.* New York: G. P. Putnam's Sons.

Corr, Charles A., and Corr, Donna M. 1983. *Hospice Care: Principles and Practice.* New York: Springer.

Cott, Nancy F. 1987. *The Grounding of Modern Feminism.* New Haven: Yale University Press.

Curran, Connie R., and Mazzie, Sandra A. 1995. "The Effect of Hospital Restructuring on Nursing: A Report on Findings from a Survey of Hospital Chief Nursing Executives." American Practice Management (APM).

Davis, Celia. 1995. *Gender: The Professional Predicament in Nursing.* Buckingham, Pennsylvania: Open University Press.

Dick, Karen. "Making a Case: Use of Strategies in Nurse-Physician Interaction." Unpublished.

Doucet, Hubert. 1988. *Mourir.* Paris: Desclée / Novalis.

Dowie, Mark. 1988. *We Have a Donor: The Bold New World of Organ Transplanting.* New York: St. Martin's Press.

Dutton, Diana B. 1988. *Worse Than the Disease: Pitfalls of Medical Progress.* New York: Cambridge University Press.

Fagin, Claire, and Diers, Donna. 1983. "Nursing as a Metaphor." *New England Journal of Medicine.* July 14.

Faludi, Susan. 1991. *Backlash: The Undeclared War Against American Women.* New York: Crown Publishers.

Farrell, James P., and Pagoaga, Jose A. 1995. "Making Change Pay." *Hospitals and Health Networks.* September 5.

Fein, Rashi. 1986. *Medical Care, Medical Costs: The Search for a Health Insurance Policy.* Cambridge: Harvard University Press.

FitzSimmons, Lorraine, et. al. 1995. "The Nurse's Role in End-of-Life Treatment Decisions: Preliminary Report from the SUPPORT Project." *Cardiovascular Nursing.* Vol. 9, no. 3.

Foley, Kathleen M. 1996. "Medical Issues Related to Physician-Assisted Suicide." Testimony to Judiciary Subcommittee on the Constitution. April 29.

Foreman, Judy. 1996. "Choosing a Good Death." *Boston Globe.* June 23.

Fox, Renee C., and Swazey, Judith P. 1974. *The Courage to Fail: A Social View of Organ Transplants and Dialysis.* Chicago: University of Chicago Press.

Fox, Renee C., and Swazey, Judith P. 1992. *Spare Parts: Organ Replacement in American Society.* New York: Oxford University Press.

Freudenheim, Milt. 1995. "Penny-Pinching H.M.O.'s Showed Their Generosity in Executive Paychecks." *New York Times.* April 11.

Friedman, Emily. 1994. *An Unfinished Revolution: Women and Health Care in America.* New York: United Hospital Fund of New York.

Gerteis, Margaret, Edgman-Levitan, Susan, Daley, Jennifer, and Delbanco, Thomas L. 1993. *Through the Patient's Eyes: Understanding and Promoting Patient-Centered Care.* San Francisco: Jossey-Bass.

Goffman, Erving. 1961. *Asylums: Essays on the Social Situation of Mental Patients and Other Inmates.* New York: Doubleday Anchor.

Gordon, Suzanne. 1991. *Prisoners of Men's Dreams: Striking Out for a New Feminine Future.* Boston: Little, Brown.

Gordon, Suzanne, Benner, Patricia, and Noddings, Nel, eds. 1996. *Caregiving: Readings in Knowledge, Practice, Ethics and Politics.* Philadelphia: University of Pennsylvania Press.

Gordon, Suzanne and McCall, Timothy. 1996. "The Price of Managed Care." *CommonWealth.* Spring.

Green, Jay. 1996. Retooling without Lay-offs. *Modern Healthcare.* February 26.

Greenwald, Howard P. 1992. *Who Survives Cancer?* Los Angeles: University of California Press.

Grollman, Earl A. 1980. *When Your Loved One Is Dying.* Boston: Beacon Press.

Hamilton, Persis Mary. 1992. *Realities of Contemporary Nursing.* United States: Addison-Wesley Nursing.

Harrington, Charlene, and Estes, Carroll L. 1994. *Health Policy and Nursing: Crisis and Reform in the U.S. Health Care Delivery System.* Boston: Jones and Bartlett.

Hartz, A., et al. 1989. "Hospital Characteristics and Mortality Rates." *New England Journal of Medicine.* Vol. 321, no. 25.

Heckscher, Charles. 1995. *White-Collar Blues.* New York: Basic Books.

Henderson, Virginia. 1961. *ICN Basic Principles of Nursing Care*. London: International Council of Nurses.

Henderson, Virginia. 1967. *The Nature of Nursing*. New York: Macmillan.

Heron, Echo. 1987. *Intensive Care: The Story of a Nurse*. New York: Ivy Books.

Heron, Echo. 1994. *Condition Critical: The Story of a Nurse Continues*. New York: Fawcett Columbine.

Heymann, Jody. 1995. *Equal Partners: A Physician's Call for a New Spirit of Medicine*. Boston: Little, Brown.

Hill, T. Patrick, and Shirley, David. 1992. *A Good Death: Taking More Control at the End of Your Life*. Reading, Massachusetts: Addison-Wesley, Merloyd Lawrence Book.

Himmelstein, David U., and Woolhandler, Steffie. 1994. *The National Health Program Book*. Monroe, Maine: Common Courage Press.

Himmelstein, David U., and Woolhandler, Steffie. 1996. "Who Administers? Who Cares? Medical Administrative and Clinical Employment in the United States and Canada." *American Journal of Public Health*. February.

Hirschhorn, Larry. 1994. The Political Economy of Nursing. Philadelphia: Center for Applied Research.

Hirschman, Albert O. 1970. *Exit, Voice, and Loyalty: Responses to Decline in Firms, Organizations and States*. Cambridge: Harvard University Press.

Hirschman, Albert O. 1982. *Shifting Involvements: Private Interest and Public Action*. Princeton: Princeton University Press.

Hirschman, Albert O. 1991. *The Rhetoric of Reaction*. Cambridge: Harvard University Press, Belknap Press.

Institute for Health & Socio-Economic Policy and Health Affairs. 1996. "Abdicating Health Care Policy to the Market." Oakland, California. April.

Institute of Medicine. 1996. *Nursing Staff in Hospitals and Nursing Homes: Is It Adequate?* Washington, D.C.: National Academy Press.

Jaklevic, Mary Chris. 1995. "Clinical Errors Humble Hospitals." *Modern Healthcare*. April 3.

Jenks Healthcare Business Report. 1996. September 24.

Jonas, Steven. 1986. *Health Care Delivery in the United States*. New York: Springer.

Jones, Anne Hudson. 1988. *Images of Nurses: Perspectives from History, Art, and Literature*. Philadelphia: University of Pennsylvania Press.

Kalisch, Beatrice J., and Kalisch, Philip A. 1982. *Politics of Nursing*. Philadelphia: J. B. Lippincott.

Kalisch, Philip A., and Kalisch, Beatrice J. 1995. *The Advance of American Nursing*. Philadelphia: J. B. Lippincott.

Kane, Nancy M. 1993. "Report on the Financial Resources of Boston Hospitals." Prepared for the Commissioner of Health and Hospitals in the City of Boston. May. Unpublished.

Kaye, Lenard W., and Applegate, Jeffrey S. 1990. *Men as Caregivers to the Elderly: Understanding and Aiding Unrecognized Family Support*. Lexington, Massachusetts: Lexington Books.

Kelly, Lucie Young. 1985. *Dimensions of Professional Nursing*. New York: Macmillan.

Kleinman, Arthur. 1988. *The Illness Narratives: Suffering, Healing and the Human Condition*. New York: Basic Books.

Knaus, W. A., et al. 1986. "An Evaluation of Outcome from Intensive Care in Major Medical Centers." *Annals of Internal Medicine*. Vol. 104, no. 3.

Krapohl, Greta L., and Larson, Elaine. 1996. "The Impact of Unlicensed Personnel on Nursing Care Delivery." *Nursing Economics*. March / April.

Larrabee, Mary Jeanne. 1993. *An Ethic of Care: Feminist and Interdisciplinary Perspectives*. New York: Routledge.

Lee, Philip R., and Estes, Carroll L. 1994. *The Nation's Health*. Boston: Jones and Bartlett.

Levit, K. R., Lazenby, H. C., and Sivarajan, L. 1996. "Health Spending in 1994: Lowest in Decades." *Health Affairs*, Vol. 15, no. 2.

Lindorff, Dave. 1992. *Marketplace Medicine: The Rise of the For-Profit Hospital Chains*. New York: Bantam Books.

Lo, Bernard. 1995. "Improving Care Near the End of Life: Why Is It So Hard? *Journal of the American Medical Association*. November 22 / 29.

Lowenberg, June S. 1989. *Caring and Responsibility: The Cross Roads Between Holistic Practice and Traditional Medicine*. Philadelphia: University of Pennsylvania Press.

Lynaugh, Joan. 1980. "The 'Entry into Practice' Conflict: How We Got Where We Are and What Will Happen Next." *American Journal of Nursing*. February.

Lynaugh, Joan. 1988. "Narrow Passageways: Nurses and Physicians in Conflict and Concert since 1875." In King, Nancy M., ed. *The Physician as Captain of the Ship: A Critical Reappraisal*. Boston: D. Riedel.

Lynaugh, Joan. 1989. "Riding the Yo-Yo: The Worth and Work of Nursing in the 20th Century." *Transactions and Studies of the College of Physicians of Philadelphia*. September.

Lynaugh Joan, and Bates, Barbara. 1973. "The Two Languages of Nursing and Medicine." *American Journal of Nursing*. January.

Marget, Madeline. 1992. *Life's Blood*. New York: Simon and Schuster.

Margolis, Richard J. 1990. *Risking Old Age in America*. Boulder, Colorado: Westview Press.

Matheis-Kraft, Carol, et al. 1990. "Patient-Driven Healthcare Works! *Nursing Management*. September.

McCall, Timothy B. 1988. "The Impact of Long Working Hours on Resident Physicians." *New England Journal of Medicine*. March 24.

McCall, Timothy B. 1989. "No Turning Back: A Blueprint for Residency Reform." *Journal of the American Medical Association*. February 10.

McCall, Timothy B. 1995. *Examining Your Doctor: A Patient's Guide to Avoiding Harmful Medical Care*. New York: Birch Lane Press.

McGarrahan, Peggy. 1994. *Transcending AIDS: Nurses and HIV Patients in New York City*. Philadelphia: University of Pennsylvania Press.

McKibbin, Richard C. 1990. *The Nursing Shortage and the 1990s: Realities and Remedies*. Kansas City: American Nurses Association.

McLaughlin F. E., Thomas, S. A., and Barter, M. 1995. "Changes Related to Care Delivery Patterns." *Journal of Nursing Administration*. May 5.

Melosh, Barbara. 1982. *"The Physician's Hand": Work, Culture, and Conflict in American Nursing.* Philadelphia: Temple University Press.

Merchant, Carolyn. 1989. *The Death of Nature: Women, Ecology, and the Scientific Revolution.* San Francisco: HarperCollins.

Merker, L. R., Cerda, F., and Blank, M. 1991. "1990 Utilization of Nurse Extenders." Chicago: American Hospital Association. Catalog No.154909.

Mezey, Mathy D., and McGivern, Diane O. 1993. *Nurses, Nurse Practitioners: Evolution to Advanced Practice.* New York: Springer.

Miller, H., and Delozier, J. 1994. "Cost Implications of the Pressure Ulcer Treatment Guideline." Columbia, Maryland: Center for Health Policy Studies. Contract No. 282-91-0080, sponsored by the Agency for Health Care Policy and Research.

Miller, Marc, S., ed. 1995. *Health Care Choices for Today's Consumer.* Washington, D.C.: Living Planet Press.

Mitchell, P., Armstrong, S., and Leutz, M. 1989. "AACN Demonstration Project: Profile of Excellence in Critical Care Nursing." *Heart and Lung.* Vol. 18, no. 3.

Morin, Edgar. 1970. *L'Homme et la Mort.* Paris: Editions du Seuil.

Morris, David B. 1991. *The Culture of Pain.* Los Angeles: University of California Press.

National Commission on Nursing Implementation Project. 1989. *Nursing's Vital Signs: Shaping the Profession for the 1990s.* Battle Creek, Michigan: W. K. Kellogg Foundation.

"New York Nurses Fight Mass Firings." 1996. AJN Newsline. *American Journal of Nursing.* July.

Nightingale, Florence. 1969. *Notes on Nursing: What It Is and Is Not.* New York: Dover Publications.

"1996 Physician Compensation Report." *Modern Healthcare.* July.

Noddings, Nel. 1984. *Caring: A Feminine Approach to Ethics and Moral Education.* Los Angeles: University of California Press.

Noddings, Nel. 1989. *Women and Evil.* Los Angeles: University of California Press.

Nuland, Sherwin B. 1993. *How We Die: Reflections on Life's Final Chapter.* New York: Vintage.

O'Connor, Bonnie Blair. 1995. *Healing Traditions: Alternative Medicine and the Health Professions.* Philadelphia: University of Pennsylvania Press.

Olmos, David R. 1995. "Kaiser Plans Cost Cutting of $800 Million." *Los Angeles Times.* September 23.

Olmos, David R. 1995. "Kaiser Seeking to Pay Bonuses to Nurses Who Help Cut Costs." *Los Angeles Times.* December 22.

Payer, Lynn. 1988. *Medicine and Culture.* New York: Penguin Books.

Pike, Adele W. 1991. "Moral Outrage and Moral Discourse in Nurse-Physician Collaboration." *Journal of Professional Nursing.* November / December.

Pohl, Mel, Deniston, Kay, and Toft, Doug. 1990. *The Caregiver's Journey: When You Love Someone with AIDS.* New York: HarperCollins.

Porter-O'Grady, Tim. 1994. "Working with Consultants on a Redesign." *American Journal of Nursing.* October.

Prescott, Patricia. 1993. "Nursing: An Important Component of Hospital Survival Under a Reformed Health Care System." *Nursing Economics.* July / August.

Proctor, Robert N. 1995. *The Cancer Wars: How Politics Shapes What We Know and Don't Know About Cancer.* New York: Basic Books.

Reinhardt, Uwe. 1996. "Spending More Through 'Cost Control': Our Obsessive Quest to Gut the Hospital." *Health Affairs.* Summer.

Reverby, M. Susan. 1987. *Ordered to Care: The Dilemma of American Nursing, 1850–1945.* Cambridge: Cambridge University Press.

Richardson, Trudy. 1994. "Reengineering the Hospital: Patient-Focused Care." In Parker, Mike, and Slaughter, Jane, eds. *Working Smart: A Union Guide to Participation Programs and Reengineering.* Detroit: Labor Notes.

Robbins, Natalie. 1995. *The Girl Who Died Twice: The Libby Zion Case and the Hidden Hazards of Hospitals.* New York: Delacorte Press.

Roberts, Marc J. 1993. *Your Money or Your Life: The Health Care Crisis Explained.* New York: Doubleday.

Robertson, John A. 1983. *The Rights of the Critically Ill.* New York: Bantam Books.

Rosen, Marty. 1995. "Experts Alarmed by Hospital Cuts." Tampa Today. *The Times.* April 9.

Rosenberg, Charles E. 1987. *The Care of Strangers: The Rise of America's Hospital System.* New York: Basic Books.

Rosenberg, Charles E. 1992. *Explaining Epidemics and Other Studies in the History of Medicine.* New York: Cambridge University Press.

Rosenberg, Charles E., and Golden, Janet. 1992. *Framing Disease: Studies in Cultural History.* New Brunswick, New Jersey: Rutgers University Press.

Rosenberg, Steven A. 1992. *The Transformed Cell.* New York: G. P. Putnam's Sons.

Rubin, Lillian B. 1984. *Intimate Strangers: Men and Women Together.* New York: Harper and Row.

Rumplik, Nancy, Gerardi, Vita, and Mayer, Laura. 1983. "To Satisfy Jesse, We Needed a 36-Hour Day." *Nursing 83.* June.

Safriet, Barbara J. 1992. "Health Care Dollars and Regulatory Sense: The Role of Advanced Practice Nursing." *Yale Journal on Regulation.* Summer.

Sankar, Andrea. 1991. *Dying At Home: A Family Guide for Caregiving.* Baltimore: Johns Hopkins University Press.

Saunders, Cicely, and Baines, Mary. 1989. *Living with Dying.* New York: Oxford University Press.

Scott, W., et al. 1976. "Hospital Structure and Postoperative Mortality and Morbidity." In Shortell, S., and Brown, M., eds. *Organizational Research in Hospitals.* Chicago: Blue Cross Association.

Siebold, Cathy. 1992. *The Hospice Movement: Easing Death's Pains.* New York: Twayne Publishers.

Siegel, Beatrice. 1983. *Lillian Wald of Henry Street.* New York: Macmillan.

Silber, Jeffrey, et al. 1992. "Hospital and Patient Characteristics Associated with Death after Surgery." *Medical Care.* July.

Skocpol, Theda. 1996. *Boomerang: Clinton's Health Security Effort and the Turn Against Government in U.S. Politics.* New York: W. W. Norton.

"Staff Cuts Left Nurses Overloaded." 1996. AJN Newsline. *American Journal of Nursing.* July.

Starr, Paul. 1982. *The Social Transformation of American Medicine: The Rise of a Sovereign Profession and the Making of a Vast Industry.* New York: Basic Books.

Stein, L. 1967. "The Doctor-Nurse Game." *Archives of General Psychiatry.* Vol. 16.

Stein, L., Watts, D., and Howell, T. 1990. "The Doctor-Nurse Game Revisited." *New England Journal of Medicine.* February 22.

Stevens, Rosemary. 1989. *In Sickness and in Wealth: American Hospitals in the Twentieth Century.* New York: Basic Books.

Strachey, Lytton. 1918. *Eminent Victorians.* London: Chatto and Windus.

SUPPORT Principal Investigators. 1995. "A Controlled Trial to Improve Care for Seriously Ill Hospitalized Patients: The Study to Understand Prognoses and Preferences for Outcomes and Risks of Treatment (SUPPORT)." Chicago: *Journal of the American Medical Association.* November 22 / 29.

Swackhamer, Annette, and Moss, Ralph W. 1986. *Caring.* Garden City, New York: Doubleday.

Tanner, Christine A., Benner, Patricia, Chesla, Catherine A., and Gordon, Deborah R. 1993. "The Phenomenology of Knowing the Patient." *Image.* Winter.

Tate, David A. 1989. *Health, Hope, and Healing.* New York: M. Evans.

Taylor, Charles. 1989. *Sources of the Self: The Making of the Modern Identity.* Cambridge: Harvard University Press.

Thorens, Jean-Benoit, et al. 1995. "Influence of the Quality of Nursing on the Duration of Weaning from Mechanical Ventilation in Patients with Chronic Obstructive Pulmonary Disease." *Critical Care Medicine.* November.

Tisdale, Sallie. 1986. *The Sorcerer's Apprentice: Inside the Modern Hospital.* New York: McGraw-Hill.

Toombs, S. Kay. 1993. *The Meaning of Illness: A Phenomenological Account of the Different Perspectives of Physician and Patient.* Boston: Kluwer Academic Publishers.

Townsend, Mary B. 1993. "Patient-Focused Care: Is It for Your Hospital?" *Nursing Management.* September.

Tsongas, Paul. 1992. "The Cancer Freed Me." *New York Times.* May 6.

Tudor Hart, Julian, and Dieppe, Paul. 1996. "Caring Effects." *Lancet.* June 8.

Twedt, Steve. 1996. "A Question of Skill." *Pittsburgh Post-Gazette.* February 11–14.

Ulrich, Laurel Thatcher. 1990. *A Midwife's Tale: The Life of Martha Ballard.* New York: Alfred A. Knopf.

Ulrich, Laurel Thatcher. 1991. *Good Wives: Image and Reality in the Lives of Women in Northern New England, 1650–1750.* New York: Vantage Books.

U.S. Department of Health and Human Services. 1992. *Acute Pain Management: Operative or Medical Procedures and Trauma.* Rockville, Maryland: Agency for Health Care Policy and Research.

Vachon, Mary L. S. 1987. *Occupational Stress in the Care of the Critically Ill, the Dying, and the Bereaved.* New York: Hemisphere.

Vicinus, Martha, and Nergaard, Bea, eds. 1990. *Ever Yours, Florence Nightingale: Selected Letters.* Cambridge: Harvard University Press.

Wald, Lillian. 1915. *The House on Henry Street*. New York: Henry Holt.

Wanzer, Sidney H., et al. 1989. "The Physician's Responsibility Toward Hopelessly Ill Patients: A Second Look." *New England Journal of Medicine*. March 30.

Watson, Jean. 1985. *Nursing: The Philosophy and Science of Caring*. Boulder, Colorado: Colorado Associated University Press.

Weber, David O. 1991. "Six Models of Patient-Focused Care." *Healthcare Forum Journal*. July / August.

"We're in the Money — Hospitals Sit on Big Cash Reserves." 1995. *Modern Healthcare*. October 23.

Woodham-Smith, Cecil. 1950. *Florence Nightingale*. Edinburgh: Constable.

Wuthnow, Robert. 1991. *Acts of Compassion: Caring for Others and Helping Ourselves*. Princeton: Princeton University Press.

Index

Index

Columbia/HCA Healthcare Corporation, 14
Columbia University College of Physicians and
  Surgeons, 300
Come, Steve, 135, 213
Connelly, Paddy, 3, 4, 5, 30, 124, 201–3, 208–9,
  240–41
Consumers for Quality Care, 254
Consumers for Quality Health Care, 291
cost cutting, 307–8
  by HMOs, *see* HMOs
  by hiring LPNs or aides, 44
  by laying off or "floating" nurses, 12–17
    (mentioned), 249–50, 261–67, 276–77, 283–86
  nurse practitioners and, 119–20
  by shortening hospital stay, 253–54, 257 (*see also*
    hospitals)
  and "team nursing," 44–45
  and workload, 216–17, 249, 277
costs
  salary, 13–14 (*see also* nurses)
  treatment of pressure ulcers, 64
CPR, 236–37
Crimean War, 33, 35–37
Critical Care Medicine (journal), 283

Dana-Farber Cancer Institute, 275
Davis, Carolyne K., 280
death and dying
  hospice movement, 206–8
  nurse's role, 143, 147–50, 187, 196–98, 201–6,
    208–15, 231–47
  patients' wishes, 231–40
  physicians and, *see* physicians
De Moro, Rose Ann, 254
Diagnostic Related Groups (DRGs), 113
Dick, Karen, 90–91, 170, 171, 175, 229, 240, 241
Dieppe, Paul, 279, 298
Diers, Donna, 19
district nurse concept, 177–79
DNR orders, 232, 233–36, 243
Dock, Lavinia, 179
doctor-nurse relationships, 18–19, 69–83, 172–73,
  198, 299–302
  and dying patient, 203, 204–5, 207
  and nurse practitioners, 182–83
  perception of nurse's role, 71–72, 75, 78, 120, 300
  and primary nursing, 47, 142–44
  "team nursing" and, 44–45
  teamwork in health care, 179–83, 249
  See also physicians
domestic violence, 302–3
Doyne (John L.) Hospital (Milwaukee), 283
Duffy, Mary, 157, 158

education. *See* nurses; physicians
ER (TV show), 14
Examining Your Doctor (McCall), 76

Fagin, Claire, 19
Focarelli, Patricia, 75
Ford, Loretta, 99, 100
Fox, Renee, 130

gender as issue, 16, 80–81, 165, 305
Gibbons, Trish, 46, 47, 278
Goffman, Erving, 134
Goldman, Leon, 81, 180–81
Gomez, Carlos, 207
Grumbasler, Kevin, 78

Haasler, George B., 283–84
Harrington, Charlene, 271
Harrison's Principles of Internal Medicine, 199
Hart, Julian Tudor, 279, 298
Hartz, A., et al., 283

Harvard Medical School, 75, 101, 199, 300
Health Affairs magazine, 253
Health and Hospitals Corporation (New York), 263
Health and Human Services (HHS),
  U.S. Dept. of, 280, 288
health care
  administration of, 285
  cost cutting in, *see* cost cutting
  FTEs, 285
  legislation on, 100, 287–91
  media coverage of, 16–17, 304, 305
  nurse practitioners and, 101
  nurses transform system, 33–38
  quality of, 298–99
  reform proposals, 119, 250–51
  teamwork in, 179–83, 249
  U.S. imbalance in, 97–98
  as women's issue, 306
  See also HMOs
HealthCare Dimensions agency, 207
Health Care Financing Administration (HCFA),
  275, 280
Health Care Patient Protection Act, 290
Henderson, Virginia, 150, 155
Henry Street Settlement, ix, 179
Herbert, Lord Sidney, 35, 36
Hershey (Milton S.) Medical Center, 207
Hill, Hester, 124, 126
Himmelstein, David, 270–71, 285
HMOs, 250, 251–52, 297
  CEOs of, 14, 252, 261, 289, 298
  cost cutting by, 253–54, 257–62 (mentioned),
    276, 279, 289, 291, 294, 296, 306
  legislation on, 289–90, 291
  sued, 276
home care, 107–9, 112–14, 170–92, 216–30
  cost cutting and, 216–17, 249
  first nurses' group, 177–79
  managed care and, 257–61
  questions or complaints, 294–95
Horvath, Kathy, 157, 158
hospice (palliative care) concept, 206–8
  origin of movement, 206
  study of, 241–42
Hospital Professionals and Allied Employees
  (HPAE), 290
hospitals
  CEOs of, 13–14, 285
  cost cutting by, 249–50, 253–54, 252–72
    (mentioned), 281
  establishment of in U.S., 37–38
  IOM report on, 265, 280–82
  medical errors in, 275–77
  mergers of, 250, 263, 278
  mortality rate of, 276, 283
  and nurses' training, 41–42
  nursing as viewed by, *see* nurses
  and "patient care services," 278, 294–95
  and "patient-focused care," 267–70
  public view of, 295–96, 297
  shortened stay in, 113–14, 249–50, 252–61, 270,
    292–96
  teaching, 72, 75
  as "total institution," 134
Hospitals & Health Networks magazine, 13
How We Die (Nuland), 160

Illness Narratives, The (Kleinman), 128
Institute of Medicine (IOM) study, 265, 280–82, 296
insurance and insurance companies
  CEOs, 14
  HMOs and, 251
  and home care, 176, 257
  intrusion of, into physician-patient relationship,
    301